Fertility For Dummies®

P9-DIJ-401

Ten Do's and Don'ts to Protect Your Fertility

- Don't have unprotected sex (use a condom — the only protection against disease).
- Don't smoke.
- Don't douche regularly.
- Don't abuse drugs or alcohol.
- Don't overexercise.
- Do maintain the proper weight.
- Do see your gynecologist regularly.
- Do assess your environment for possible fertility busters (see Chapter 3).
- Do try to reduce stress levels.
- And if you're a guy — don't wear tight underwear!

Five Most Important Fertility Tests

- Semen analysis
- Baseline blood tests
- HSG
- Thyroid levels
- Midcycle blood tests (to make sure you're ovulating)

See Chapter 7 for more about tests.

Normal Blood Test Results during a Menstrual Cycle

- Estradiol day 2 or 3 of menses: 25–75 pg/ml
- Estradiol midcycle (about day 14): Greater than 150 pg/ml
- Progesterone day 2 or 3: Less than 1.5 ng/ml
- Progesterone postovulation: Greater than 15 ng/ml
- LH day 2 or 3: Less than 7 mIU/ml
- LH midcycle (around ovulation): Greater than 20 mIU/ml
- FSH day 2 or 3: Less than 13 mIU/ml

See Chapter 7 for more about blood tests.

Common Terms Used by Fertility Online Support Groups

AF: Aunt Flo (don't ask), also known as your menstrual cycle.

B/W: Blood work.

BB: Bulletin board.

BBT: Basal body temperature.

BCP: Birth control pills.

BD: Baby dance, also known as intercourse.

beta: A blood test to measure the amount of hCG in the blood. Done as the "gold standard" of pregnancy tests.

BFP, BFN: Big fat positive, big fat negative. In reference to the results of an HPT or beta test.

blast or blastocyst: An embryo that has matured past the point of 32 cells.

CD: Cycle day. Cycle day 1 is considered the first day of your menstrual cycle.

cycle buddy: Another woman whose cycle coincides with yours and who will be trying to conceive at the same time.

DD/DS: Darling daughter or darling son.

DE: Donor egg.

Fertility For Dummies®

Cheat Sheet

Common Terms Used by Fertility Online Support Groups (continued)

DH: Darling husband (sometimes referred to as darn husband, dumb husband — you get the picture).

donor: Woman who is donating her eggs.

DS: Donor sperm. Not to be confused with darling son! Context should differentiate.

E2: Estrogen.

embies: Embryos. The fertilized egg.

FET: Frozen embryo transfer. Refers to the transfer of embryos that were frozen following a previous cycle or a donor egg cycle and then thawed at a later time and transferred back into the uterus.

follies: Follicles that contain a woman's eggs.

FSH: Follicle-stimulating hormone.

GIFT: Gamete intrafallopian transfer. Similar to IVF except the egg and sperm are not fertilized outside the body but instead transferred back into the fallopian tube (rather than the uterus) to fertilize naturally.

hCG: Human chorionic gonadotropin. The pregnancy hormone measured in a pregnancy test. Also used as part of a stimulated cycle to trigger the start of ovulation.

HPT: Home pregnancy test.

IUI: Intrauterine insemination. A medium-tech procedure that can be done with or without fertility medications.

LH: Luteinizing hormone.

M/C: Miscarriage.

MDL: Microdose Lupron. A drug used in stimulated IVF cycles.

multiples: Refers to twin, triplet, or higher pregnancies.

NC-IUI or NC-IVF: Natural cycle IUI or IVF, that is, without the use of fertility medications.

O: Ovulation.

OPK: Ovulation predictor kit.

P4: Progesterone.

PG Ment'd, Child Ment'd: The text mentions a pregnancy or a child. Considered Internet etiquette to alert readers.

+++: Positive result.

RE: Reproductive endocrinologist or fertility doctor.

recipient: The woman who is the recipient for the donor eggs (embryos).

retrieval: The part of the IVF process when the eggs are removed from the woman's body to be fertilized with the sperm.

stims: Fertility medications that stimulate the ovaries to produce eggs.

3-day transfer, 5-day transfer: The amount of time the fertilized eggs (embryos) are allowed to divide outside of the body before being returned to the uterus. Five-day transfers generally signify the "return" of blastocysts.

transfer: The part of the IVF process when the fertilized eggs (embryos) are put back into the woman's uterus.

2WW: Two-week wait. Describes the period between ovulation and the pregnancy test.

U/S: Ultrasound.

YO: years old, as in 32 YO.

ZIFT: Zygote intrafallopian transfer. Similar to IVF and GIFT except that the egg and sperm are fertilized in the lab but returned to the fallopian tube (rather than the uterus) prior to any division of the embryo.

Copyright © 2003 Wiley Publishing, Inc. All rights reserved.

Item 2549-2.

For more information about Wiley Publishing, call 1-800-762-2974.

For Dummies: Bestselling Book Series for Beginners

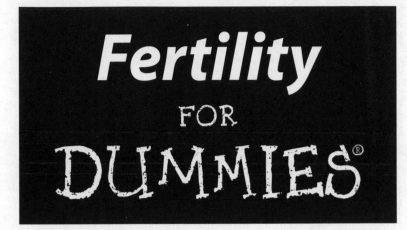

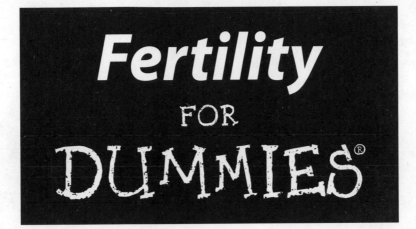

by Jackie Meyers-Thompson
and Sharon Perkins, RN

WILEY

Wiley Publishing, Inc.

Fertility For Dummies®

Published by
Wiley Publishing, Inc.
909 Third Avenue
New York, NY 10022
www.wiley.com

Copyright © 2003 by Wiley Publishing, Inc., Indianapolis, Indiana

Published simultaneously in Canada

About the Authors

Jackie Meyers-Thompson is managing partner of Coppock-Meyers Public Relations/For Your Information Communications and a "professional" fertility patient.

It's been said that we make plans . . . and the gods laugh. Jackie has heard that laughter often. It took her longer than she expected, and yielded more than a few laughs, and tears, before she met her husband-to-be, Darren Thompson. But by 35, she was newly married and deliriously happy and felt that the rest of the story would soon fall into place. Jackie can be a slow learner.

Nonetheless, she's an industrious worker. She loved writing and, as a result, carved her path in marketing and public relations. She had a loving husband and a successful business, so the only things left to add were a few cherubic children and her own Great American Novel. Two years and a slew of physicians later, Jackie had more than a few doubts whether her future would ever include children. But her persistence and focus paid off. *Fertility For Dummies* is, in part, Jackie's story of the journey that landed her a book and a baby, and a lot more interest in and knowledge of the incredible yet inefficient process known as human reproduction.

When not writing, working, or sharing stories online, Jackie spends her time making plans. Some things never change.

Sharon Perkins is the nurse coordinator for the Cooper Center for In Vitro Fertilization in Marlton, New Jersey, one of the largest infertility centers in the United States, and has worked as an infertility nurse for the last six years. She previously worked as an RN in labor and delivery and neonatal intensive care, so her nursing experience covers every aspect of conception, pregnancy, delivery, and newborn care. She lives with her husband, John, an Air Force pilot, and a varying number of children, depending on which of her five children is living at home at the moment. This is her first book, although her children have been nagging her for years to stop telling them all the crazy things that happen in nursing and write them down.

Dedication

From Jackie: This book is dedicated to my Darling Husband (DH!), Darren Thompson, who has loved me and believed in us, through it all. And to my mother, Larissa Meyers, and my father, the late Leonard Meyers, who taught me early and well that I could climb any mountain.

From Sharon: This book is dedicated to my father, who always believed I could do anything.

Authors' Acknowledgments

From Jackie:

My indoctrination to the field of fertility came after a failed in vitro fertilization cycle, a few unreturned phone calls by a disinterested doc, and a tearful after-midnight discovery of online bulletin boards and chat rooms devoted to providing people like myself with information and support. This wonderful network of women propped me up emotionally and spiritually and led me to an excellent and compassionate doctor, nurses, and a clinic that eventually brought me the pregnancy I had struggled for three years to achieve.

In keeping with our online anonymity, I thank Tricia, AndreaD, AS, Liz, Irene, Robin, Janet, KarenNJ, SusanM, and the dozens of other women who walked with me on my path, and continue to do so to this day. They are proof of the strength of human spirit and the power of coming together in the face of any hardship. I wish for them all the joy and success that they deserve.

I don't believe I would have gotten to this point (pregnant *and* writing a book!) had it not been for the wonderful care and treatment that I received through Dr. Jerome Check and the Cooper Center for In Vitro Fertilization in Marlton, New Jersey. Dr. Check and his colleague, Dr. Jung Choe, tirelessly helped us overcome both physical and emotional hurdles as we recovered in their care from two years of misinformation and overmedication. They proved to us that there still exist doctors totally devoted to the success and well-being of their patients, even at the expense of their own bottom line. It was also at the Cooper Clinic that I met my writing partner and friend, Sharon Perkins. Her humor, caring, and expertise make her as great a nurse as they do a writer.

Apart from the virtual world, I have so much to be grateful for in the support of family and friends. Cousin Sandy searched and researched and learned as much about fertility as his own field of medicine in helping us through the maze of doctors and protocols. The Thompsons, the Jaffes, the Cicecklis, and the Perlsteins also helped and supported us every way they knew how. Melissa, Camille, Suzanne, Courtenay, Susan, Leslie, Sharon, and Nancy were unfailing in their encouragement and always provided a shoulder to cry on or a voice to laugh with.

In the writing of this book, a number of professionals became friends as well. Stephanie Smart, licensed acupuncturist and Chinese herbalist, and Jennifer R. Bloome, occupational therapist, health and wellness counselor, and resident of Anji, Inc. provided us with great insight into the power of mind and body when trying to conceive.

From Sharon:

I started writing books in the third grade, but writing books and selling them are two different things! This book would never have gotten to market without the incredible sales ability of my coauthor, Jackie Meyers-Thompson, who not only never doubted for a minute that we could do this, but never let anyone else doubt it either.

Families put up with a lot when one member is writing a book, and I give my husband, John, enormous credit for not only listening day and night to every idea that went through my head but also for reading every word and telling me when I was writing over everyone else's head. He knows more about infertility than he ever wanted to! Thanks also to my children, John, Matt, Kim, Greg, Cindy, Ben, and Molly, for providing a constant cheering section and also some distraction from work and writing! And special thanks to Matt and Kim for the gift of Matthew Ryan, the most wonderful grandson in the world, who brings joy to my heart every single day.

My mother, Lois Orchard, is not only the best mother on the planet but also the most supportive. Her encouragement from my first book of stories to this one has never faltered. My sister, Sue Collins, is my lifelong best friend, and I appreciate her support always. Ditto for my sister-in-law, Louise Kalmouni, whose artwork around my home reminds me every day of the importance of family. To all I didn't mention individually, I love you all and appreciate every one of you.

My father, father-in-law, and mother-in-law would all have loved to see this book become a reality. As my mother says, they're having a book party in heaven!

I never could have written this book without the knowledge gained from working at the Cooper Center for six years. Dr. Check, Dr. Choe, Dr. Nazari, Dr. Krotec, you've all taught me more than I ever thought I would know about infertility, and it's been a privilege to work with you. Unlike many nurse managers, I'm fortunate to work with some of my best friends. Carol, you make me laugh every day. And when I'm not up to laughing, you cry with me. I'm grateful to *all* the IVF nurses for putting up with my frantic moods, rewrite irritability, and constant book conversation for the last year. I work with wonderful people, from embryology to the front desk, and I appreciate you all. And to all the wonderful patients I've met over the years, this book is really for — and because of — you.

Our thanks to our technical advisor, Dr. Marguerite Shepard, who made sure that we were accurate in everything we said, and to our illustrator, Kathryn Born, who made it all more vivid.

Finally, if not for publisher Diane Steele and acquisitions editor Kathy Cox at Wiley Publishing, this book would never have been written by these authors! Both Diane and Kathy believed in our vision and ability and gave us the opportunity to share our voices. They confidently placed us in the capable hands of our project editor Norm Crampton and copy editor Tina Sims, who helped bring this book to life, and we thank you both. Through your editing, we learned that red ink is not a dirty word! Your skills have made this a better book without changing its direction or focus. To everyone else behind the scenes at Wiley, the people who do their jobs without an individual mention, we thank you all for doing things we didn't even know about but that were essential to the publication of this book.

Publisher's Acknowledgments

We're proud of this book; please send us your comments through our Dummies online registration form located at www.dummies.com/register/.

Some of the people who helped bring this book to market include the following:

Acquisitions, Editorial, and Media Development

Project Editor: Norm Crampton

Acquisitions Editor: Kathleen M. Cox

Senior Copy Editor: Tina Sims

Technical Editor: Marguerite K. Shepard, MD

Editorial Manager: Christine Beck

Editorial Assistant: Melissa Bennett

Cover Photo: © Dave Teel/Corbis

Cartoons: Rich Tennant, www.the5thwave.com

Production

Project Coordinator: Dale White

Layout and Graphics: Beth Brooks, Jennifer Click, LeAndra Johnson, Micheal Kruzil, Kristin McMullan

Special Art: Kathryn Born

Proofreaders: Laura Albert, TECHBOOKS Publishing Inc.

Indexer: TECHBOOKS Publishing Inc.

Special Help: Chrissy Guthrie

Publishing and Editorial for Consumer Dummies

   Diane Graves Steele, Vice President and Publisher, Consumer Dummies

   Joyce Pepple, Acquisitions Director, Consumer Dummies

   Kristin A. Cocks, Product Development Director, Consumer Dummies

   Michael Spring, Vice President and Publisher, Travel

   Brice Gosnell, Publishing Director, Travel

   Suzanne Jannetta, Editorial Director, Travel

Publishing for Technology Dummies

   Andy Cummings, Vice President and Publisher, Dummies Technology/General User

Composition Services

   Gerry Fahey, Vice President of Production Services

   Debbie Stailey, Director of Composition Services

Contents at a Glance

Table of Contents

Introduction

• •

This book was born during Jackie's in vitro fertilization egg retrieval, when she woke from anesthesia to see Sharon smiling at her. Normally, the first thing a nurse would tell a patient after an egg retrieval would be how many eggs she got, but Sharon had another agenda. "I didn't know that you were a writer. I've always wanted to write a book," she said. So while no baby was born from that particular egg retrieval, this book was.

Infertility is a medical problem for more than 6 million Americans, but treatment is out of reach financially for some people and a tremendous personal strain on most people. Many people (the "just relax and you'll get pregnant" crowd) misunderstand fertility, and a few (the "take this magic pill and you'll get pregnant, guaranteed!" group) even exploit it. The medical aspects of infertility are making great gains, yet the emotional side is often ignored.

Fertility For Dummies was conceived by combining Jackie's knowledge of infertility from a patient's viewpoint, Sharon's wealth of information as an infertility nurse, and both of their personal experiences. We wrote this book so that patients dealing with infertility will know that they're not alone. We hope it finds its way to the bookshelves and nightstands of every patient who needs it to help find their road to their baby. And, as Sharon and Jackie found out along the way, anything can happen!

About This Book

You can't pick up a magazine or turn on *Oprah* without hearing it: the great fertility debate over when women should have babies. Unfortunately, much of the information is inappropriate or just plain inaccurate.

Meanwhile, for the 6 million infertility patients (1995 Vital Statistics) being *treated* in the United States alone (which doesn't take into account the many people who haven't sought or can't afford formal treatment), the question is not "when?" but "if?" Will they ever be able to conceive, carry, and deliver the child they are seeking, paying up to $20,000 for the privilege of being told "Sorry, the test was negative."

This book is our attempt to help those of you who want to walk into the doctor's office and not walk out feeling foolish and out of control of your fertility. Our vision is to provide fertility patients — both those at the starting line and those close to the finish — and the people who love them with as much information as we can on the options available to them. We discuss topics ranging from the scientific to the spiritual. Just as others have been available to help and teach *us,* we're here for you, providing a thought, an idea, or just a laugh. Maybe we just serve as a reminder that "It ain't over until the fat lady sings" (and not to worry, as she's still bound and gagged in a fertility patient's basement somewhere).

You can read through this book from front to back and feel confident that you can find the answer to just about any fertility issue, from natural family planning to cloning. But if you're like most people, you'll probably look through the table of contents, zero in on the chapters that affect you, and jump directly to them. This book is meant as a resource, which means that you can go back to it whenever a new issue or question arises, and find the answer you need without reading through everything that goes before. This book is meant for people with every degree of fertility expertise, from the novice to the jaded, been-there-done-that patient. The no-tech and low-tech fertility chapters come first, so you can skip them if you're already a veteran and move right into high-tech and *really* high-tech stuff found in the second half of the book.

We intersperse personal stories throughout the book; these (hopefully!) make interesting reading from the viewpoint of either Sharon (an infertility nurse) or Jackie (an infertility patient). If you skip them, you won't miss any essential information, although you may miss a few humorous sidelines or "I did it, so you can too" stories.

Conventions Used in This Book

To help you pick out information from a page, I use the following conventions throughout the text to make elements consistent and easy to understand:

- ✔ Any Web addresses appear in `monofont`.
- ✔ New terms appear in *italics* and are closely preceded or followed by an easy-to-understand definition.
- ✔ **Bold** highlights the keywords in bulleted lists.
- ✔ Sidebars, which look like text enclosed in a shaded gray box, consist of information that's interesting to know but not necessarily critical to your understanding of the topic.

How This Book Is Organized

Fertility For Dummies is divided into six parts. If you're just beginning to think about getting pregnant, you may want to start with the first chapter. If you're familiar with infertility treatment, you may want to skip to the sections that apply to your current treatments, or to those you may be moving up to in the future. If you want to read through the entire book, you'll be well informed on all the latest infertility issues and the newest technological advances in the field.

The following sections explain the organization of this book:

Part 1: The No-Tech Road to Baby

If you're a newcomer to the wonderful world of baby making, we suggest that you start reading here. In this part, we explain male and female anatomy (including everything you ever wanted to know about reproductive organs), look at the logistics of getting pregnant, and review behaviors you should change — or not — before trying to get pregnant.

Part 11: The Low-Tech Road: Expecting a Pregnancy

This part helps you fine-tune your conception efforts by using methods to predict ovulation, and helps you understand how complicated getting pregnant really is. We also guide you through your initial gynecology visits for simple infertility treatment and help you understand and deal with loss of pregnancy. We also take a look at some alternative approaches to pregnancy, from herbs to acupuncture.

Part 111: Medium-Tech Baby Making: Finding the Problem

This part explains the tests you may be doing to find out why you haven't gotten pregnant yet; we explain what the tests are and what the results may mean. We also accompany you on your first visits to a doctor who specializes in infertility, help you make sure this doctor is the one for you, and help you decipher what the doctor tells you, including the treatments that are prescribed. We also describe the common fertility medications and give you support for getting through the dreaded injections.

Part 1V: The High-Tech Highway: Moving Up to In Vitro Fertilization

This part explains what in vitro fertilization is, what it involves, and how to deal with the costs of high-tech treatment. We guide you through the complicated maze of finding the right clinic and take you through the stimulation process and the egg retrieval itself. We visit the embryology lab after your egg retrieval and give advice on how to get through the "two week wait" for your pregnancy test without losing your mind.

Part V: The Road Less Traveled . . . So Far!

This part guides you through third-party reproduction — the use of donor eggs, sperm, or embryos to get pregnant. We also discuss parenting for the nontraditional family (gays, lesbians, and singles) and discuss adoption for every kind of family. Last but not least, we look at what's down the road for fertility, from controversial new treatments to cloning.

Part VI: The Part of Tens

Want to know the ten most annoying things people say when you're trying to get pregnant? Want to know where to find fertility medications for reasonable prices and find out exactly what a gonadotropin is? This is the part for you.

Icons Used in This Book

If either of us has a personal story that is funny, informative, inspirational, or otherwise interesting, we identify it with the Personal Story icon. These anecdotes are never essential reading, but they're usually entertaining!

If something's really important for you to keep in mind during your fertility treatment, we mark it with a Remember icon.

If something's interesting from a technical standpoint but not really essential to know, you see the Technical Stuff icon.

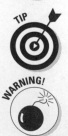

The Tip icon highlights practical information that may make the road to baby somewhat smoother.

If you see the Warning icon, pay special attention. It tells you about potential problems or difficulties.

Part I
The No-Tech Road to Baby

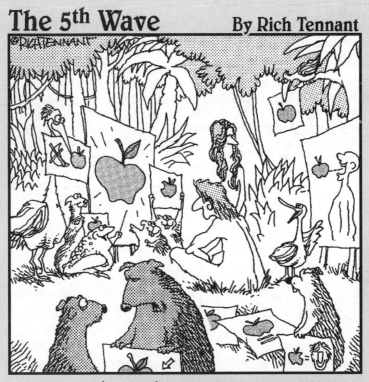

The 5th Wave   By Rich Tennant

"We're getting nowhere – send in the snake."

In this part . . .

You may not have given much thought through the years to the difficulties of getting pregnant. More likely, your focus has been more on *not* getting pregnant. Once you make the decision to have a baby, however, it's time to look at all the factors that go into having a successful pregnancy, from health issues to lifestyle changes. In this part we look at questions you should ask before trying to get pregnant, and we give you some basic information on how human reproduction works and how it can best work for *you*.

Chapter 1

In the Beginning

*I*n the beginning, there wasn't much to say about having a baby because there weren't any babies yet. Imagine Adam and Eve's surprise at the first appearance of Cain. You have to wonder how many children they had before they caught on to exactly where they were coming from, or did God give them a little instruction manual about the care and making of new humans? At any rate, they didn't need to worry about getting pregnant, or staying pregnant, because they had no idea how they got pregnant in the first place or how long it might take a baby to appear. They also didn't have the stress of dealing with parents hanging around asking them when they were ever going to give them grandchildren. Lucky Adam and Eve.

This state of affairs didn't last forever. A few generations later, their descendant Abraham wanted a little Abe, but his wife wasn't getting pregnant, so his wife Sarah gave him her maid Haggar so he could have a child with her. Infertility had arrived in paradise, along with surrogacy. Now 5,000 or so years later, you're ready to start a family and probably thinking it's going to be easy. You want to have a baby — so have one! And that's exactly what may happen — no problems. But it's a fact that 10 percent or more of the childbearing population all over the world, including 6.1 million Americans, have problems getting pregnant or staying pregnant.

In this chapter, we look at some of the genetic realities you should be aware of as you think about adding to your family tree, and we discuss some personal and financial matters, too.

Making Babies: An Inefficient Process at Best

You may think of Mother Nature as a pretty efficient woman, but the truth is, the path to pregnancy is an inefficient one even under the best of circumstances. For example, out of 100 couples under the age of 35 trying to conceive, only 20 will get pregnant in any given month, and of those 20, 3 will miscarry. In other words, if you're under 35, every month you have a 17 percent chance of walking out of the maternity ward with a baby nine months later. Obviously, nature is not as efficient as people think.

The good new is that 80 percent of couples under 35 will be pregnant within one year of trying. Of the 20 women not pregnant after a year of trying, 10, who may be subfertile or have mild infertility issues, will be pregnant after two years of trying without medical intervention. That leaves the other 10 percent, who may never get pregnant without some help from the medicine man. High-tech infertility treatments, such as in vitro fertilization, claim a success rate of about 50 percent for those under age 35, which means 5 out of 100 women will not become pregnant, even with medical intervention. Part IV of this book is all about in vitro fertilization (IVF).

If you're over 35, you're in good company; 20 percent of all first-time moms in the United States are over 35! Despite this, Mother Nature doesn't make it easy to get pregnant past age 35. By your late thirties, only 10 percent of you will get pregnant in any given month and 17 percent will miscarry. If you're over 40, the pregnancy rate, per month, slips to 5 percent, with 34 percent miscarrying. By age 45, your chance per month of conceiving is less than 1 percent, and 53 percent will miscarry.

Why the decrease in pregnancy and rise in miscarriage as you get older? It's because of the increase in chromosomal abnormalities in your eggs as they age. At age 20, your chance of having a baby with a chromosomal abnormality such as Down syndrome (also called Trisomy 21), or Trisomy 13 or 18 (these usually result in newborn death shortly after delivery), is 1/526. By age 30, the risk is 1/385; by age 35, 1/192; by age 40, 1/66; and by age 45, 1/21. The following minitable pulls all the numbers together.

Age	Under 30	30–35	36–40	41–45	Over 45
Percentage of women who have difficulty conceiving (trying to conceive naturally for one year without success)	20%	20%	33%	66%	95%
Miscarriage rate	15%	15%	17%	34%	53%
Rate of chromosomal abnormalities	1/526	1/385	1/192	1/66	1/21

Does your racial background affect your chance for pregnancy? There is a slight difference in infertility rates, with Hispanic women under 35 experiencing a 7 percent infertility rate, Caucasians a 6.4 percent infertility rate, and African American women recording a 10.5 percent rate of infertility. These differences could be due to socioeconomic factors, such as poverty, poor nutrition, or lack of physician care, rather than strictly racial issues.

Whatever category you fall under — whether it's "easy to conceive," "not so easy," or "what's it gonna take to get me pregnant?" — we're here to help you have the baby of your dreams in the shortest time possible for you and to help keep you sane while you wait.

How Aging Affects Fertility

Whether you're dealing with fertility or fitness, age *does* play a role. Whether you *feel* like you're 15 or 50, whether you look your age or not, your body knows how old you are, and your ovaries do too.

Calculating your fertility odds at different ages

For women, optimum fertility occurs when you're about 18 years old. It stays pretty constant in the early part of your 20s and then begins a gradual downward turn. By the time you turn 35, the process has accelerated. When you hit 40, the slide becomes even more dramatic; 33 percent of women over 35 have some difficulty getting pregnant, and 66 percent of women over 40 have infertility issues.

Men have it a little easier (don't they always?). Their peak fertility generally remains constant throughout their 30s. It does begin to decline over time, but at a slower pace than their female counterparts. Recent studies, however, do show a rise in chromosomal abnormalities in men over 35, and by age 50, most men show a 33 percent decrease in the number of sperm produced. So although their problems may be less obvious when it comes to conceiving, the effects of age may play a significant role down the road.

You can keep yourself in better baby-making shape (and better overall health) through good self-care, including nutrition and exercise. We touch on these topics in Chapter 2. But ultimately, you can't fool Mother Nature.

Now you may respond with the story of your 18-year-old cousin who couldn't conceive, your 45-year-old sister who did, or the 80-year-old movie star bouncing the newborn on his knee. Anything is possible. However, statistics provide information on the *likelihood* of conception, a healthy pregnancy, and babies. These numbers are a resource for determining the best plan of when and how you will conceive. But they're not a reason to review your life so far and regret not having your first baby in high school, spending too long with Mr. Wrong, or choosing to travel the world before settling down.

Second-guessing will get you no closer to your goal of baby than accepting your choices thus far and doing the best with where you are now.

Understanding how much age itself matters

We say this often throughout this book: Human reproduction is a very inefficient process *at any age*. When a woman is 35, one out of four embryos is abnormal; this number increases to one out of two at age 40, and five out of six at age 45. Although these statistics certainly show that age is a factor in conceiving, remember that you're an individual, not a statistic, and your odds may be better or worse than the statistics.

If a 40-year-old woman gets pregnant easily and gives birth to healthy child after healthy child, the statistics on age have little bearing on her life! Conversely, if a woman has trouble conceiving and/or maintaining a healthy pregnancy, even if time is on her side, the statistics don't appear to be important either. Ultimately, *you* are the only statistic that counts when you're trying to conceive. Again, the statistics provide probable outcomes, not facts. And if you remember only one piece of information in the field of fertility, it is that there are always exceptions. Consider that for all the reasons (including age) why you may not get pregnant, 20 percent of women are diagnosed with unexplained infertility. This statistic certainly shows that while much is known, much is still not understood.

This said, by no means are we encouraging you to wait for Medicare to kick in before trying to conceive. This approach will likely (very likely) cause you many problems. However, trying to turn Mr. Right Now into Mr. Right so that you can hit the 35-year-old cutoff is not sane thinking either. Use age as a suggested guideline. Fertility, most often, decreases *over time*. You will not become infertile overnight. Indeed, studies have shown that many women experience *perimenopause* (the stage prior to menopause) and subfertility for as long as five to seven years before the onset of actual menopause (which *generally* signifies the end of your reproductive years). The average age of menopause is 51. You can still become pregnant during perimenopause, although it may be more difficult and/or require medical intervention because you ovulate less frequently and the quality of your remaining eggs is not as good as it once was.

Separating Fact from Media Myth

You can't pick up *People* magazine or turn on *Oprah* without hearing it: the great fertility debate over when women should have babies. Unfortunately, much of the information is inappropriate and just plain inaccurate. Recent statistics report an approximate 5 percent chance in a given month for a woman over 40 to conceive. This number sounds frighteningly low, until you compare it with the statistic that shows that a healthy couple in their 20s has only a 20 percent chance of success during any given month. This comparison is seldom brought up because the one isolated, surprising statistic often sells better than the facts. Our advice: Be a careful consumer.

Over time, most people become fairly desensitized to the latest surefire cures or health warnings used to sell everything from the scientific to the supernatural. Apply the same approach when weeding through the information on fertility. You wouldn't take medical advice from your car mechanic, so don't just assume that everyone who offers up an opinion, even a public one, knows anything more. Instead, ask your doctor, ask your nurse, or read a book (like this one) written by someone actually in the field. Although the media may provide you with a source of information, make sure that you qualify that source. More often than not, you'll find that the information presented has a mere modicum of truth in it surrounded by a lot of hype designed to get your attention. Ignore the hype. The next big story will take its place in no time.

Examining the State of Your Union

When it comes to baby making, sooner is often better than later, but keep in mind that this is from a biological perspective. And although you may hear the biological clock ticking away, ready-or-not is not the best way to make your decision about when to conceive. The state of your union is an issue we revisit throughout this book as it is one of the most important aspects in dealing with fertility, infertility, and baby makes three (or more). And although biology is a key issue in deciding when and if you're ready to conceive, maturity, financial security, and stability are equally important, whether your challenge is trying to get pregnant or trying to raise said baby in a difficult and expensive world.

Many couples are anxious to seal the deal with a baby. This approach is fine for some couples, but others find that they need an adjustment period in the marriage before introducing someone new. Start out by talking with your partner about your hopes and expectations for children. Some couples find that although both partners want children, their timing may be different. You may need to negotiate (an oft-used tool in any working partnership) so that your partner can still fulfill his dream to see the world, all the while planning for a baby before your biological clock stops ticking altogether.

The quality of your partnership is the foundation for your family. Take the time to make sure that it's solid before moving on to the next level.

Don't just assume that a baby is the next logical step in a marriage. Babies are cute and cuddly *at times* (ask any parent about the alternatives of cranky and unmanageable), but they also require an enormous commitment of emotions, time, and money. If you or your partner struggle with the demands of your existing relationship, a baby will only make things more difficult. If both of you have trouble with joint decisions, finances, or future plans, a baby will more than likely exacerbate those differences, *not* diminish them. Teamwork is essential in raising Junior. Now is a good time to practice working together.

Some couples ease into the new addition by starting with a pet. Fido and Fifi can serve as good indicators of your (and your partner's) sense of responsibility, discipline, and sacrifice. If you find yourself at each other's throats over whose turn it is to feed, walk, or bathe the dog, you may have a little work to do before upping the ante to baby.

Just keep talking! As with all other areas, communication is key in the decision to add on to your family. If you find yourselves to be at an impasse, enlist the help of an outside party; a member of the clergy, a therapist, or a physician may be better able to guide both of you toward a decision that will ultimately benefit your entire family, however large or small that may turn out to be.

Second-guessing a two-year honeymoon

My husband and I (coauthor Jackie) married when I was 34 years old. We decided to settle in to our marriage for a few years before trying to conceive. When I was 36 years old, we began our quest for a baby. Three years later, we found ourselves still trying. I second-guessed myself endlessly: "Maybe we _should have_ started trying right away" or "If only I had those extra two years." After much personal torment and a fair amount of soul-searching, I came to the conclusion that had we started trying earlier, one of two things would have happened:

✔ We would have gotten pregnant . . . and would not have been ready, neither individually nor as a couple. Our first few years of marriage allowed us to enjoy one another, discover ourselves and each other, and learn how to be a team. Those two years also gave us the opportunity to pay off joint debt, further establish ourselves financially, and even begin saving for the future!

✔ We wouldn't have gotten pregnant . . . and would have faced the problems and stress of infertility and treatments two years earlier in our marriage, robbing us of the joy we experienced together during that time. As fledglings in our new partnership, we were ill-equipped to handle the roller coaster ride of infertility, a ride we were better prepared for a few years later in our marriage.

In other words, telling yourself "I should have" or asking yourself "What if?" is useless, whether reflecting on your own decisions or those you make with your partner. This type of hindsight only causes undue stress in your partnership.

Getting Sick in the Executive Washroom: Pregnancy and Work

How will getting pregnant affect your job? Thanks to the Pregnancy Discrimination Act, part of the Civil Rights Act of 1964, employers can no longer refuse to hire women who are pregnant; women who are pregnant are also entitled to the same leave period as anyone with a physical illness. As long as you're able to perform the main functions of your job, you can't be fired or not hired.

Thanks to ten years of discussion about the "mommy track," it's a pretty well-established fact that women who are pregnant or have small children are often at a disadvantage when it comes to promotions; the workplace perception in many companies is that a mother will put her family before her job. And in most cases, that's a pretty logical assumption! So if you're a fast-track person who wants to stay on the fast track, you may have to do a real tap dance act to convince your employer that your commitment to the job isn't going to change after you have a child.

 Even though you may feel strongly *now* that your commitment to your career isn't going to change after you have a child, your feelings may change considerably after the baby arrives. One issue that may affect your situation is child care. Good day care isn't always easy to find. Your working hours and the sitter's availability may not mesh, or the sitter's children may get sick, leaving you without a sitter. The possibilities for disruption of even a well-planned child-care system are endless!

If you have a job commitment that is completely inflexible — if you're in the military, for instance — you may be *required* to submit a child-care plan that shows who will care for your child if you suddenly get sent overseas. Military child care is pretty good, but the military won't keep your baby for six months! You may think that your mom, sister, or best friend would be happy to watch your child for a short time, but you better get it in writing!

On the other hand, more executives are becoming attuned to the amazing fact that women own half the talent, intelligence, and ambition in their company. Consequently, management is making a real effort to offer on-site day care, flex time, and liberal maternity leave to keep the talent they have. Hopefully more companies will change their mind-set about working mothers and offer improved family benefits for working moms *and* dads.

Recognizing That Babies Don't Fix Life's Problems

 Just as Junior's appearance will not repair a partnership in peril, it will also not put you on the personal road to happily ever after. Your child will not and *should not* be your antidote to a bad job, bad marriage, bad childhood, or bad life. This thinking sets up unrealistic expectations and virtually guarantees disappointment, both for yourself and your offspring. A baby will not fix what ails you, and such an expectation has a negative impact on your child's emotional development as well. A baby brings not only joy but also sadness, anger, and all the emotions that you experience in your own daily life. Your child will come into this world with his or her own destiny and dreams to fulfill, not yours.

 If your life is miserable without a child, chances are it will still be miserable after your child is born.

So if you're looking to salvage your life by creating another one, consider making the changes you need to in order to create your own happiness *today*. Your future child, and everyone else, will thank you for it tomorrow.

Figuring the Cost of a Baby in Dollars and Sense

The Department of Agriculture says that today's middle-class family needs between $10,000 and 20,000 a year to raise a child to age 18 (and you thought the department only counted cows!). Because few parents kick their children out at college age, you can plan to spend at least $20,000 for a state college education, and the sky's the limit if the kid goes to Harvard. You may think that these numbers are unbelievable, and that you can do it for much less with a borrowed crib and three years of breast-feeding. Sit down one night when you're in a contemplative mood and add up what you will realistically need to spend per year to raise a child. Don't forget the toys that light up and play music when your baby kicks them with his foot, because if he doesn't have that stimulation, he'll be way behind in preschool! All kidding aside, raising children is expensive. Unless you're independently wealthy, you'll need to make financial trade-offs.

If you both work outside the home, you'll have both financial and emotional factors to consider:

- Will you (usually the mother, but not always) stay home for a few years?
- Will you use day care?
- Will your mothers baby-sit?
- How will you feel if your baby cries for the sitter to pick him up rather than you?
- How will you deal with your mothers giving the baby too many cookies or putting too many clothes on him?
- How will you find an in-home sitter and how do you know that you can trust him or her?
- Can you afford not to work at all?

Ah, you say, but my child will go to school in a few years and then I can go back to work! Yes, but do you know how many days a year school is *actually* in session? Do you know how often your kid will get sick, fall down on the playground, or have a crisis at school requiring a "team meeting" (yes, you're part of the team and need to be there)? Do you understand that T-ball practice starts at 4 p.m. and that every other child in kindergarten is on the team? Do you know that children sometimes miss their bus and need to be picked up or dropped off at school?

How about the preteen years? Will you leave your child home alone for a few hours? Do you have any idea what two 12-year-old boys think is a really neat thing to do with the cat and your washing machine? Can you trust your 14-year-old daughter not to bring home her new friend Basher, who is 17 and has two lip rings and a large motorcycle? How hard do you think it is to find an after-school sitter for an 11-year-old, and how much of a fuss do you think said 11-year-old will kick up about being baby-sat?

And if you think parenthood ever ends, well, think again. Your grown children get divorced, lose jobs, have drug or alcohol problems, or enter the military and need a place to leave their baby for a few months. Parenthood is a lifelong job. That adorable, cuddly, blond newborn could turn into a green-haired, multipierced, loudmouthed punk before you know it, and you can't take this child back to the store, unlike other things you've acquired and decided you didn't care for! And you wouldn't want to, because you'll love him — so much that it hurts sometimes, so much that his problems will break your heart, so much that you would give your life for his. That's what parenthood is.

Make sure that you're prepared for the job of parenthood before you sign up.

Timing Your Baby: The Big Picture

Timing is a major baby-making factor in several ways. We get into the nitty-gritty later (and specific timing tools in Chapter 3), but for those of you who want to know some baby stats:

- ✔ **How long will I be pregnant?** You probably think that nine months is the correct answer, but pregnancy is actually counted as 40 weeks, or ten months. This isn't as long as it seems. The first two weeks don't count, because they're the weeks before you ovulate, and the next two weeks are the weeks before you expect your period, so they don't really count either.

  Want to know what your due date will be? Take the date your last period started, count back three months, and then add one week. For example, if the date your last period started was July 1 and you count back three months, to April 1, and then add one week, your due date is April 8.

- ✔ **What is the most popular month for conception?** The most common months for *delivery* are July, August, and September, so it stands to reason that the most common conception months are October,

November, and December. You may think that people would be too busy during the holiday season, but apparently not.

- ✔ **What time of the day are most babies born?** This information is for you who want to organize your yearly planners ahead of time. Although it seems that most babies arrive after midnight, thereby upsetting everyone's life from the get-go, most are actually born during the day. The most popular day for deliveries is Tuesday.

- ✔ **Am I equally likely to have a boy or girl?** As far as conception, boy babies outnumber girl babies 130:100, but by the time of birth, this ratio drops to 105:100, signifying the higher rate of miscarriage for baby boys.

Pulling these stats together in a practical way, if you're looking forward to your child going to school, you may want to plan for a delivery early in the year, around January to March, especially if you're hoping to have a boy (more on sex selection later in this section and in Chapter 19). That way, you won't have to make the difficult decision on whether to put your child in kindergarten before he turns 5 or hold him back until he's a year older. *Him* is the right word in this case: Boys are more commonly held back than girls.

Now that you're planning ahead, you want to know about the timing of . . . well, sex. We touch on this a few more times, but the way to get pregnant is to have sex a day before or the day of the release of your egg, a process known as *ovulation* (we tell you in Chapter 2 how to figure out when that is). That gives the sperm time to get to the egg and meet in the fallopian tube. Sperm, by the way, are pretty long-lived; they can hang around two or three days. Eggs, on the other hand, are more fragile; 24 hours is about their life expectancy.

Want a boy? Or a girl? One theory is that boy sperm (those that carry the Y chromosome, which, combined with the woman's X chromosome, creates a boy baby) are shorter lived but faster swimmers; girl sperm (those that carry the X chromosome to create a girl) live longer but are slower. So if you want a girl, have sex two days before ovulation; if you want a boy, try to hit the day of ovulation straight on. (We discuss sex selection more in Chapter 19.)

Understanding the Long-Term Effects of Birth Control

You may not be quite ready to start baby making yet; you may want to wait for your medical benefits to kick in, your sister's wedding to be over, or your new house to be built. In the meantime, you want to use birth control, but you don't want to use it if it's going to make it harder for you to get pregnant later. So what method should you use?

Birth control pills

The good news is that birth control pills aren't likely to impair your long-term fertility at all. Today's pills contain a fraction of estrogen compared to pills from the 1960s. Most doctors say that you can start trying to get pregnant immediately after stopping the pill without any problem. The pill is not advised for women over 35 who smoke, as it may increase the chance of blood clots and stroke.

Intrauterine devices

Intrauterine devices (IUDs) have gotten lots of bad press over the years, and with reason. They can increase the chance of *ectopic pregnancy* (a nonviable pregnancy that develops in the fallopian tubes instead of the uterus) and can cause infection, sometimes quite serious. (We talk more about ectopic pregnancy in Chapter 6.) For this reason, an IUD is not the best choice if you want to become pregnant soon, especially if you have *endometriosis,* an outgrowth of uterine tissue into other parts of the abdominal cavity, or if you have a history of vaginal or cervical infection. (You can read more about endometriosis and infections in Chapter 7.) In fact, some doctors recommend against using an IUD if you've never had children, because an IUD-related infection may make it harder for you to become pregnant. And if you do get pregnant with an IUD in place, there's a 50 percent chance that you'll miscarry.

You've always got rhythm!

The old rhythm method now goes by a few other names, such as the Billings Family Planning Method, but the basic premise is the same: Avoid having sex on your ovulation days. This method is actually pretty successful, as long as you use it religiously. If you really, seriously, absolutely don't want to get pregnant right now, however, use a more reliable method.

The old standbys — condoms and barrier devices, such as the diaphragm — are still fairly effective, at least 90 percent if used consistently and correctly. Although they're not necessarily as easy or unobtrusive to use as the pill or an IUD, they don't have the side effects of their higher-tech cousins.

Looking at the Family Tree: Mr. Green Genes and His Kin

Before trying to get pregnant, you'll want to know whether any diseases occur more than once on your family tree. This disease may be caused by a dominant gene that you could pass on, if you carry it, even if your partner doesn't carry it. Depending on how open your family is, finding out this information can be difficult. Many families don't discuss anything related to pregnancy, especially not problems getting pregnant, pregnancy losses, or genetic defects. Just a few generations ago, parents of children with genetic abnormalities were encouraged to put them in a home and tell the relatives the baby had been stillborn.

 Ask the most talkative member of your family for a family "birth history." You may be surprised what you learn. And remember, sometimes a vehement denial, such as "there's never been any problem in *our* family," may be a clue to dig a little deeper and find out why everyone is so defensive.

Researching your family history can provide valuable information. For example, you may learn of family genetic tendencies that could cause problems on your own reproductive road. Or you may find out that everyone in your family took six months to get pregnant, a fact that may put your mind at ease, particularly around month number five of trying without success.

 If your family tree does hold a genetic problem or a birth defect that shows up more than once, you'll probably want to have genetic testing done. A gene map, which can be done from a blood test, will show whether you carry abnormal genes that could cause problems for your child.

If you're a known carrier of a disease such as Tay-Sachs disease, sickle cell anemia, or cystic fibrosis, you'll probably want to have your partner tested as well. These diseases are carried on recessive genes and are inherited only if both partners are carriers. Sometimes the only thing you learn from family records is nonspecific, such as "all the Smith boys died young." Try and pin down why they all died young: Did they have hemophilia or muscular dystrophy, or did they all fall out of the same apple tree?

 If you do uncover a "bad" or questionable gene through testing, don't panic. This is the reason for testing in the first place. Before you make out a will or go hunting down your mother, father, or great-great-aunt to give them a piece of your mind, remember this:

✔ Not all gene mutations are disease causing. Some are merely benign changes. These differences are what make us all unique individuals.

✔ If you're a carrier of a recessive genetic disorder, you're carrying only one gene and will not get the disease. You're simply a potential conduit.

Sometimes your search for family information can lead you to some unpleasant truths. It's not unheard of, even today, for people to be unaware that they're adopted until a family crisis occurs and the information comes out. You may be surprised to learn that both your grandmother and great-grandmother were hospitalized with mental illness or that three of your uncles were a little "slow" and/or spent time in jail. Many syndromes have been diagnosed in the last 50 years, and what may have been called a family trait may actually have been a (recently recognized) chromosomal or genetic defect.

You may also want to ask your mother whether she took any pills during her pregnancy, or whether her doctor gave her anything to prevent miscarriage. Women whose mothers took DES, a synthetic estrogen hormone, to help prevent miscarriage may have a T-shaped uterus, which may make it difficult to carry a pregnancy. Almost 5 million women were given DES by their doctors between 1938 and 1971, and as many as 50 percent of their daughters may have infertility issues related to DES exposure. Studies are now beginning to be done on problems that affect DES sons and their fertility. The following male problems may be linked to DES:

✔ **Varicoceles:** An enlarged vein in the testicles that can affect sperm production

✔ **Undescended testicles:** Testicles that fail to descend into the scrotum

✔ **Hypospadias:** A misplacement of the opening on the end of the penis

The good news about inherited diseases

When it comes to inherited diseases, you have options your grandmother and mother never did. You can receive pre-pregnancy genetic counseling or have early pregnancy testing of the fetus for abnormalities. Your grandmother, who may have had children well into her 40s, was more likely to have a baby born with chromosomal abnormalities. Such problems are more common in women over 35, and there was no way to test for them during pregnancy in earlier generations. Your mother may have been afraid to have more than one child if she knew there was a family history of cystic fibrosis or muscular dystrophy. The problem that your aunt had during pregnancy from an inherited bleeding disorder is now a condition that can be diagnosed and treated during pregnancy, increasing your chances of having a healthy full-term baby. Rh factors may have caused fetal death just two generations ago, but they can now be easily prevented by an injection of RhoGAM, which prevents the growing fetus from having its blood cells attacked in utero.

Don't be too hard on Mom for not telling you everything. Many women aren't even aware that they took DES until their children enter their reproductive years and begin experiencing problems. Asking the doctor what was in the pills he gave you wasn't something many women did in the 1950s and 1960s.

If you and your partner are blood relatives, it is especially important to see a genetic counselor before getting pregnant. You may carry more of the same abnormal genes than unrelated partners would, which may make you more likely to have a child with a genetic problem. The risk for serious birth defects is 1 in 20 for second cousins and 1 in 11 for first cousins.

Getting Pregnant: More Difficult Today than Yesterday

Sometimes things seemed easier in Grandma's day. Large families were common, and it appeared that everyone had children. In fact, getting pregnant may be harder today, for several reasons:

- People are having children later in life. Over age 25, there is a slight but definite decrease in fertility in women, a decrease that increases dramatically over age 35. Men are also less fertile at older ages.

- Due to better medical management, people are living longer and getting pregnant (or trying to) despite the presence of serious chronic disease, such as diabetes or lupus. In the past, just the *presence* of these conditions would have precluded the possibility of pregnancy.

- Male infertility, related to decreased sperm counts, has increased. Many theories circulate as to why this is occurring, with environmental factors being carefully studied.

- The incidence of sexually transmitted diseases has increased. Some of these diseases, such as chlamydia, cause serious damage to the reproductive organs.

- More men and women have had either a vasectomy or a tubal ligation at a young age and then decided to have another child. Needless to say, they immediately face fertility issues due to their previous choices.

- It may seem as if everyone had children years ago, but start asking questions and you'll get a different story. You may find out that Uncle Charlie wasn't really Aunt Jo's son; he was her sister's child, whom she raised after his mother died young, and on and on. Everyone may have been raising children, but many of those children may have been extended family members.

✔ People today talk more. Just because you never heard about your grand-mother's stillborns or your mother's miscarriages doesn't mean they didn't happen. Pregnancy talk today is big business, and everyone in the world seems to be in the news talking about their babies, lack of babies, adopted babies, and how they got pregnant. This focus puts a constant in-your-face emphasis on pregnancy. It also makes you feel, when you're trying to get pregnant, like everyone else is doing it — and doing it better than you are!

Relax, this is only the beginning for you, and we do our best to help you start baby making with the best of them.

Chapter 2

Baby Steps

Okay, its official . . . you're trying to get pregnant. You've checked out the family tree and checked yourselves out financially, emotionally, and physically, and you're ready to get started. Undoubtedly, you think that you know how to get pregnant. Doesn't everybody? Our goal is to show you how to get pregnant in the shortest amount of trying time (not that trying isn't fun!) with the healthiest possible pregnancy. We take a close look at behaviors and habits (both good and bad) that can help or hinder your baby quest. In this chapter, we review a little basic biology and give you a list of do's and don'ts, along with some interesting pregnancy folklore suggestions that you may want to try for fun . . . or results!

Biology 101: Reviewing Male and Female Anatomy

Were you paying attention in Biology 101? If you were, you probably learned hardly anything about reproducing one of your own kind, though you probably became well versed in the reproduction of worms or frogs. Most likely you suffered through the mandatory sex ed class (which usually rotated with drivers ed and gym), but because you were busy picking lint off your sweater and blushing (if you were a girl) or poking your buddies and guffawing (if you were a guy), you probably didn't retain much. You probably took a quick peek at the film on the miracle of birth and announced loudly to all your friends, "Eww, gross, I'm never having kids!" And yet here you are, some undisclosed number of years later, completely changing your mind and wishing you had paid more attention back then. Don't worry; we're here to fill in the gaps in your reproductive education.

The human body has the basics and the accessories — just like at Macy's! When you buy an outfit, you can be dressed with just the basics, but the accessories really pull your outfit together. When you're trying to have a baby, the parts that you don't see — the "accessories" —determine whether you can get pregnant.

Looking at the female accessories (besides shoes)

A naked woman is pretty unrevealing, from a reproductive viewpoint. You can't see the organs that count in childbearing, so you can't tell at a glance whether yours are present and functioning. Here's a look at what should be inside every woman, starting from the outside and working your way up. (See Figure 2-1.)

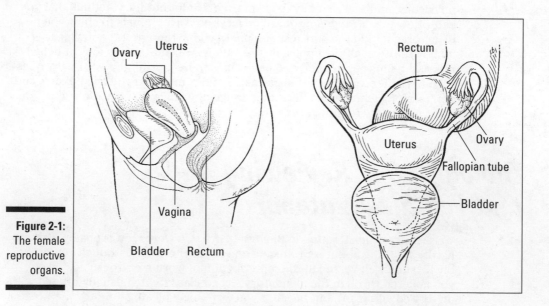

Figure 2-1: The female reproductive organs.

The vagina

The vagina mostly serves as a passageway, first for the penis to deliver sperm up near the opening of the uterus, and later for the delivery of the baby. If you have a very small vagina, intercourse may be uncomfortable. If your vagina is large, as it may be after having a baby, sex may be less pleasurable. Neither condition, however, should affect your ability to get pregnant.

The vagina contains glands that secrete fluid during sexual arousal; this makes it easier for a penis to enter the vagina — and a lot more enjoyable!

Some women are born without a vagina; usually the uterus is also missing in these women. The formal name of this syndrome is Rokitansky-Kuster-Hauser-Mayer, and it's the second most common cause of *amenorrhea,* or lack of periods starting by age 16. This condition is usually diagnosed when you don't start your periods in your teens.

The *hymen* is a nonfunctional piece of circular tissue found at the entrance to the vagina; the bleeding many women have the first time they have sex comes from the tearing of the hymen. The hymen is not a solid piece of tissue; 99 percent of baby girls already have openings, or perforations, in the hymen. An *imperforate hymen,* one that has no holes, can cause blood to back up behind the small opening; this blood can be forced back up into the fallopian tubes. Women with an imperforate hymen have a higher incidence of endometriosis. (See Chapter 7 for more on endometriosis.)

The cervix

The *cervix* is the lower part of the uterus. It keeps the baby from falling out of the uterus when you're pregnant because it's a tight, musclelike tissue. The cervix also guards against infection because it's filled with mucus that forms a barrier between your vagina and the inside of the uterus. If you have an *incompetent cervix,* it means that the cervix doesn't stay tight and closed when you're pregnant but starts to open up from the weight of the growing baby. An incompetent cervix is usually stitched with a suture called a *cerclage* in early pregnancy to keep the baby where it belongs.

The uterus

The *uterus,* or womb, is a pear-shaped organ designed to hold and nourish a baby for nine months. Every month the lining of the uterus, called the *endometrium,* thickens to make a nourishing bed for an embryo. If you don't get pregnant that month, the lining breaks down and is shed as your *menstrual flow,* or *period.*

If your body isn't making enough of the hormone estrogen, your lining may not grow very much, and you may not have much flow. Even though it may seem as if you pass buckets of blood each month, the average amount of blood lost with each cycle is only about four tablespoons. If you're a real gusher, you may lose as much as a cup, in which case you should check your hemoglobin (iron levels) to make sure that you're not anemic from a heavy flow.

Many women have a uterus that doesn't conform to the standard upside-down pear shape you've all seen in pictures marked "this is your uterus." If you're one of these women, your uterus is flopped forward, toward your pubic bone. Twenty percent of women have a tipped or retroverted uterus, which does not cause problems getting pregnant.

Around 2 to 3 percent of women have an abnormally shaped uterus. The most common variation is a *septate uterus,* which means that a band of tissue *(septum)* partially or completely divides the inside of the uterus. This tissue can be surgically removed. A T-shaped uterus is often a side effect of your mom's taking DES, a drug given from the 1940s to the 1960s to prevent miscarriage. *Bicornuate* (two-horn) and *unicornuate* (one-horn) uteri have either one (uni) or two (bi) narrower-than-normal cavities. Women with T-shaped, bicornuate, and unicornuate uteri have higher-than-normal miscarriage rates.

It's also possible to have two separate uterine cavities, called a *didelphys uterus;* such women usually also have a second cervix. You may need to have a cesarean section (a surgical delivery) if you have a double cervix, meaning that more isn't always better. In addition, you could quite possibly get pregnant with twins, one developing in each uterus.

Even if the shape of your uterus is normal, it may contain some unwanted "accessories" — growths such as polyps and fibroids — which may decrease the chance that a fetus can implant and grow in your uterus. Polyps are easily removed and don't cause any complications after they're gone. Removing fibroids is more complex; sometimes they can't be removed without damaging your uterus. Removing fibroids can leave scar tissue in the cavity that can make it harder to get pregnant because the fetus won't be able to implant in the scarred area. You may also need a cesarean section after fibroid removal. Scar tissue can also form in your uterus after a dilation and curettage (D&C for short). If there's a lot of scar tissue, nearly filling the uterus, it's called Asherman's syndrome. This scar tissue can also be removed surgically to make it easier for you to get pregnant.

The ovaries

Most women have two ovaries, which contain the most important accessory of all — eggs! How many eggs? Well, to look at a newborn baby girl, you would never guess that her ovaries already contain about 1 million eggs — and that's after a loss of 2.5 million eggs in the last three months before her birth! Every single day of your life, many eggs are lost through *atresia,* which means that they die off because they're not being stimulated to mature. By puberty, only 300,000 to 400,000 eggs remain, and every month, 500 to 1,000 are lost, along with the one or possibly two eggs that mature and are released each month. By age 50, only 1,000 or so eggs remain, and many are abnormal because the "good" eggs get used up first.

What makes an egg develop and mature? The process goes like this:

1. Follicle-stimulating hormone (FSH) is released from your pituitary gland.

2. In the ovary, 10 to 15 eggs begin to grow. The tissue surrounding each egg forms a follicle, a fluid-filled sac. Each follicle contains one egg.

3. Luteinizing hormone (LH) is released from the pituitary gland. The follicle begins to produce estrogen.

4. One follicle becomes dominant, growing faster than the others.

5. As the dominant follicle grows, it produces more estrogen. The amount of FSH released decreases, and the smaller follicles stop growing.

6. A large amount of LH is released as the estrogen rises. This makes the egg inside the dominant follicle mature.

7. The follicle bursts, and the egg is released.

8. The leftover part of the follicle, now called the *corpus luteum,* produces progesterone to help an embryo implant.

What exactly is in this egg?

You may wonder what eggs contain to make them into your potential screaming newborn. The answer is chromosomes — 23 chromosomes, to be exact. Each chromosome contains the genes that determine whether your baby is tall or short, blond or brunet, and, to some extent, fat or thin. (See Chapter 1 for more information on chromosomes and genes.)

Of course, there's more to an egg than chromosomes. Three protective layers surround the egg, starting with the *cumulus layer.* That's the nourishing and protecting fluffy layers of cells that completely surround the egg. Moving inward, you'll see the *corona radiate,* the protective single layer of cells covering the *zona pellucida,* the "shell" of the egg. A mature, ready-for-fertilization oocyte, or egg, has a small attachment called a *polar body,* which is the remnant left after the egg divides (a process called *meiosis*) so that it contains only 23 chromosomes.

All cells in the human body besides eggs and sperm have 46 chromosomes. Eggs and sperm have 23, so the baby they create has 46.

If you have only one ovary, either because you were born that way or because one was surgically removed, your one ovary usually takes over egg making each month.

Determining whether it's a good egg

Making a mature, healthy egg is essential to getting pregnant. How do you know whether you're making good eggs? You can't be sure whether any month's egg is Grade A, but a properly matured egg, released at the right time of the month, when the lining of the uterus is ready to receive it, is needed for pregnancy to occur.

How can you tell whether you have eggs at all, much less good eggs? One sign of good egg production is a regular menstrual cycle. If you're very irregular, skip months, or have periods closer than three weeks apart, you may not be making good, mature eggs. Your periods should start about two weeks after your egg is released from the ovary (ovulation).

But how do you know when you ovulate? Some women always know, but others need the help of an ovulation predictor kit to be sure. We discuss ovulation predictor kits more in Chapter 3, but if you're lucky, your best sign of ovulation will be pain.

The fallopian tubes

You should have two fallopian tubes, one near each ovary. Tubes are kind of like a pickup bar — a place where sperm and egg should meet and hopefully go on to create something bigger and better: a baby! When an egg is released from the ovary, little projections called *fimbriae* on the end of the tube move back and forth to "entice" the egg into the tube. Once in the fallopian tube, the egg needs a few days to shimmy down to the uterus. Hopefully along the way it meets Mr. Sperm and fertilizes, thereby transforming into an embryo by the time it reaches the uterus. Damaged tubes, usually damaged from infection but sometimes from endometriosis or surgery, are a very common cause of infertility. We talk about this in depth in Chapter 7.

The breasts

Breasts aren't necessary for getting pregnant; women who have had breasts removed can get pregnant. The normal number of breasts, of course, is two. Nipples are a different matter. As many as 1 in 20 people have more than two nipples. The extras may be nothing more than a reddish brown, rough piece of skin, often found in line with the main nipples. Check yourself out!

Ouch! I think I ovulated

About 20 percent of women have pain called *mittelschmerz* (German for "middle pain") when they ovulate. The pain seems to be caused by blood and fluid irritating the tissues around the ovary after it releases from the follicle. Sometimes a small amount of vaginal bleeding occurs with ovulation too.

Putting all the parts together: Your menstrual cycle

The ovaries, uterus, and fallopian tubes all need to function together for you to get pregnant. Here's what happens:

- **Days 1 to 5:** In the ovary, an egg begins to mature. This is called the follicular phase of the ovary. In the uterus, the old lining breaks down and passes through the vagina as your menstrual flow. This process takes one to five days.

- **Days 6 to 13:** In the ovary, one egg-containing follicle is growing and producing estrogen. In the uterus, the estrogen produced by the ovary is making the lining thicken. This is called the *proliferative phase*.

- **Ovulation (around day 14):** In the ovary, the follicle bursts, and the egg is released. It begins to travel down the fallopian tubes. This journey takes several days. The uterus is now thick enough to support the growth of an embryo.

- **Day 14 (approximately) to day 28:** In the ovary, the leftover remnant of the follicle, the *corpus luteum,* produces progesterone. This is called the *luteal phase* of the ovary. The embryo floats in the uterus for several days and then implants in the thickened uterine lining and starts to grow. This is called the *secretory phase.* If you're not pregnant, the lining will break down two weeks after ovulation, and your cycle will begin again.

Hanging out with the guys

Compared to women, guys let it all hang out, reproductively speaking. That's a good thing because "hanging out," at least as far as testicles are concerned, is necessary to keep the developing sperm from getting too warm. Take a look at what every guy should have. See Figure 2-2 for a graphic portrayal of your average man.

The penis

The number-one guy concern is probably related to penis size: How do I compare to everyone else? For those obsessed, here are the standards: normal length when flaccid, or limp, 3.9 inches; stretched (still limp), 4.8 inches; erect, 5 to 7 inches. Hopefully that made most of you fellows feel better. A small penis, less than 1.9 inches limp, is usually able to impregnate as long as it can get the sperm into the vagina, up toward the cervix. Size is rarely an issue in infertility.

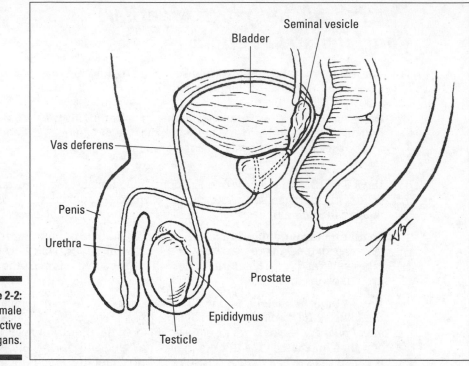

Figure 2-2:
The male
reproductive
organs.

Size may not matter, but function does. If you watch Viagra commercials, you may be comforted to know that even athletes and famous men have problems with erectile dysfunction, also known as impotence. As nice as it is to know that you're not alone, this condition can be an embarrassing detriment to getting pregnant. *Impotence,* the ability to have or sustain an erection, is more common as men get older; as many as 50 percent of men between the ages of 40 and 70 have had problems with impotence. Impotence can be caused by diseases such as diabetes or by chronic conditions, such as alcohol abuse, or it can be a side effect of medications. (We discuss impotence in Chapter 7.)

The opening that lets both urine and sperm out of the penis should be at the tip of the penis, located dead center. Two types of variations can cause problems getting pregnant. One in around 300 men has *hypospadias,* which means that the opening is on the underside of the penis. In 20 percent of cases, this problem is hereditary. In *epispadias,* the opening is on the top of the penis. Both conditions are associated with an unusual curvature of the erect penis; it curves up in epispadias and down in hypospadias. Both conditions can prevent the sperm from getting exactly where they need to be. Surgical correction is possible.

The testicles

Testicles are the sperm production and warehouse site. Here, as in many other places on the human body, nature has been generous and given two testicles, in case something happens to one. Testicles first develop inside the abdomen and gradually descend outside the body by the time a baby boy is born. At birth, about 4 in 100 boys have undescended testicles, properly called *cryptorchidism.* Testicles need to be kept a few degrees cooler than 98 degrees for sperm to develop properly, so to prevent future infertility, doctors usually recommend surgery to lower the testicles outside the body as soon as the baby is a year old.

The testicles are contained in a pouch of skin called the *scrotum.* In about 80 percent of men, the left testicle is bigger and hangs lower. Sometimes the testicles are abnormally large, which can be caused by a *hydrocele,* which is a collection of fluid inside the scrotum, or by a *varicocele,* which is the condition of dilated or varicose veins in the testicle. These conditions can be surgically corrected. If left alone, they can raise the temperature of the testes and cause infertility.

Sperm are produced every day, but it takes about 70 days for the new sperm to fully mature. Sperm production starts in the testes. FSH and LH, the same hormones that develop eggs, are needed to begin sperm production. LH stimulates production of testosterone, another male hormone. The sperm mature in the epididymis and travel through the vas deferens, where they're bathed in the fluid known as semen. They're then ejaculated through the urethra during male orgasm.

Sperm — 200 million of them!

Here comes one egg — or maybe two eggs, if it's a good month — tooling down the fallopian tubes. The egg is about the size of a pencil point dot — in other words, barely visible. All of a sudden the egg meets up with about 200 sperm, the sole survivors of an ejaculate of over 100 million sperm a few hours before — talk about an embarrassment of riches. The sperm are much smaller than the egg, so small that all the sperm needed to repopulate the earth could sit on an aspirin tablet. There's enough room for all of them to attach their heads to the egg and try to beat down the door. Ideally, only one will succeed, and the others will be shut out immediately.

Why are there so many more sperm than eggs? Because it's a *long* way through the uterus and up the tubes, and because only 50 percent (of a *good* sperm sample) of the sperm know how to swim forward, *and* because some of them are barely moving, a tremendous number of sperm are needed to ensure that a few hundred will get through to the egg. Their journey is like one of you trying to swim across the Pacific Ocean. If there were 200 million of you, maybe a few hundred would make it. Imagine if you had to fertilize an egg when you finally got there! (We talk about sperm much more in Chapter 7.)

Putting Male and Female Parts Together: Having Sex (At the Right Time)

Now that you know how all your parts work, are you ready to have a baby? Yes? Then it's time to have sex. No, not right now. It's important to have sex when the timing is right. How do you know when the timing is right? This is more than just mood lighting and foreplay. To get pregnant, you need to be close to ovulation.

You may be able to tell that you're ovulating in a few simple ways, just by watching the calendar and being observant about your bodily functions.

If you're an on-the-dot, regular-as-clockwork type, with 28 days between each period, you probably ovulate around day 14. You're also rare as hen's teeth. Few women are that regular; most women usually have a few days' variation from month to month. But if your periods are regular, you can figure that you're ovulating about two weeks before your period starts, so if you have 32-day cycles, you ovulate around day 18.

Usually the mucus from your cervix increases around the time of ovulation. It also becomes very thin, clear, and stretchy; you can easily stretch it out a couple of inches. Rising estrogen levels from a developing follicle create this mucus, which is easier for sperm to swim through than your usual thicker mucus and also has an alkaline pH, which helps the sperm live longer. At other times of the month, cervical mucus is acidic. Be sure that you're not confusing cervical mucus with semen from previous sex or increased secretions from sexual arousal.

If you're taking antihistamines, you may not notice a change in cervical mucus. Antihistamines, usually found in cold medications, dry up mucus everywhere, not just in your nose and chest.

If you have no objection to feeling around inside your vagina, you'll also notice that your cervix becomes softer, slightly open, and easier to locate with your fingers when you're about to ovulate. At other times of the month, the cervix is found farther back in the uterus, feels firmer to the touch, and is tightly closed.

Some women have headaches around the time of ovulation, and others complain of bloating or breast pain. You're probably already aware of your personal ovulation indicators, but you may have just never paid much attention to them. Now you should. They're a big help in choosing when to have baby sex.

Conceiving a Baby: How Sex Should Work

The time is right, the moon is bright, and it's time to get pregnant. Here's what needs to happen:

1. It's near ovulation; an egg is about to release from its follicle.

2. You and your partner become aroused. Your vagina produces secretions that make it easier for the now erect penis to enter the vagina.

3. During the man's orgasm, several million sperm are forcefully ejaculated into the vagina. As they pass through the cervix into the uterus; the cervical mucus "washes" the sperm so that they're ready to penetrate an egg.

4. Your egg releases from the follicle and enters one of your fallopian tubes.

5. The sperm swim through the uterus up to the fallopian tubes; half choose the wrong tube to enter.

6. The next day your egg meets up with several hundred sperm in the fallopian tube, and they all attach themselves to the egg, trying to beat down the door.

7. One sperm breaks through the outer layer of the egg, and the egg immediately becomes impenetrable to the rest of the sperm.

8. The genetic material of the egg and sperm combine, and the newly created embryo drifts down the fallopian tube to the uterus.

9. The embryo implants in the uterine wall and grows, and you miss your period.

10. You're pregnant! Congratulations.

 After sex, just lie there for a while. Don't jump up and go to the bathroom right away. Let gravity help those little swimmers get to where they need to be. Some doctors advocate placing a pillow under the hips during sex to give gravity a little edge in directing the sperm where they need to be. Doing so probably isn't necessary. Of course, the missionary position, man on top, is also an aid to gravity.

Figuring Out How Often to Have Sex

When you're trying to get pregnant, you need to strike a balance between too much sex and not enough. Too much sex decreases sperm counts, but if you have too little sex, you may miss the right moment for conception. Not having sex for more than five days may raise the number of sperm but decrease their motility (the active movement). Sex less than two days apart may decrease the sperm count. So how do you figure out when the right time is?

When you're close to ovulating, have sex at least every other day; some doctors recommend the two days before and the day you ovulate as the best time for conception.

Making Sure That You're Healthy — Before Conception

Even though you're probably anxious to get started on baby making, take a little time to make sure that you're in the best possible condition for conceiving a healthy baby. This means making sure that you're not carrying an infection that could harm you or your baby and taking a look at your lifestyle habits, good and bad.

What you can't see: Common infections that may cause problems

The onset of the sexual revolution in the 1960s caused a lot of fallout, and some of it fell on future fertility. Sexually transmitted diseases, or STDs, have increased dramatically in the last 20 years. More than 13 million Americans each year are affected, and many STDs pack a major antifertility wallop for both sexes. You may not even know that you have a sexually transmitted disease. Some STDs cause a vaginal or penile discharge, others cause itching or small sores, but some cause no symptoms at all. Most are easily treated with antibiotics. The problem is that many women don't realize they have an infection because most have no clear symptoms. The following sections describe a few of the most damaging STDs and provide some statistics about the diseases in the United States.

Chlamydia: The most common STD

Chlamydia is the most common sexually transmitted disease in the United States. The bacterium *Chlamydia trachomatis* is responsible for the infection. Both men and women can be infected, and both male and female fertility can be damaged. Chlamydia is easily tested by swabbing the penis or vagina and sending the swab to a lab for testing. A new test using urine is also being developed. Chlamydia is easily treated with antibiotics.

Here are some facts about the disease:

- About 4 million new cases of chlamydia are diagnosed every year.

- Approximately one in ten sexually active adolescents has been exposed to chlamydia.

- Women with untreated chlamydia have a 40 percent chance of developing pelvic inflammatory disease (PID), a major cause of damaged fallopian tubes.

- Women with PID are seven to ten times more likely to have an ectopic pregnancy, a pregnancy that grows outside the uterus, usually in the tubes. (For more about ectopic pregnancies, see Chapter 6.)

- Most women (75 percent) have no symptoms of infection; symptoms include lower abdominal pain, burning with urination, and vaginal irritation.

- Twenty five percent of men have no symptoms from chlamydia; 75 percent have a discharge from the urethra, or pain and burning on urination.

- Men with untreated chlamydia can develop *epididymitis,* an infection in the testicles, where sperm are developed. This condition can lead to low sperm counts.

- Each year, 100,000 women become infertile from chlamydia. With a first infection, 12 percent of women become infertile; a second case increases infertility to 40 percent. Eighty percent of women who have had chlamydia three or more times are infertile.

- Fifty percent of people with chlamydia also have gonorrhea.

- Untreated chlamydia when you're pregnant can lead to blindness in your child.

Gonorrhea

Gonorrhea is caused by the bacterium *Neisseria gonorrhoeae,* which can infect the genital tract, mouth, or rectum. It can be carried by males and females and can be cured with antibiotics. Here are some other facts about gonorrhea:

- Each year, 650,000 new cases of gonorrhea are diagnosed.

- Gonorrhea is diagnosed second only in frequency to chlamydia.

- Like chlamydia, gonorrhea in women can cause PID, leading to tubal damage. Most doctors test for gonorrhea and chlamydia before doing common fertility tests such as a *hysterosalpingogram* (HSG), in which dye is injected into the uterus and fallopian tubes to see whether there are any irregularities. (We discuss HSGs in more detail in Chapter 7.) If you have gonorrhea or chlamydia and push dye into the tubes and uterus, you may push the infection up also and end up with more tube or uterine damage than you had to begin with.

✔ Men with gonorrhea usually have a discharge from the penis and a burning sensation; women may have no symptoms.

Syphilis

Syphilis is caused by the bacterium *Treponema pallidum*. The bacterium can be transmitted through genital, oral, or anal contact. Syphilis is easily cured with penicillin. Contrary to folklore, syphilis can't be caught from a toilet seat. But consider the following:

✔ Syphilis can cause stillbirth, blindness, mental retardation, or chronic syphilis in your unborn child if you have this disease while pregnant. Syphilis is treated with antibiotics.

✔ Lest you think syphilis is a thing of the past, 35,000 cases were reported in the United States in 1999, with 556 cases of congenital syphilis in newborns.

Ureaplasma and mycoplasma

Ureaplasma and mycoplasma are microorganisms that can affect different parts of the body, depending on the strain. The genital tracts of both sexes can carry mycoplasma or ureaplasma. The following list gives some other information about the diseases:

✔ As many as 40 percent of women and men are carriers of bacteria called *ureaplasma* or *mycoplasma*.

✔ Some controversy exists about whether certain strains of ureaplasma and mycoplasma cause problems in getting pregnant; some studies show that they increase the incidence of miscarriage and/or problems with the embryo implanting in the uterus. This seems to be related to either partner having the infection, which is easily passed between partners.

✔ New studies are questioning whether these bacteria really cause infertility or miscarriage; more studies will probably be done.

✔ As with other STDs, both partners are easily treated with a 14-day course of an antibiotic, such as doxycycline. Both partners must take the drug, or they'll probably continue to reinfect each other.

Genital herpes

Genital herpes is caused by the herpes simplex type 2 virus. The cold sores some people are prone to on their lips are caused by the herpes simplex type 1 virus. Scientists are working on a vaccine against herpes, which would work only for those not already infected with the virus. Here's some more information:

✔ Sixty million Americans are infected with genital herpes, with 500,000 new cases diagnosed each year.

✔ If you have an outbreak of genital herpes at the time your baby is ready to be delivered, you'll need to have a cesarean section; if you deliver vaginally without treatment, your baby may suffer from mental retardation or may die.

✔ Herpes can't be cured; outbreaks are treated with antiviral medications.

HIV

Human immunodeficiency virus (HIV) causes the disease AIDS (acquired immune deficiency syndrome). At present, there is no cure for AIDS, although antiviral medications may keep the disease under control for some time.

✔ Women with HIV can become pregnant and carry the pregnancy to term, but they risk transmitting HIV to the baby.

✔ The risk of transmission is about 25 percent if you're untreated and may be as low as 8 to 9 percent if you receive AZT, an antiviral drug, while you're pregnant.

✔ Some doctors believe that the stress of pregnancy may cause your symptoms to worsen.

✔ You may reduce the risk of transmission of the disease to your baby if you have a cesarean section rather than a vaginal delivery.

✔ You must wait 3 to 18 months after delivery to find out whether your baby is HIV positive, because during pregnancy your antibodies are passed to the baby. This means that all babies of HIV-infected moms will test positive at birth. It can take as long as 18 months for all your antibodies to disappear from your baby's blood. After your antibodies are all gone, if the baby tests positive, it means he or she is infected with the virus.

You can be tested for sexually transmitted diseases, including HIV, before trying to conceive. If you suspect that you may have an STD, or have been exposed to one, you need to rule out this potential danger to your fertility and your unborn child.

Making healthy lifestyle changes

"Everything in moderation" is certainly a good motto for habits, good and bad. Too much exercise can have a less than desirable effect, while coffee, drunk in moderation, can be benign. But, before you say yes to things that are better left in the no category, consider that some things are best eliminated entirely, particularly when you're trying to conceive.

Giving up smoking

Smoking is bad for you. You all know it. Yet 30 percent of women in the United States still smoke. Need some good reasons to quit? Here are a few:

- ✔ Smokers are 50 percent more likely to miscarry.

- ✔ Smokers are two to four times more likely to have an ectopic pregnancy (one that implants in the fallopian tube rather than in the uterus, a topic we discuss in detail in Chapter 6).

- ✔ Smokers go through menopause earlier, decreasing the number of years pregnancy can occur.

- ✔ Smokers' eggs have more genetic abnormalities.

- ✔ Smokers' eggs are prone to *polyspermy,* where two or more sperm enter an egg. The embryos that result are chromosomally abnormal and will not grow.

If you've quit but your partner hasn't, he may want to consider the following:

- ✔ Men who smoke have a lower sperm count.

- ✔ Men who smoke have a 20 percent decrease in sperm motility.

- ✔ Smokers' sperm have more abnormal shapes. Abnormally shaped sperm have a higher rate of chromosome abnormalities.

Eliminating alcohol

Studies show that heavy drinkers (more than three drinks a day) have more trouble getting pregnant. Continuing to drink while pregnant increases the chance for miscarriage and also can cause fetal alcohol syndrome (FAS). FAS babies have learning and behavioral problems and typically have small heads, a flat midface, small eye slits, and a low nasal ridge.

Saying no to drugs

Undoubtedly you know that illegal drugs are taboo when trying to become pregnant! Here are the problems that some common drugs can cause when you're trying to get pregnant.

Cocaine

Cocaine causes constriction of the blood vessels, which can result in early miscarriage, preterm delivery, and problems with the *placenta,* the organ that nourishes the baby. In addition, cocaine can cause menstrual irregularities, possibly making it harder for you to become pregnant.

Marijuana

Marijuana lowers sperm count, decreases sperm's motility or ability to move forward, lowers the amount of testosterone in males, and results in an increased number of abnormal eggs and sperm.

Cutting back on caffeine

Caffeine is controversial, but several studies have shown that drinking several cups of coffee a day may increase the risk of developing *endometriosis,* abnormal tissue growth that can affect your uterus or fallopian tubes as well as cause increased difficulty becoming pregnant and early miscarriage. A cup of coffee contains twice the caffeine in one can of soda. Limit caffeine to less than 300 mg, which is three cups of coffee, or, better yet, cut it out completely! Teas also contain caffeine, but much less than coffee— 12 to 100 mg per cup.

Staying out of the hot tub

Anything that raises the temperature of a man's testicles can decrease sperm production and motility. Hot tubs, saunas, steam rooms, and tight underwear are out for men! And in case you're thinking of jumping in the tub without him, high temperatures have also been associated with egg damage and miscarriage. Find another way to relax when you're pregnant or trying to be.

Exercising with caution

So your partner decided to work out stress by bicycling or playing rugby. This exercise should be a good thing, right? Wrong! Prolonged cycling can cause damage to the groin from constant pressure of the bike seat, and contact sports can lead to injury to the testicles and can damage sperm production.

Women who exercise heavily may find that their periods have stopped. This condition is called *amenorrhea* and is common among women who are very thin and exercise daily. Obviously, you can't get pregnant if you're not having periods; you're not making any eggs. So what can you both do to reduce stress that won't cause fertility problems? Knitting is nice. If knitting isn't enough for you, exercise in moderation is fine — for both of you!

Avoiding anabolic steroids

Some studies show that as many as 6 to 7 percent of all males have used anabolic steroids before age 18 to build muscle mass. Anabolic steroids suppress the body's ability to make testosterone, which is necessary for normal sperm production. This damage can be permanent, so stay away from the steroids.

Dumping the douche

Douching is a bad idea whether you're trying to get pregnant or not. Women who douche regularly have a 73 percent increase in pelvic inflammatory disease (PID), which can cause damage to the fallopian tubes and uterus. The ectopic pregnancy rate is about 75 percent higher in women who douche regularly. Thirty-seven percent of women between the ages of 15 and 44 douche, and their risk of developing cervical cancer is about 80 percent higher than those who don't. Dump the douche!

Behaving Yourself When Trying to Conceive

Because the best parents generally practice what they preach, setting up some good habits even *before* conception occurs is as good of a start as any! Good nutrition is important at every stage of your life, but particularly when you're trying to conceive and maintain a pregnancy and ultimately deliver a healthy child. Although a perfectly tuned body isn't a necessity for having children, it certainly provides an ideal starting point. Nurturing your mind and heart is equally important. The following sections offer some tips on keeping your entire self in tiptop baby-making shape.

Getting the proper nutrition

Although vitamins provide good supplementation, get as many nutrients and minerals as possible from the food you eat. So before ingesting supplements ranging from vitamin A to zinc, start instead with your diet. Eating three square meals a day, plus a snack, is a good place to begin. What should those meals be made of? If you consider chocolate a food group, read on.

Look at your fertility diet in the shape of a pregnant woman's body. See Figure 2-3 for a visual of a pregnant you as a food chart. At the top, the smallest spot (your head) should be reserved for fats, oils, and sweets. This category includes jam, mayonnaise, margarine, candy, and so on. Use these foods sparingly.

The next step down on the chart consists of two slightly larger categories: the milk, yogurt, and cheese group and the group that includes meat, poultry, fish, dry beans, eggs, and nuts. It is recommended that you consume two to three servings from the milk, yogurt, and cheese group. In this category, a serving is considered 1 cup of milk or yogurt or 2 ounces of processed cheese. Two to three servings (ounces) are recommended in the group that includes lean meat, poultry, fish, eggs, dry beans, and nuts. This level provides you with calcium, riboflavin, protein, iron, and B vitamins.

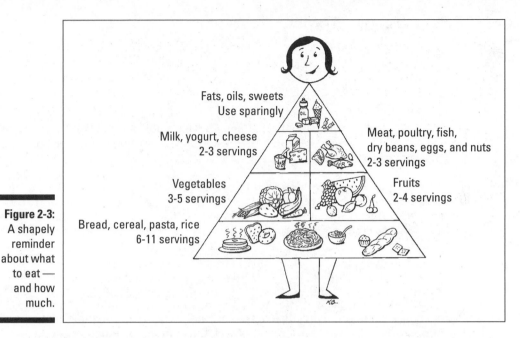

Figure 2-3:
A shapely
reminder
about what
to eat —
and how
much.

Fats, oils, sweets
Use sparingly

Milk, yogurt, cheese
2-3 servings

Meat, poultry, fish,
dry beans, eggs, and nuts
2-3 servings

Vegetables
3-5 servings

Fruits
2-4 servings

Bread, cereal, pasta, rice
6-11 servings

The next level calls for three to five servings of vegetables and two to four servings of fruit. A serving size of vegetables consists of 1 cup of raw leafy vegetables, ½ cup of cooked vegetables, or ¾ cup of vegetable juice, and a serving size of fruits consists of one medium apple, banana, or orange, ½ cup of chopped cooked or canned fruit, or ¾ cup of fruit juice. Notice that the recommended servings have increased from the higher level of this food chart. Pay attention to this recommendation. Vegetables and fruits are your most important source for fiber, vitamin A, vitamin C, and carbohydrates.

At the bottom of the pregnant woman food chart, you find the largest food group, which contains bread, cereal, rice, and pasta. Consider this the abdomen! The recommendation is that you eat six to eleven servings of this group per day. But before you wolf down a plate of pasta, remember your serving sizes. A serving in this group consists of one slice of bread, half a bagel, 1 ounce of ready-to-eat cereal, ½ cup of cooked rice or pasta, three to four small, plain crackers, or one 4-inch pancake.

If this seems like any other food plan you've ever seen, there's a reason for it — it is! Healthy eating is a standard practice. There are few tricks to eating healthy. When trying to conceive, eat enough but not too much and use your calories for healthy foods and not empty ones (such as chocolate). If you're not lactose intolerant, you may want to up your dairy intake; if you're *lactose intolerant*, which means that you can't properly digest milk products, you can get calcium from oral supplements.

Be careful of health foods such as soy, sunflower seeds, or herbs such as Vitex that promise to raise your estrogen level. (You can read more about herbs in Chapter 5.) Your body — more specifically, your ovaries — should be producing estrogen. By introducing an exogenous (outside) source, you're not assisting your body in manufacturing its own supply; you're only supplementing it artificially. This addition does not change the quality of your eggs or their output of estrogen. It only confuses any measurement of estrogen, as it's impossible to distinguish what your body makes on its own from that which you gain from outside sources. Skip any supplement or food that claims to increase your estrogen level.

Another practice to avoid is dieting, particularly fad diets. Conception is an act of incredible balance and timing. You don't want to throw your body off with the latest diet that promises to help you lose five pounds fast. More than likely, such a diet is a method that probably won't help your weight or your health any more than it will help your fertility.

If you're significantly overweight or underweight, you may want to consult your physician first (an Ob/Gyn will do). Either extreme can cause problems in fertility, particularly if your weight is symptomatic of another condition such as diabetes, polycystic ovary syndrome (PCOS), or amenorrhea. Twelve percent of all infertility is a result of weighing either too much or too little. The good news is that 70 percent of all women diagnosed with infertility related to being overweight or underweight conceive spontaneously when their weight normalizes.

If weight loss or weight gain is in order, consider addressing this matter before trying to conceive. Check with your physician and ask for a healthy diet and exercise plan. If you must embark on a weight adjustment program simultaneously with your baby-making efforts, make sure that your physician is aware of *both* goals.

In an Australian study of 3,500 women, very obese women were half as likely to conceive when compared to their healthier peer group. The researchers also concluded that it was no good being underweight either: Women who were below moderate weight also had less of a chance of becoming pregnant.

Ways in which extremes of weight can affect fertility include menstrual disturbance, disturbance to the lining of the uterus, inability to ovulate (anovulation), and increased risk of miscarriage.

Taking vitamins

Multivitamins are a good way to supplement your diet, but they're not a substitute for good nutrition. While you're trying to conceive and when you get pregnant, you need both. Much has been written about the importance of folic acid in early pregnancy. It has been shown to diminish certain birth defects, such as spina bifida.

Most garden-variety multivitamins contain adequate amounts of folic acid and suffice while you're trying to conceive. While you pursue no- and low-tech means to conceive (read: natural), you may want to ask your general practitioner to prescribe prenatal vitamins instead. Some fertility doctors cite a slightly lower conception rate among women using prenatal vitamins, but as of this writing, this belief is unproven. If you want to play it safe, opt for a standard multivitamin. Your Ob/Gyn can switch you to prenatal vitamins as soon as you become pregnant. As with everything else, moderation is key. Mixing and matching individual vitamin supplements can result in too much of a good thing, which translates into *not* such a good thing. Let the drug manufacturers figure out the dosages. Just stick with the basics.

Turning to books and the Internet for information

Reading is good. Reading about pregnancy is better, particularly if you choose books and other materials that focus on areas that you *do* have control over, namely nutrition, exercise, and good self-care. Take the time to read about and make the changes that you can to create a healthier you, which in turn will make you a healthier *two*.

Books are always a great source of information, but the Internet can also provide an abundance of resources. Log on to a search engine such as Google or Yahoo! You'll be rewarded with a plethora of possibilities on everything to do with pregnancy and then some. Be a careful consumer, however. When visiting a Web site, check out the source providing the information. Chat rooms are wonderful for support and referrals, but act on medical advice only from a professional.

Talking to friends

Ooooooh, a toughie! Support is a wonderful thing, but pressure is not. If you decide to share with your friends that you're trying to conceive, don't turn your efforts into a quest or a competition. You may want to inform your friends that you're trying and that you'll let them know if and when you succeed. This approach can help prevent the "Are you there yet?" questions that are asked in the right spirit yet often result in a feeling of pressure, albeit unintended.

Friends who have had children or have tried to conceive can be incredibly helpful in lending perspective to your monthly challenge and can also offer suggestions on everything from doctors to diapers, reading materials to relaxation techniques. You may also find an enormous amount of support from friends who are neither married nor with children. Those faced with the challenge of searching for Mr. or Ms. Right may turn to the same elements of luck and timing that also apply to making a baby. Single friends can be incredibly supportive in relating along these lines.

Through my own journey, I (coauthor Jackie) have forged new and valuable friendships. Some of these friendships came about due to our shared struggle of trying to conceive, and others were the result of realizing just how supportive and loving an acquaintance, neighbor, or colleague really can be. These friendships proved to be the blessings in disguise that pointed me toward wonderful women whom I otherwise may not have gotten to know. Although old friends may be your foundation, you may be surprised by the other nice people you find along the way.

Listening to the Old Wives

The good news about letting your friends and family know that you're trying to conceive is that everyone has an idea. The bad news is . . . everyone has an idea. And although most of these ideas are well meaning, many of them also weigh in at downright wacky. As my husband and I (coauthor Jackie) traveled the long road to baby, we tried to take these suggestions in the spirit that they were given and actually tried a few along the way. And although not one of these tales bears any medical significance, women have claimed success with many of them, often when other methods have failed.

So if you're game for a different approach, you might give an old wives' tale a whirl. If you'd rather stick with the more proven track, you may still enjoy reading about some of the superstitions and stories that others swear by. If doing so only gives you cause to smile, just remember another old adage: Laughter is the best medicine.

Here are some ideas from several old wives:

- ✔ Honeymoons are a really good time to become pregnant . . . with twins! You may think this outcome is related to sex, but no, according to one tale, a couple will have twins if they see a movie during the first three days of their honeymoon or go swimming on the first day of their marriage.

- ✔ If you can't manage a honeymoon just now, you might consider having a messy friend come to your house and leave a diaper under a bed. Doing so is supposed to ensure a birth in your house.

- ✔ If you'd rather be the one leaving things about, go to a strange house and lay your coat or hat on a bed there; doing so is also supposed to help you get pregnant. Maybe you could visit all the open houses in your area and lay your coat all over town to make *sure* that this method works.

- Consider becoming a member of the local Welcome Wagon. If a woman is the first to visit a newborn, she'll have the next child, according to another tale.

- Eating peanut butter during the last two weeks of your menstrual cycle helps an embryo to "stick."

- Sniff! Sniff! Smelling behind a pregnant woman's ear will cause you to conceive.

- Caffeine before sex increases a woman's fertility.

- Holding a newborn baby for a day will bring about your own baby.

- "Crawl around on the floor like a baby before you have sex," a friend whispered to Jackie at a family dinner. "My grandmother says it works every time . . . well, at least the two times she tried it."

- Some people swear by this method: After sex, stand on your head for ten minutes or so. It's doubtful this really gets the sperm to the egg any faster, but it may be fun if you're the athletic type.

None of the stories in this section has any scientific basis whatsoever. They remain mysteries wrapped in faith and coincidence.

A real "believe it or not!"

One of the most famous far-out remedies for infertility comes from none other than Ripley's Believe It or Not. In 1993, Ripley's acquired two African fertility statues from the West African nation of Cote D'Ivoire, the Ivory Coast. Carved of ebony, the statues stand 5 feet tall and weigh over 70 pounds each. The man, a king, holds a short sword in one hand and a mango, a common African symbol of fertility, in the other. The woman, his wife and queen, holds a new-born infant.

Initially, the statues were placed like sentinels in the headquarters of Ripley Entertainment, where they were an interesting conversation piece but nothing more. Then, unexplainably, an extraordinary number of women working in the Ripley office became pregnant. *The Wall Street Journal* ran an article, and soon the statues became national news and, soon afterward, international celebrities.

Ripley's decided to take the statues on a world tour. To date, the ebony figures have been around the world twice, seen by millions of people, and featured in magazines, in newspapers, and on television. Hundreds of women claim to have become pregnant after touching the statues — believe it or not!

Your humble authors can attest only that a good friend had tried without success to conceive for more than five years — trying everything from no-tech to high-tech. As a last-ditch effort before beginning the adoption process, she convinced her skeptical husband to make the eight-hour car trip to Niagara Falls, where the Ripley statues were on display. One month later, with no medical intervention whatsoever, she was pregnant and, at the time of this writing, has just given birth to her first child, a daughter.

Part II
The Low-Tech Road: Expecting a Pregnancy

The 5th Wave   By Rich Tennant

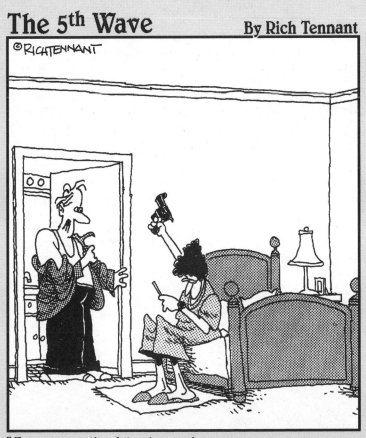

"I never realized trying to have a baby would mean replacing the soft music and candle light with an ovulation strip, a thermometer, and a starter pistol."

In this part . . .

If pregnancy doesn't occur immediately, you may want to look at some simple methods of improving your chances, as well as some alternative choices such as herbs or acupuncture. If pregnancy does occur but is followed by miscarriage, you may be very concerned about your chances of having a healthy baby. In this part, we address ways to increase your chances by better predicting ovulation so you'll get pregnant. We also give you emotional help in handling a pregnancy that ends too soon, and explain why miscarriages may happen.

Chapter 3

We're Trying! We're Trying! (to Get Pregnant)

After you start trying to get pregnant, you expect results — that's human nature. But Mother Nature isn't always on your timetable, and you may find yourself still trying after a few months, and anxious to step up the pace a bit with some scientific aids. In this chapter, you can find out about some low-tech but helpful methods of trying to pin down an elusive positive pregnancy test.

A number of testing methods are available to help you pin down exactly when you're ovulating; they test everything from urine to saliva. Some have been used for decades, and others are brand new.

You also get a look at how all this planning may affect the romance in your relationship, and we give you some ideas for keeping the spark alive.

Predicting Ovulation: Kits, Sticks, and Software

Maybe a month of trying to get pregnant has gone by — or maybe two, three, or four months — and you're beginning to feel frustrated and even a little scared that you're never going to get pregnant. Go back and read the statistics in Chapter 1 to remind yourself that nature is inefficient, and remember that everyone in your family took six months to get pregnant. You may be thinking, "That's all well and good to read about," but you want to do something *now*.

There must be something more scientific and more successful that you can do. You thought that you hit all the "right" days to have sex for the last few months, but maybe you're missing the right day or misinterpreting your body's ovulation signs. This section covers a few ways to monitor your ovulation cycle that are more "scientific" than stretching cervical mucus (we explain what that's about in the section "Using TesTape," later in this chapter) and counting calendar days. Hopefully, one will work for you!

Ovulation is the monthly release of an egg from your ovary. Ovulation is the one time during the month that you can actually get pregnant. Your window of opportunity is approximately two to three days.

Using an ovulation predictor kit

Ovulation predictor kits (OPKs) are a popular way to test if and when you ovulate. The tests measure the amount of LH (luteinizing hormone) found in your urine. LH generally rises 24 to 36 hours before ovulation; the rise of LH is called your *LH surge*. You should have sex the day or two before ovulation and the day of ovulation to improve your chance of getting pregnant.

OPKs are easy to find; every drugstore carries them. They use your urine, a cheap and abundant substance, to test for ovulation. The sticks are small enough to carry around with you.

The OPKs, or "pee sticks" as they're called, have some drawbacks. Certain women, such as women with polycystic ovaries (see Chapter 7), may have a high LH all the time, so the kits will always be positive. Women over 40 or those in premature ovarian failure (POF) may also have a higher than normal LH, because LH and FSH (follicle-stimulating hormone) both rise in POF. Some tests are also difficult to read, require several steps that need to be carefully done for good results, or start to show positive only when the LH reaches 40mIU/ml, the International Standard for an LH surge.

Some women may not have a surge that registers as high as 40mIU/ml; look for kits that register positive at 20mIU/ml.

Most kits show a positive as a line as dark as or darker than the control line. Read the test at exactly the time indicated; sometimes the lines darken over a few hours, but that doesn't mean you're having a surge.

The kits are harder to use if you don't have regular cycles; unless you know approximately when you ovulate each month, you may use up a lot of sticks trying to figure out when your surge starts. If you have regular cycles, you can start testing about 16 days before you expect your next period, but if your cycles are irregular, you need to test every few days to make sure that you don't miss the big O day. Table 3-1 can help you determine when to start testing.

Table 3-1	Counting Days, Saving Sticks
Length of Normal Cycle	*Start Testing This Many Days After Your Last Period*
40	23
39	22
38	21
37	20
36	19
35	18
34	17
33	16
32	15
31	14
30	13
29	12
28	11
27	10
26	9
25	8
24	7
23	6
22	5
21	4

OPKs aren't cheap; they cost about $14 for five sticks. You'll use one stick each time you test, and you need to test every 12 to 24 hours around the time of ovulation to accurately "catch" your surge. Resist the urge to buy the cheaper kits. They may not register lower LH levels, and they may be much harder to read. As a result, you use up more sticks because you're showing all your friends and asking their opinion on which line is darker. In addition to using up a lot of sticks, you may use up a lot of friends, too!

Positive levels of some urine OPKs

Many brands of urine ovulation predictor kits are available. The ones listed below are just a sampling. The number listed is the amount of luteinizing hormone needed to make the stick register a positive surge.

- ✔ **Assure:** 35mIU/ml

- ✔ **ClearPlan Easy:** 30mIU/ml

- ✔ **LH 1 Step:** 25mIU/ml

- ✔ **Midstream LH:** 20mIU/ml

- ✔ **Ovuquick:** 40mIU/ml

- ✔ **SureStep:** 25mIU/ml

OPKs register only when your surge has begun, so you won't be able to time sex as accurately for the two days immediately before ovulation. Also, the strips must be stored at temperatures between 59 and 86 degrees F to ensure their accuracy, so carrying them around in a purse can be problematic unless you live in a totally climate-controlled world.

Last but not least, OPKs tell you only when you're *about* to ovulate — they can't show you whether you've actually released an egg. Women with LUFS, or luteinized unruptured follicle syndrome, may produce an egg, have an LH surge, and yet not release the egg. Of course, you won't get pregnant if the egg doesn't release.

Adding computer power with a fertility monitor

If you want to go a little higher tech than the OPKs, you may be interested in a fertility monitor. A fertility monitor works a little differently than the standard OPK. These devices are actually small computers that store data about your cycle to tell you when you're going to ovulate. They're more labor intensive; you need to start testing the first day of your period and test every day around the same time. Morning is the most recommended time to test. Because they test both estrogen and LH levels, fertility monitors can better predict ovulation about five days before it occurs, giving you a better chance to have sex two days before ovulation.

The fertility monitor can be used if you're taking fertility medications, unlike some of the one-use OPK urine tests. It also "sets" itself to your cycle if you're somewhat irregular.

These monitors are expensive — about $200 — and you also need to buy the sticks. Like the less expensive kits, they may not be accurate if you are menopausal or breast-feeding, have polycystic ovaries (see Chapter 7) and a normally higher than normal LH level, or are taking tetracycline antibiotics, so they won't be able to tell if you've released an egg.

Just spit here — the saliva test

This is one of the newest and most interesting ovulation prediction tests out there; it tests your saliva for a rise in salt content, which rises as your estrogen rises. This method has several advantages:

- ✔ The tube that holds the lens you place saliva on and the tiny lighted microscope you look through are all contained in what looks like a tube of lipstick, so carrying this around isn't too conspicuous.

- ✔ Because the lens can be washed and reused, this is a one-time purchase.

- ✔ According to the U.S. Food and Drug Administration, this method is about 98 percent accurate.

- ✔ Unlike ovulation kits, which use urine, these can be used any old time, not just when your bladder is full. Peeing on demand can be hard, but you always have saliva. Plus, you can use the saliva kit on the bus, which is out of the question with urine-based OPKs!

Disadvantages to this method include the following:

- ✔ It's fairly expensive, about $60.

- ✔ It's slightly more complicated to use. You have to take the lens out and put it back properly or you won't read it correctly. You also risk the possibility of breaking or scratching the lens.

- ✔ Also, as with OPKs and TesTape, this tells you only when you're about to ovulate. It won't confirm that you did actually release an egg.

The saliva test can be done every day starting at day one of your cycle; at first you'll see only little dots (of salt) when you look through the viewing piece. As ovulation gets closer, you'll see what look like ferns (see Figure 3-1); when the ferns cover the whole slide, you're about to ovulate. It takes about five minutes for the slide to dry so you can accurately read it.

The saliva tests have an advantage over urine-based OPKs, which will only give you a yes or no answer as to whether you're ready to ovulate. The saliva test gives you more advance warning that ovulation is coming. With the saliva test, you can also avoid some of the false positives from LH kits and the fluctuations in temperature that can throw off results of the basal body temperature method (see "Taking your morning temperature," later in this chapter).

Even though the saliva test is initially expensive, it may be cheaper than buying ovulation predictor kits every month. And if you do get pregnant, you can use it after you deliver to *prevent* pregnancy until you want another baby! This method of birth control is approved by the Catholic Church and is much more accurate than the rhythm method of counting days to avoid pregnancy.

Saliva monitors that store and analyze data, just like the urine monitors, are now available. These are quite expensive, however — over $200.

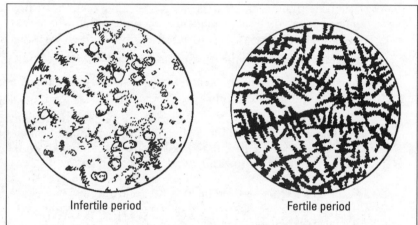

Figure 3-1:
Ferning appears on a saliva test when you're close to ovulation.

Infertile period

Fertile period

Saliva tester brands to check

Two nonelectronic saliva tester products are widely available. One goes by the name Donna (*Doña* in Spanish-speaking countries). It looks like an ordinary lipstick tube and is very easy to carry with you. The other is Lady Q, which also looks like a lipstick container and is easy to use anywhere.

Going higher tech, you may want to take a look at OvaCue II, an electronic saliva tester. It comes with a spoon-sized sensor that you place on your tongue for eight seconds in the morning, so it's not quite as portable as the lipstick-sized tubes. It also comes with a vaginal probe, which you can use in addition to the oral probe for even greater accuracy. Obviously, this isn't a product to use on the bus or in the office. It's manufactured by Zetek.

If you already have a microscope and slides hanging around the house from a leftover science project or something, you can test saliva at home without any of the expensive packaged equipment. Put some saliva on a slide and take a look!

Tracking your fertility with software

You really should keep track of all the information about your menstrual cycle, but maybe you write everything down on little pieces of paper and keep losing them. Of course, you may have a fertility notebook by now. If you'd like a more scientific approach, however, books and software are available that are specifically designed for keeping track of all kinds of fertility information.

Two software titles available on the Internet are TCOYF (Taking Charge of Your Fertility) Software found at `www.tcoyf.com` and CycleWatch, found at `www.cyclewatch.com`.

Lifecycle online and Fert Friend let you download software to chart your basal body temperature, cervical mucus, and cervix changes to let you know that you should "have sex now," as the software puts it. If you have an OvaCue II saliva tester, you can buy software to use with it that will let you download your information, chart it, graph it, and print it out.

Taking your morning temperature

Recording your basal body temperature (BBT) is one of the oldest methods of predicting ovulation. I (coauthor Sharon) remember doing this before getting pregnant with my son, who is now 30 years old! A basal body temperature is just a long-winded way of saying your individual normal temperature. You use the same type of thermometer you do whenever you take your temperature to find out whether you have a fever when you're not feeling well.

This method of predicting ovulation is simple but requires a certain amount of determination and a good memory. You need to remember to take your temperature every morning *before* you get up. Most doctors recommend that you not get up, eat, drink, or smoke before taking your temperature because any activity at all will raise your temperature, and eating or drinking will raise or lower it, depending on what you had.

The baby dance: It's not just sex anymore

baby dance (bay-bee danse): also known as BD'ing; traditional method for conceiving a baby, sexual relations; very popular prior to the turn of the century and the emergence of the field of fertility.

Believe me (coauthor Jackie), I never thought I'd have to warn my husband of impending sex. But trying to conceive, along with its host of physical and psychological issues, does bring it back home . . . and right into the bedroom.

There's nothing like a stranger in your sex life, even if that stranger is only the instruction manual on the ovulation predictor kit, directing you to have sex around the time that the second purple line appears. It seems simple enough — even sounds like fun. However, after that purple line has appeared for the *fourth day in a row,* even newlyweds feel a bit put upon.

"Again?!" my husband would ask incredulously when I called him into "service" for the sixth day in a row. I explained, patiently at first, that I wasn't quite sure exactly *when* I had ovulated, so this way we were covering all the bases. This wasn't exactly a romantic proposition for him, nor did I ever expect that I would have to cajole someone into "one more day" with the promise of the next week off.

As time wore on, my husband began to take the attitude of "close enough," while I became more intent on pinpointing the exact *second* that my egg might release, and timing sex accordingly. As our attitudes went their own separate ways, so did our desires. Compromises, such as "only

during halftime," arose, and we began distinguishing between baby sex and making love. Unfortunately, sometimes one man's baby sex was another woman's making love and vice versa. And as we began to up the ante on fertility treatments, our schedules (well, my schedule actually) became more crowded with ultrasound appointments, blood tests, and doctor visits, allowing precious little time for the basics: food, water, and, of course, the baby dance.

After one year of trying to conceive, I had arrived at two amazing conclusions: 1) Sex had become something to finish in order to get to something better, much like homework and broccoli had been back in the time when I looked forward to having a sex life. 2) More advanced methods of fertility treatments, such as in vitro fertilization, were actually seeming more attractive, in that any sex necessary would take place in a petri dish and require neither the presence of my husband nor myself.

I didn't feel that I could share these thoughts with my husband, who, much to his credit, always gave it the old college try. I was so focused on everything getting to where it needed to go in the time it needed to get there that pleasure seemed like a fringe benefit that we would have to do without. I remember speaking with a friend of mine who had just learned that she was pregnant with twins. When she sighed to me, "And we never have to have sex again," I realized that these thoughts are often shared by couples from sea to shining sea who are trying to conceive.

Some doctors also recommend buying a special BBT thermometer, which has larger numbers and reads only up to 100 degrees or so. Each one-tenth of a degree is much easier to read on this type of thermometer. You don't need a BBT thermometer, but it's nice to have if your temperature doesn't fluctuate much or if your eyesight is going.

Many charts are available to help you chart your temperature, but you can easily make one yourself. All you do is mark down your morning temperature to the exact one-tenth of a degree and then connect the "dots." You're looking for a subtle drop in temperature, followed by a sustained rise in temperature, meaning a rise for more than three days. Your temperature should rise at least 0.5 degrees. The drop occurs around ovulation, and the rise indicates an increase in your progesterone levels — progesterone increases only after you've ovulated.

This method has a few drawbacks. The most obvious one is that you need to be scrupulous about taking your temperature and recording it so that you don't forget it. Also, you have to keep your chart for the whole month. If you're the type who loses things easily, keep a few copies of the chart around in case you lose one.

Factors other than hormones can cause an increase or decrease in your temperature. If you're sick, even small temperature fluctuations may make your chart inaccurate, and you'll think you've ovulated when you actually have the flu. Alcohol, too little or too much sleep, and subtle illnesses can all change your temperature.

Your BBT can give you an idea of whether you're pregnant. If your temperature stays elevated more than 15 days, there's a good chance that you're pregnant — unless, of course, you have the flu. If your temperature starts to drop after ten days or so, you may have a *luteal phase defect,* which means that your progesterone may be too low to sustain a pregnancy.

If you're prone to losing paper charts, you may be interested in a digital thermometer that stores your previous temperature. This device is handy in case you forget to write your temperature down one morning. Digital thermometers are a little more expensive than glass ones, but not more than $7 or $8 for a good one. And you can "store" your last temperature even with a glass thermometer by *not* shaking it down immediately after using it. This tip is especially convenient if you don't have time to record your temperature right away. The mercury will stay at your temperature point until it's shaken down.

Using TesTape

TesTape, another method of predicting ovulation that I (coauthor Sharon) remember from the 1970s, is another way of testing cervical mucus. As with "stretching" your mucus (discussed in Chapter 2), you need to be comfortable putting your fingers into your vagina. You tear off a piece of yellow TesTape, which is sold over the counter in drugstores (diabetics use it to test sugar levels in urine), and hold it to your cervix for a second. Then you bring out the piece of paper and watch to see whether it turns color. It will first turn an olive color a few days before ovulation and then turn dark green or blue when your cervical mucus is alkaline, as it is right before you ovulate. If you have no idea how to find your cervix, it's pretty easy. You just *carefully* insert your finger into your vagina until you feel a bump. That's your cervix. You'll notice that your cervix also changes at different times of the month; around ovulation, it becomes softer and feels slightly open in the center.

Sperm testing at home

This method won't give you detailed information, but it will let you check out two semen samples to see whether the concentration of sperm meets the accepted fertility level of 20 million/ml. The brand name is FertilMARQ. You can purchase this product online and have it sent directly to your home, to avoid an embarrassing trip to the drugstore. Two Web sites that sell the sperm test are www.babyhopes.com and www.completefertility.com; both also sell basal digital thermometers, home pregnancy tests, and OPKs.

Coming Full Circle: Why Baby Sex Can Be a Good Thing

After a while of waiting for a baby, you may find that you and your partner settle into a comfortable and — dare we say — fun pattern of accommodating whatever fertility ritual you're facing.

Realize that you're not alone . . . in the greater sense of the word! Knowing that most other couples deal with these periods of boredom with their sex life helped us feel a lot more normal, even in less than normal circumstances. Hearing and sharing about what others do to put the dance back into their baby dance may give you something to laugh about, if nothing else.

Realize that your circumstances, and thus your feelings, are temporary. No matter how things turn out, you will *not* be struggling to have a baby ten years from now. "This too shall pass" may make your less-than-enthusiastic attitudes a bit more bearable, for yourself and each other.

Relax. With each month, you'll come to realize that the timing, although important, isn't everything. Many factors come into play in the business of baby making, and they all have to be working in order to succeed. There is no exact right moment, and you haven't missed your only opportunity. The realization of this fact, along with an increased ability to trust that whatever was meant to happen will indeed occur, will help you be less dependent on that little purple line as the ultimate stopwatch for the rest of your life.

Looking for a Positive — Home Pregnancy Tests

If you think that you used a lot of ovulation predictor sticks, wait until you start using the home pregnancy tests (HPTs)! They're widely advertised on TV, depicting a couple excitedly waiting for the good news or a tense woman alone hoping for the happy news that she's *not* pregnant. Home pregnancy tests have been available since the 1970s; earlier tests had to be done in the doctor's office. The earliest tests were available in the late 1920s and gave rise to the sweetly whispered phrase, "The rabbit died," in movies for the next 40 years. The urine was collected in the doctor's office and then sent off to the lab, where it was injected into a virgin rabbit. A day or two later, the rabbit was killed and her ovaries examined to see whether they contained bulging masses called *corpora hemorrhagica.* If they did, you were *enciente,* as they said on the TV show *I Love Lucy* in the 1950s, when the word *pregnant* couldn't be said on TV. As you can see, the rabbit *always* died in the very early testing years. Later, medical science found a way to not only keep the rabbit alive but to use it for more than one test! So if you think you feel bad killing multiple boxes of home pregnancy tests, imagine how you'd feel if each of them were a rabbit!

The first tests done without the help of rabbits required you to bring a container of urine to the doctor's office. I (coauthor Sharon) will never in my life forget the look on the receptionist's face when I plopped down on the counter a recycled 32-ounce applesauce jar filled with urine. "You only needed a little, dear," she whispered as I ran, red faced, from the office, devoutly wishing home pregnancy tests had been invented.

The first home tests were available in the 1970s, and everyone probably would have been a little more squeamish about leaving them in the fridge next to the milk if they had known that they contained prepackaged red blood cells. These tests were very sensitive to movement, so you had to put them someplace quiet and leave them alone for a few hours. When you finally peeked into the fridge, you looked for the dark ring at the bottom of the tube — that's what appeared if you were pregnant. The clumping together of red blood cells if you were pregnant is what formed the ring.

All the tests, from the 1920s on, measured hCG (human chorionic gonadotropin), the hormone released by the implantation of the embryo and the growing placenta. The newest tests are very sensitive; the most sensitive tests of the 30 or so brands on the market claim to detect concentrations of 25mIU/ml, which usually occur around the time you would miss your first period. Others don't test positive until the hCG level is 50 or even 100mIU/ml, so read the box before you buy. Some tests claim to be accurate a few days *before* your period is due, but a negative test at that time may not be accurate. You may have had a late implantation, or you may have ovulated a day or two after you thought you did. Another test should be done a few days later if your period still hasn't started.

The average level of hCG ten days post ovulation is 25mIU/ml; it is 50mIU/ml 12 days post ovulation, and 100mIU/ml 14 days after you ovulate. Keep in mind that these numbers are averages; your number may be higher or lower and still be perfectly normal.

Blood tests can also measure hCG, detecting concentrations less than 5mIU/ml. (We talk about pregnancy blood tests more in Chapter 15.) Blood tests give an exact number, so only with blood tests can you tell whether your hCG levels are doubling every two to three days, as they do in most normal pregnancies.

Home pregnancy tests are available in every drugstore, so if you're buying in bulk because you're a compulsive tester, you can hit every grocery store and drugstore in town, and no one will know that you're compulsive — er, anxious to know! These tests give fast results, usually in two to five minutes. Most tell you to not urinate for four hours before you test so the concentration of the hormone will be high. Some kits suggest that you urinate in a cup and dip the wand into it, and other kits suggest peeing directly on the stick. Some show a positive as a little + sign; others want you to drag all your friends back in to the bathroom (if you still have any friends left after ovulation) and have them compare the control line to the test line to see whether they match. Usually a positive is indicated by a test line that's as dark as or darker than the control, and many women drive themselves mad staring at the line trying to determine its exact shade of purple. Don't let the test sit around before looking at it, as some test results will change after an hour or two and will not be accurate. See Figure 3-2 for positive and negative results on a home pregnancy test.

Dealing with a false positive

False positive results are rare in home pregnancy tests. You may have a false positive if

- ✔ You're taking injections of the hormone hCG to induce ovulation or for any other reason; it takes 14 days for 10,000U of hCG (a standard dose) to completely clear your system.

- ✔ You recently had a miscarriage or ectopic pregnancy, and the hCG levels have not dropped to a negative range yet.

✔ You have developed a rare cancer called a choriocarcinoma. This cancer usually follows a full-term birth, miscarriage, or other pregnancy loss. Sharon's sister developed this cancer in the 1970s, after a normal full-term delivery; her doctors initially thought she was pregnant again and miscarrying due to heavy bleeding. This is a fast-growing cancer, so if you recently had a pregnancy loss of any kind and have a positive home pregnancy test and heavy bleeding, you *must* see a doctor immediately. This cancer is usually treated with methotrexate. Sharon's sister was one of the first women to receive this treatment rather than a hysterectomy and delivered a healthy boy five years later.

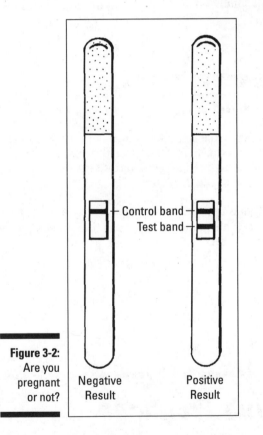

Figure 3-2:
Are you pregnant or not?

Negative Result — Positive Result

Control band — Test band

We list here the common brands of home pregnancy tests and the lowest number they claim will register a positive result. Sensitivity is measured in units called *mIU,* which means milli-International Units per milliliter.

✔ **AimStick:** 20mIU
✔ **Answer:** 100mIU

> ✔ **Clearblue Easy:** 50mIU
>
> ✔ **ClearPlan Easy:** 50mIU
>
> ✔ **Confirm 1 step:** 25mIU
>
> ✔ **CVS cartridge:** 50mIU
>
> ✔ **Drug Emporium One Step:** 50mIU
>
> ✔ **e.p.t.:** 40mIU
>
> ✔ **Equate** (Wal-Mart): 25mIU
>
> ✔ **First Response Early Result:** 25mIU
>
> ✔ **One Step:** 50mIU

Including OPKs and semen and pregnancy tests in one kit

Some enterprising manufacturers have marketed kits containing about seven ovulation predictor sticks and one or two HPTs. Of course these are more expensive than buying just the home pregnancy tests, but it certainly cuts down on all those embarrassing trips to the drugstore.

> ✔ **First Response Pregnancy Planning Kit:** This kit contains seven ovulation predictors, one HPT, and some Tums antacids! We guess this process is *supposed* to give you acid indigestion!
>
> ✔ **Baby Start:** This kit contains six ovulation predictor sticks and a sperm testing kit good for two uses. They should put an HPT in there, too.
>
> ✔ **Web Womb:** This Web site (www.webwomb.com) sells a kit with 12 spreadsheets to chart your BBT, and also a home pregnancy test.

It's That Time of the Month Again: The Pain of Not Getting Pregnant

It's negative . . . again. I (coauthor Jackie) always added that last word to every negative home pregnancy test or blood test I took. That word seemed to remind me, and everyone else, of just how hard I was trying and how frustrated I had become. In the beginning, the negative results were easier to take, and I looked at the next chance of success as only a few days away. But, as time passed and negative results accumulated, the process of getting back on the horse grew more difficult.

I spent many a dime (forget that — try dollar!) on every different type of home pregnancy test available. Maybe one of them would finally register that second pink line, the victory sign for those trying to conceive. As the months wore on, I found myself considering adding strobe lights in the bathroom to better illuminate what could be a very faint positive. Another friend who was also trying to conceive bought four different tests to compare faint lines. When she went two for four, she decided to pay a visit to the doctor, where her pregnancy was confirmed. Another friend got a negative result and then another one. A week later, her period hadn't arrived, and she tested again. The result was negative again. She too visited her local physician, whose test found her to be absolutely pregnant.

Yes, sometimes the drugstore-variety home pregnancy test can be wrong. And although the preceding stories keep many of us staring at HPTs with magnifying glasses, they are rare indeed. Most positive results are picked up by these simple tests. So how do you deal with those results that are less than positive? Here are a few suggestions to make the process a little easier:

✔ Don't test on the morning of a big presentation, your wedding, or other such auspicious event. A negative, or positive, result can wait the extra day. It's not worth spoiling a special occasion with a foul mood.

✔ Test once and forget it. Our bodies are beautifully timed in that if you are indeed pregnant, you'll know soon enough. Although not every pregnant woman misses a period, other symptoms and signs pop up. If you're still not sure, test again in a week (not to be confused with an hour). If you're truly not satisfied then, call your doctor and request a more formal pregnancy test (also known as a *beta,* which we discuss in Chapter 14).

✔ Try not to drown your sorrows in copious amounts of alcohol or drugs or engage in other reckless behavior. You still may be pregnant, and that type of negative celebration is not the best way to welcome your new addition. Even if you're not pregnant, you want to stay in tip-top shape so that you can get there. A glass of wine is fine; a bottle is not.

✔ It's okay to be sad and to share this news with friends and family. It feels like a loss, and for some women, it is. Just remember that you have done nothing wrong. Human reproduction is a gamble. This month, you were on the opposite side of the odds.

Looking at drugs and your work environment for answers

Have you overlooked something that could be interfering with your getting pregnant? Think back a few months, especially when thinking about sperm production; the sperm being ejaculated today have been over two months in the making, so anything your partner was taking a few months ago could be affecting his sperm count today. Ask yourself the following questions about a few possible deterrents you may not have thought about:

- Has your partner taken antibiotics, such as erythromycin or gentamycin, or antifungal medications, such as ketoconazole, or been treated for psoriasis with methotrexate? Has he been on anabolic steroids? These medicines can all affect sperm production.

- Does your partner have high blood pressure? Sometimes, when you've been taking a medication for a long time, you almost forget that it can have serious side effects. Men who take certain types of antihypertensives called calcium channel blockers may produce sperm that can't penetrate eggs well; may have *retrograde ejaculation,* a condition in which the semen is pushed backwards into the bladder instead of being ejaculated out; or may have an inability to get and sustain an erection. Other antihypertensive drugs are available that don't have these effects. Suggest that your partner talk to his doctor about switching medications if possible.

- Are you using a vaginal lubricant for sex? Even though substances such as KY Jelly, Astroglide, and Replens don't contain spermicides, they can slow down sperm in their race to the egg. If you have to use a lubricant, try plain baby oil.

- Where do you work? Think about substances that you're exposed to at work. For instance, if you're a home remodeler, bridge painter, welder, or solderer, you may be exposed to large amounts of lead. You run the same risk if you're remodeling an old house and scraping old paint off the walls. Lead exposure in men has been linked to low sperm count and decreased motility of sperm. In women, lead exposure may cause low birth weight in babies, high blood pressure during pregnancy, damage to the baby's nervous system, and developmental delays.

Healthcare workers are exposed to a number of potentially dangerous drugs, as are pharmacists; exposure to chemotherapy drugs, radiation from X-rays, or inhaled anesthetics used in the operating room all can contribute to infertility.

Changing your job isn't always easy, but you do need to consider potential exposure to dangerous substances and take steps to protect yourself from them.

Considering religious practices

You may not have thought much about your religious practices causing problems with fertility, but at times, religious practices can interfere with your getting pregnant. For example, if you're an observant Jew, you may go to Mikvah, the cleansing bath, every month after your period ends, to cleanse yourself before having intercourse again. You have to wait seven days after all blood flow has stopped to go to Mikvah. If you have heavy, long periods, you could easily be missing ovulation if your cycles are short (25 or 26 days). You may be a member of another religious sect that has restrictions on when you can have intercourse; just remember that not everyone ovulates on day 14, and skipping days before day 12 may mean that you miss your fertile time each month.

Adjusting your calendars to be together

In today's age of conflicting schedules, many of you may find that you and your partner are spending far more time apart than together. This type of schedule is fine for ships passing in the night, which aren't responsible for making baby ships. But for those trying to conceive, being in the same place at the same time is critical.

If you're not one of the few women whose ovulation is both predictable and consistent, traveling partners can be a problem. You're not alone. Couples who are separated by work/travel schedules or who find themselves on different work shifts have an inherent difficulty in baby making. Because of these erratic schedules, determining whether the problem is timing or something more serious is often difficult. Many couples end up in their doctor's office when the only adjustment they need is to their day planner.

Ever wonder why so many women get pregnant on vacation? Sure, relaxation is part of it, but for others it may signify the rare occasion of being with your significant other at just the right time.

If you fall into this "too busy" category, figure out, as best you can, when you might ovulate, and schedule a time for you and your partner to be together then. OPKs, basal body temperature, and other predictors can help you pinpoint the time of ovulation. However, as far as being in the same place at the right time, you may need a little more creativity. Joining your partner on an ill-timed business trip, even for a night, may be just what it takes. An afternoon rendezvous, rather than lunch, can also bridge the gap. Finding time together — alone — may not only get you on the road to parenthood but also give you plenty of practice for it along the way!

Chapter 4

Seeing a Doctor — and Keeping Your Cool

Two classic Norman Rockwell drawings show a family on vacation in the station wagon. In the first scene, the daughter's braids dance in the wind, and everyone is in clean new outfits and wearing big smiles. The second scene shows the return from vacation — everyone is dirty, bedraggled, and grumpy, and Dad looks like he's ready to drive the whole group over a cliff.

You may have started toward pregnancy in the vacation mode, thinking "Can't wait to do the nursery," "What kind of maternity clothes should I get?" and "I wonder who'll give me a baby shower?" After a few months with no pregnancy, you may resemble the return group, worn out and testy, wondering why you ever thought any of this was a good idea and how you went from being a regular person to being a potential fertility patient.

In this chapter, we look at the first tentative steps toward being a fertility patient and help you to cope with family, friends, and your partner at this difficult point.

Deciding When You Should Make an Appointment with Dr. Basic

Conventional medical opinion says that you should consult a physician if you haven't gotten pregnant in one year if you're under age 35, or six months if you're over 35. These guidelines must have been written for very patient people. If you're under 35 and patient enough to wait for a year — a *year* — before talking to a doctor about getting pregnant, you must be a saint.

Seeking professional help is a big step. Here, you always thought you were an average sort of person, and now you find that you're part of the 20 percent of women who don't get pregnant in a year of trying. For the first few months, you could pretend it wasn't a big deal, but now, well, open the phone book. It's time to call Dr. Basic.

When not to wait — even a few months

Sometimes even Conventional Wisdom, that conservative soul, says not to wait six months or a year before seeing a doctor about not getting pregnant. If you're a woman over age 38, you should see a doctor before even trying to get pregnant. You may want to do more thorough testing before trying; you have fewer months to spend trying than your younger "sisters" because your aging ovaries are making fewer good eggs.

You'll also want to see a doctor from the beginning if you've had a previous ectopic pregnancy or have pelvic inflammatory disease. You may have damage to your fallopian tubes, which may make surgery necessary. If you're not getting your period, or getting it very irregularly, you may need help regulating your cycles so that you produce an egg every month. Lastly, if you have very painful periods, you may have endometriosis (see Chapter 7 for more discussion of all of these conditions) and may need treatment to get pregnant.

You may want to have your partner do a semen analysis early on if he has a history of trauma to the testicles, had undescended testicles, or knows that he had mumps as a child. Any of these conditions may have caused damage to his sperm.

Of course, if you've had your tubes tied or if your partner had a vasectomy, you need to see a specialist to discuss either reversal of the surgery (see Chapter 7) or in vitro fertilization (which we discuss in detail in Part IV). If you need to use donor sperm, you'll also probably want to see a specialist who can tell you how to order the sperm.

Choosing between a family doctor and an Ob/Gyn

So who *is* Dr. Basic when you're trying to get pregnant? The average doctor has about nine initials after his name, so how are you supposed to know which one you should see when you're trying to get pregnant? Some of the more common abbreviations you may see include the following:

- **M.D.:** Medical doctor trained in traditional medicine with four years of medical school after college and a residency length varying with specialty. After that, residency can be from two to ten years, depending on the specialty.

- **D.O.:** Doctor of osteopathy. These doctors used to be more trained in manipulation and homeopathic methods, but today's osteopaths train in programs virtually identical to traditional medical schools.

- **OB:** Obstetrician. This specialist is trained to take care of pregnant women and handle labor and delivery. OBs are also gynecologists but may specialize in pregnancy.

- **GYN:** Gynecologist. This physician is trained to take care of women's health. Obstetricians and gynecologists all start with the same four-year residency training after medical school, but they may choose to specialize in one area of the specialty.

- **RE:** Reproductive endocrinologist. This doctor is a graduate of an Ob/Gyn program who has chosen to specialize in infertility. After medical school, these doctors complete three years of additional training, called a fellowship, to take tests to become certified for this specialty.

- **FP:** Family practitioner. These doctors have chosen to specialize in the health of the entire family. In some parts of the country they, rather than OBs, handle many women's health problems, including pregnancy and deliveries.

- **FACOG:** Fellow of the American College of Obstetricians and Gynecologists. A doctor who has FACOG after his name is board certified and is a member of this national society.

You may also come across these terms when doctor-shopping:

- **Board eligible:** These doctors have completed two years of practice in their specialty and can now take the tests to become board certified.

- **Board certified:** These doctors have practiced their specialty for two years, taken the tests necessary to be certified, and have passed them.

If you live in a remote area, you may need to start with your family doctor because specialists may not have offices in your area. Also, you may feel more comfortable starting with a doctor who already knows you, such as your Ob/Gyn or family doctor. If your doctor believes that your case is more complex than he is qualified to treat, he'll probably refer you to someone more experienced in your particular situation. When you're just beginning treatment, you can probably safely assume that your regular doctor or Ob/Gyn can handle your case, unless you already have reason to suspect that you have tubal issues or that your partner has sperm problems requiring high-tech intervention.

Bringing your partner to the Ob/Gyn office

Back in the olden days of gynecology, say before the 1960s, you *never* saw a man at the Ob/Gyn waiting room. Oh, yes, a man might show up there if his wife had just had surgery and he had to drive her to the appointment. Even then, he probably stayed in the car. Few places made men more twitchy than the obstetrician's office — not a decent magazine in sight, women in every stage of pregnancy, wailing infants, and a pink-and-blue decorating scheme. Today, however, the situation is different; some men accompany their partner to every Ob/Gyn visit. The magazine categories have been improved, and the decorating scheme doesn't scream "Rock-a-Bye Baby." Many doctors even specifically request that you bring your partner to a visit so that you can all get to know each other.

So should you encourage your partner to attend your first why-aren't-we-pregnant visit? That depends on a few things:

✔ Will he feel horribly out of place, not pay attention, or say something you'd rather he didn't?

Some men — no, make that most men — don't like to go to the doctor, ever, for anything. Whether it's the loss of control, the digging into what they consider their personal business, or just discomfort in the face of an authority figure, many men are not assets at the doctor's office. You probably know by now whether your partner will do well at the doctor's office. If you're going to sit there (half naked, no less) worrying about what embarrassing thing he might say or do, go by yourself.

On the other hand, if your partner is the person in your twosome who remembers detail, writes things down correctly, asks sensible questions, and provides moral support, by all means, take him to your first doctor visit. If you don't get pregnant right away, he'll probably need to have his own testing done, so he may as well get familiar with the doctor right from the start.

✔ Are you going to have to impart information that you don't want your partner to know?

For example, did you have an abortion, give a child up for adoption, have a sexually transmitted disease, or do any other thing you'd rather your partner didn't know about? Then go to the first visit by yourself, frankly explain the situation to your doctor, and take your partner to the *next* visit.

✔ Are you going to be embarrassed about undergoing an examination with your partner there?

Even today, in this let-it-all-hang-out age, some of you aren't comfortable having other people, even your partner, present for a gynecological exam. If this situation is going to make you uneasy, maybe your partner can wait in the waiting room until the exam is over and then come in when you're dressed.

Making a list of questions for your first visit

Whether you go alone or as a team to your doctor's appointment, prepare a list of questions ahead of time so that you won't forget anything. Here's a starter list. You'll probably have other questions specific to your own situation.

- Do you treat many patients trying to get pregnant?

  Obviously, you don't want to have a doctor taking on your case whose practice mostly consists of gynecological surgery on women over age 50.

- Will you do any testing before we start treatment?

  Some doctors just start you on medication for a few months before putting you through more invasive testing. Other doctors do blood work, semen analysis, and ultrasounds before starting you on medicine.

- Will you monitor me if I'm on Clomid (a pill to help you ovulate)?

  Many doctors do no monitoring when you're taking Clomid (we discuss Clomid in the section "Take two Clomid and call me in three months," later in this chapter). Other doctors want you to have blood work and ultrasounds while on Clomid, because there is a small risk of multiple pregnancy while on Clomid.

- Will my insurance cover any testing?

- What do you think my chance for success will be?

  Obviously, your doctor doesn't have a crystal ball but should have some general idea, based on your age and history, of what your chance of getting pregnant is.

- How long should we try this before we do further testing?

  If your doctor shrugs and gives you the impression that she would do simple methods forever, you may want to find another doctor.

Dr. Basic is going to have some questions for you, too. He'll want to know the following, so come prepared with the answers:

- How long you've been trying to get pregnant

- How often you have sex

- Whether you use any lubricants

- Whether you engage in any unusual practices that could affect your fertility

- How long your periods last

- How long your cycles are from day one of one cycle to day one of the next

✔ The date of your last period

✔ Whether your periods are painful

✔ Whether your periods are heavy

✔ How many pads or tampons you use a day

✔ Whether sisters or other close relatives have children

✔ Whether there are any known genetic factors in your family

✔ Whether you used ovulation predictor kits and what they showed

Dr. Basic may have a lot more questions aimed specifically at you. If you're heavy and have adult acne or facial hair, he may wonder if you have polycystic ovary syndrome (PCOS). PCOS patients often don't ovulate on their own. If you're very thin, he may be concerned about your not getting periods due to overexercising, anorexia, or poor nutrition.

You may wonder why the doctor doesn't want to go all-out on your first visit, doing lots of testing to make sure that you don't have a problem that will require high-tech fertility treatments, such as in vitro fertilization (IVF). The fact is, most patients who see a doctor because they're not pregnant have fairly simple problems, such as lack of ovulation (releasing an egg), or just bad timing of sex, and won't need the high-tech stuff. Despite the emphasis today on high-tech methods, only a small percentage of infertility patients, less than 5 percent, actually do IVF. Your doctor may do an ultrasound to see whether you're developing any follicles, or he may check your blood work to see whether your FSH (follicle-stimulating hormone) level is elevated, which could indicate perimenopause. But, remember, many doctors won't do any invasive monitoring until they've tried some simple things first.

Trying conception over the counter: Baby aspirin and cough syrup

If your doctor is a laid-back type whose philosophy is to try the simple stuff first, he may suggest trying baby aspirin and cough syrup for a few months. Although this advice may have you thinking you've wandered into the pediatrician's office by mistake, these suggestions may have some merit.

Baby aspirin is given to post-heart-attack patients because it decreases the normal clotting of the blood, keeping blood flowing more easily through the blood vessels. Some doctors believe that giving baby aspirin to infertility patients may increase blood flow to the uterus, giving the embryo an improved lining in which to implant. If you've had more than one miscarriage, baby aspirin may be recommended to counteract certain antibodies that can cause excessive clotting and decreased blood flow to the placenta.

Cough syrup is a little more controversial. Around ovulation, the cervical mucus should be thin and stretchy; in some women, the mucus doesn't thin enough for sperm to get through it. The theory is that cough syrup, which must be pure cough syrup or guaifenesin, thins all the mucus in the body, not just the mucus in your chest. The sperm then have an easier time getting through the vaginal mucus.

If you haven't bought your first basal thermometer yet, you may also be instructed to start charting your daily temperature before getting up or going to the bathroom. Your doctor may also want to check your basal body temperature (BBT) charts (see Chapter 3 for more information about temperature charting) to see whether your temperature shows a pattern of ovulation. If no pattern indicates that you're ovulating on your own, your doctor may bring out the prescription pad and write you your first infertility medication.

"Take two Clomid and call me in three months"

The prescription Dr. Basic hands you (if you can decipher it) may say "Clomiphene citrate 50 mgm qd X 5 days, #10. Refills 3." Or it may simply say "CC 50mg qd d 3-7." What does this mean?

Clomiphene citrate, more commonly called Clomid or Serophene (two brand names), is given to help you make an egg or to help you make a *better* egg; it may also help sustain a pregnancy with higher progesterone levels. Normally, you take Clomid for five days. Some doctors start you on it on day three of your cycle, and others start you on day four or five. The exact timing isn't important; the point is to start it before your ovaries start to develop one dominant follicle.

Usually doctors give you one pill a day the first month or two and then move up to two or three tablets a day if you still don't seem to be ovulating regularly. Clomid comes in 50 milligram tablets, so if your doctor starts you at a higher dose, 100 to 150 milligrams per day, you'll need to take more than one. After you stop taking the pills, you can check for ovulation by using your old friends, the basal thermometer and the ovulation predictor kits.

Clomid works by fooling the body into thinking it's not making enough estrogen. When your hypothalamus thinks that you're low on estrogen, it releases GnRH (gonadotropin-releasing hormone), which stimulates the release of FSH (follicle-stimulating hormone) into your blood. The FSH stimulates the ovary to produce estrogen, so that a follicle will begin to grow. Eighty percent or so of women taking Clomid ovulate in response to this stimulation.

Clomid works best for those whose ovaries are capable of functioning normally but need a little tuneup. If you're already ovulating a mature follicle regularly, Clomid probably won't help you get pregnant.

You doctor may tell you to try Clomid and come back in three to six months if you're not pregnant yet. Most pregnancies from Clomid occur in the first three to six months, so if you're not pregnant by that time, your doctor will want to investigate why you're not getting pregnant.

Clomid has a few drawbacks, including the chance for multiple births. Between 5 and 10 percent of all Clomid pregnancies are twins, 1 in 400 is a triplet pregnancy, and 1 pregnancy in 800 results in quadruplets. Obviously, you may be delighted to have a twin pregnancy, but triplets or quads may not be so thrilling. Higher-order multiples (triplets and above) have a very high rate of premature delivery and significantly higher than normal maternal and infant complications. Multiples result from Clomid working too well and stimulating more than one follicle to grow.

Some doctors monitor you with ultrasounds while you're on Clomid to be sure that you're not making too many eggs. If you're making a large number of eggs, you may develop ovarian hyperstimulation syndrome, which can cause a very high estradiol level, making hospitalization necessary. If you're on Clomid and feel very ill, with a sudden weight gain, severe bloating in your abdomen, or abdominal pain, call your doctor immediately. This is a rare side effect of Clomid.

Clomid also has some less serious side effects. Because your body has been fooled into thinking that it doesn't have enough estrogen, you may have some of the same symptoms women have when they enter menopause and their estrogen drops: hot flashes, headaches, nausea, or blurred vision. Let your doctor know if you have these symptoms. Some doctors may give you estrogen to decrease your symptoms.

Clomid can also interfere with your production of cervical mucus because it locks into all the estrogen receptors, including those in your cervix, so they don't make mucus in response to rising estrogen like they normally do. Because estrogen also builds your uterine lining, some women on Clomid don't make a thick lining. If you have either of these side effects, you may need to take estrogen after you start making a follicle.

Dealing with a Difficult Doctor, Partner, or Family Member

Trying to keep your emotions on an even keel is hard enough. Keeping control is even harder when the people you count on for support don't seem to understand what you're going through. Here are some suggestions for dealing with the people you need most when they're supporting you the least.

When Dr. Basic doesn't get it

Although we would all like to think otherwise, the letters M.D. after a name don't automatically make a person a compassionate or thorough medical practitioner. Sure, just like the rest of us, your doctor may have bad days that have nothing to do with you — she may have had a difficult surgery or a patient may have died. But if your doctor is consistently too casual or unconcerned about your infertility, you may want a "divorce" from him or her.

Infertility is hard enough to deal with even with a supportive partner and doctor. When your doctor thinks you're overreacting, too emotional, or making too much of your situation, it's time to find a new doctor.

What you're looking for in a doctor may not be what your best friend is looking for. Some people want to know everything about their medical condition, and some people don't want to know anything. Some women want the paternalistic, leave-it-to-me kind of doctor. Some women do better with a jokester, while others are offended by humorous approaches to what they see as a very serious problem.

Some doctors also do better with a patient who deals humorously with her situation, while others don't take a patient with a sense of humor seriously. Some doctors are offended by a patient armed with 24 infertility books, and others welcome an informed patient. Don't feel like your first choice of a doctor has to be your last. Maybe he's great with Pap smears but not so great with infertility. Move on if your relationship isn't working for either of you.

Considering your partner's feelings

Not all partners are into the baby thing as much as you may be. Few things cause more upheaval in a relationship than one partner being more interested in having a baby than the other. Divorce is not uncommon in infertility patients, even after they become pregnant.

Your partner may have been willing to have a baby, as long as it wasn't too much trouble for him. But when the pressure to do further testing starts or when he's asked to evaluate one too many ovulation predictor kits strips, he may begin to get testy. Don't immediately assume that he's not interested in having a baby. Some men react to medical events by becoming uncooperative because they feel uniformed or left out or are worried about what lies ahead.

On the other hand, your partner may be trying to tell you something important. The drive to have a child isn't always as intense in men as it is in women, and he may feel ambivalent about the process. In other words, if you get pregnant, great, but if you don't . . . well, he could live with that too.

Sometimes the help of an outside person, such as a counselor or your doctor, can help both of you decide whether the pursuit of pregnancy is going to damage your relationship and, if it is, whether it's worth continuing to try to get pregnant. This is a difficult decision, but many couples have opted out of the baby chase at this point and thought about adoption or child-free living. If you're picking up negative signals from your partner at this point, stop and listen. Other options are available besides pursuing higher-tech methods of getting pregnant, and you may want to think about them . . . together.

Coping with meddling relatives

Sometimes your doctor is wonderful and your partner is a rock, but your mother, sister, or best friend is a royal pain in the proverbial you-know-what, wanting to know all the details of how things are going, how you're feeling, how your partner is reacting, and so on.

The obvious way to handle this situation is to just tell everyone to stay out of your business, but as you well know, this is much easier said than done. Like it or not, these people are usually important to you or you wouldn't let them interfere in your lives this way, and you *do* want your potential child to have a grandma, aunt, or godmother some day.

Some families consider this sort of interference as sort of a family right. Inquiring into your reproductive plans may have started the minute your relationship with your partner began. A polite "I'd rather not discuss it" isn't going to work in this kind of family. Before you know it, the whispering has begun, and the word is out in the family that something is wrong with you.

How much you tell is up to you and your partner. Usually your partner isn't as eager to blab the details to one and all as you may be, but you may want to consider that even the most prying parents and friends may turn out to be a real source of support after they know what you're going through.

You can try, nicely but firmly and hopefully unemotionally, to let relatives know that their concern is welcome but their advice and opinions are not. Most often, you'll find they don't really want to know all the details. They just want to feel like they're an important part of your life and that you care enough about them to include them in what's going on.

Managing Your Frustrations

Unfortunately, at times, even the greatest minds in medicine (also known as your doctors) don't know why you're not pregnant yet. They're doing the best they can to find out. Your job is to stay sane through the process.

If your rose-colored glasses seem to have faded to black, the best way to clear your vision and your mind is to stop. Your body will not be rushed, and trying to rush things can often create further problems, both psychologically and physiologically.

Getting pregnant is not a goal. Having a baby is.

A watched pot never boils; the same thing applies to a watched uterus.

Consider taking a month off from your position as baby maker wannabe. More often than not, the continued stress of trying and trying and trying harder doesn't add up to better results. Breaking the pattern, even for a month, can give your mind and body the rest they need. Think of fertility as a marathon, not a sprint.

I (coauthor Jackie) am the kind of person who runs late to almost everything. The later I am, the more uneasy I become. This uneasiness quickly turns into a frantic feeling. When I'm frantic, I experience the feeling that the whole world is out to make me even later than I already am; every pair of pantyhose in my closet has a run, green lights turn to red, and I end up putting lipstick on my nose in an effort to apply makeup and drive at the same time. If I'm lucky, I manage to avoid an accident, but one way or another, I arrive at my destination irritable and nervous — not exactly the best way to begin. Trying to conceive is much like this. The more you go through the process, the more you may feel that you want — no, *need* — to have a baby *now*. This stress leads to frustration, fear, and the urgency brought on by the (generally false) belief that each cycle may represent the last chance (not a medical term). Left untreated, this belief leads to baby panic, a condition in which everything in life begins to feel colored by the unsuccessful effort to conceive, and you become increasingly more irritable and unreasonable (albeit for good reason).

Human reproduction is an inefficient process. Eighty percent of the healthiest and youngest women need a minimum of six months to conceive. Pace yourself, as you'll need your energy later. Persistence pays off. Panic doesn't.

Keeping on keeping on

Consider an attitude readjustment. Fighting with your fertility is a battle best won with kindness, toward yourself and your partner. Here are our suggestions for marking time:

✔ Take the time to appreciate good health — it's not a guarantee, whether you conceive or not.

✔ If you don't have a baby to love yet, direct that energy toward the children and adults who *are* in your life today. Doing so involves no risks, and the rewards will carry you through this difficult time.

✔ Are you angry? Makes sense to us. Perhaps you can channel that anger into a letter to your congressman lobbying for better coverage for fertility patients.

✔ Do you feel it's unfair that people you consider undeserving parents get to have the children that you dream of? Step up to the plate and volunteer to be a Big Sister or Big Brother for a child who will truly benefit from your good parenting skills.

✔ Pamper yourself and your body. Get a massage, enjoy fine (and healthy) dining, read a good book, go for a walk, or play with a puppy.

✔ Create a support network. While your old friends are like gold in getting you through this, no one can truly comfort and sustain you quite like another person experiencing the same thing. You'll find plenty of other women and men out there struggling with fertility.

A good friend once said that even the most optimistic of us experience those times when our hope switch is stuck on "off." Like fertility, this is a temporary, albeit painful, condition. Rebooting your emotions can go a long way toward resetting your physical condition as well.

Sound too Pollyanna-ish? (Pollyanna was a fictional character who always saw the bright side of everything.) Perhaps, but the effects from this self-care will result in a calmer, happier, healthier you, the kind of you who will make a great parent someday.

Making your partner feel part of the team

You need to consider another person here, and your partner may have a host of feelings all his own. Keeping the lines of communication open, wide open, is the only way to avoid the land mines that come from assuming one another's feelings, or lack thereof. The person going through treatment often has better resources because that person is more in touch with the doctors, nurses, and other patients who may provide a shoulder, an ear, or a piece of advice. The partner, who may receive little or no treatment, may have less of an understanding of or comfort level with the entire process. While the fertility patient learns firsthand of every test and result, the partner gets only a secondhand account, often a jumbled reconstruction of the facts in broken medicalspeak. Your partner may be interested in what's going on, but he may be intimidated as well. Instead of pulling out *Cliffs Notes on Reproductive Endocrinology,* you may decide to arrange for you and your partner to visit the doctor together or to schedule a phone consultation with the doctor, to help keep both of you in the loop about any problems.

You may also find that you, as the patient, have a greater desire to talk out every possibility that may or may not *ever* happen. Your partner may not have this need. In order to respect these wishes, occasionally glance at your partner to see whether he's still conscious. When you notice his eyes rolling back in his head, consider this your cue to stop talking.

Respecting the difference of the sexes

While one partner's emotions may often rise and fall with each test result, the other person's feelings may not. One common view of partners is that the proof is in the baby, not in the myriad details. Instead of accusing your partner of hiding feelings under a shroud of optimism or pretending that he's not worried about your latest estrogen level or egg count, consider this difference in your reaction as a wonderful example of balance. As you move along on your road to baby, you may become more grateful for this balance and less likely to try and shake your partner down for a buried feeling. Who knows? The score of the Super Bowl may actually have a greater impact on your life than the level of your follicle-stimulating hormone!

Finding fertility-free time

The partner of the fertility patient is the one who primarily faces the problem of loneliness resulting from the pursuit of a baby. While one partner is trying to cope with the possible loss of fertility, the other partner is dealing with a loss of a different sort: the loss of a partner immersed in the facts, figures, and minutiae that can become all-encompassing when trying to conceive. For the fertility patient, the struggle with fertility may bring a great deal of fear and pain, but it can also deliver new friends (real and cyber), enough reading and research to fill a lifetime, and a litany of emotions to sort through. A woman may find herself so busy with these activities that she doesn't even have time for a quiet night with her partner in front of the television.

To help solve this problem, we recommend "fertility-free zones," times and places where the subject is off-limits. Although detaching from what appears to be such a looming issue may be hard, the space created by these mini-vacations allows you to recharge yourselves as a couple and remember what brought you together in the first place.

PERSONAL STORY

Reacting to news of others' pregnancies

I (coauthor Jackie) married at 34 and began the quest for baby by 36. When my best college friend, Leslie, got married at 39, I was still trying. She and I had discussed fertility at great length. We were the same age, and she too anticipated being faced with the same uphill battle. She decided to start trying right away, and I walked her through the ovulation predictor kit and the tale of the little purple line. Although I would never wish it upon her, I fully expected that soon she would join me in the waiting room of a reproductive endocrinologist's office somewhere. Two months later, after recounting our latest high-tech fertility strategy, I asked her how her low-tech attempts were faring. The long pause was what got me. "Jackie," she said, her voice breaking, "I'm pregnant." I couldn't believe it. Hadn't she gotten married only 15 minutes ago? I managed to blurt out, "When?" struggling with the conflicting emotions of wanting to congratulate her and wanting to cry. "I'm six weeks along," she replied. "It happened the second month." Thank God for call waiting. When the other call beeped in, I quickly wished her all the love and luck in the world and cut the conversation short. That poor telemarketer. Talk about making the wrong call at the wrong time.

I love my friends and wish them the best. And despite this, Leslie's success seemed to be my failure, even more so than the unsuccessful years of trying. Luckily, I had my network in place. A call to my friend Susan, who was also experiencing infertility, quickly salved my wounds, at least temporarily. "Don't you hate it when that happens?" she said with a sigh. She proceeded to share her stories of a sister-in-law who conceived every time her husband walked in the room. Susan, on the other hand, had spent the last five years in low-, medium-, and high-tech fertility treatments with no baby to show for it (although by the time of this writing, she had just given birth to a healthy baby girl, who came about in a completely unplanned, non-technological way!). Susan's ability to immediately understand helped me to begin to put the situation in perspective. Sharing with the newly pregnant Leslie that I felt happy for her *and* jealous also eased the pain. I remembered how difficult it was when I lost friends who couldn't deal with the fact that I was getting married while they remained single. I knew I didn't want to give up my friendship no matter how difficult it felt. Instead, I committed to working through it by continuing to communicate with the same honesty and sensitivity that I was seeking. When all else fails, I try to see another's pregnancy as my chance to observe just what I'm getting myself into. I hope to put this more intimate knowledge of the pros and cons of being pregnant to good use in the future.

Talkin' it out

One of the most difficult emotions that many fertility patients deal with (and subsequently subject their partners to) is the overwhelming sense of guilt that they're denying their partner a child of their own. Left untreated, this thought process can move on to the assumption that your partner is as equally bereft over the lack of a baby and perhaps angry to boot. This type of "stinking thinking" is a dangerous example of assumptions gone wrong. The result can be the emotional absence of one partner and the peace of mind of the other. Instead, have the courage to confront your partner with your fears and believe that you are loved, despite your reproductive system. Doing so helps to forge a bond that really does make for a stronger relationship.

There is no *i* in *team*. Infertility is no one's fault, regardless of where the problem lies, or where you think it may be. Fertility can be the result of a number and/or combination of causes, some of which have yet to be determined. It's a challenge that you and your partner face together.

Surviving the holidays

Holidays bring their own special challenges to almost everyone, but those trying to conceive may be particularly affected. The summer holidays always seem to be the perfect setting for family picnics, reunions, and other get-togethers where carefree children frolic and nosy relatives coyly ask when you will be eating for two. Winter provides little relief as Thanksgiving, Hanukkah, Christmas, and Kwanzaa all seem to focus on extended family, talk of Santa, the latest children's toys, and holiday newsletters that share every painstaking family detail, from birth to potty training to Junior's first car accident.

Some of this family updating is normal, but you may be especially sensitive to the topic while you're trying to conceive yourself. Try as best you can to determine whether the conversation is the speaker's way of trying to connect or reconnect with family and friends or whether you're face-to-face with an insufferable boor. If you discover the latter, realize that you can't do much to guard against people like this, whether they're related to you or not. Even when you do have children of your own, they're little protection in this situation. Those who want to prattle on endlessly about themselves and their families will do so anyway, with little notice given to whether you're with child or without. In such situations, the art of the smile, the nod, and the hasty exit will serve you well.

If you plan on spending extended time with your extended family, consider cluing in a few folks about your situation. They can be helpful in deflecting family or friends who are notorious for ill-timed comments. Arriving late and/or leaving early is another way to minimize your contact with difficult people and situations. You may want to plan something special for you and your partner or a friend after your family affair. This activity will give you something to look forward to throughout the family function.

I (coauthor Jackie) was certain that, after attending family functions solo for years, my discomfort would end if and when I was married. How was I to know that there was still another hoop to jump through? What I did learn was that there will *always* be another obstacle, if I allow it. Even if I were to arrive with my perfect family in tow, some new challenge would always await.

Holidays can become a time for comparison rather than a time for joy, if you choose to compete. Instead, consider meeting those ill-timed comments and people with a hug and an expression of good wishes. Your grace may just stop the others in their tracks.

For those who truly are interested in you and your life, share some of the positive things from the past year. They may truly appreciate the chance to connect, much more so than a bouncing baby story.

Rather than ignore the children playing with their new toys, get in there and play with them. Doing so is wonderful practice for the future. And in the meantime, you may just discover some of the fun of being with children and sharing their joy, before giving them back to their rightful owner after the excitement wears off! Consider this your gift of the holiday season.

Declining invitations

If a family member or friend is expecting, you may find it difficult to be expected yourself at any gathering that this pregnant woman attends. Don't chide yourself for your absence. A little denial can go a long way toward helping you gracefully deal with a painful situation. You may decide to bow out of a family dinner or two or 'fess up with the truth and count on the understanding of those who love you. Either way, you'll preserve your integrity and that of your family relationships by not forcing yourself to handle even one bit more than you think you can. This too shall (and will) pass.

Forecast: Baby showers likely

Definition of a baby shower: A seemingly benign tradition that can wreak havoc in the hearts of infertile women everywhere (many men claim this as well, no matter what the circumstances). Here's some advice on the topic:

- If you choose to attend (and remember you don't *have* to), don't go it alone. Sometimes that may mean sharing your situation with the pregnant guest of honor. Although it is *her* day, a little bit of knowledge goes a long way toward sensitivity.

- If you don't choose to confide in the lady of the hour, hang with a friend. Face it: Baby showers can be very emotional, but they can also be very, very humorous, particularly when shared with someone who understands your situation and can help you see the (inevitable) comedy of errors that often surrounds the pregnant population. This tactic can help you to laugh your way through situations that you may have spent months dreading. Remember though, be nice — isn't that how you want to be treated when you're pregnant?

✔ If no allies are in attendance, the telephone can be a wonderful thing. Try to make a difficult situation tolerable by calling a trusted friend before, after, and sometimes during (that's what bathrooms are for!) the event. Cellular phones are wonderful for this purpose and have helped many a pregnant woman through a tough spot. Consider turning down the ringer and/or putting your phone on vibrator mode if you expect a "cavalry call" to help you through. This way, you can get the support you need and not disrupt the party.

✔ If you're going solo to the shower, you can always use the bathroom, the porch, or your car for temporary refuge . . . or for a good cry if you need it.

✔ You don't have to stay until the last present is unwrapped either. Making an appearance is sufficient, particularly when you're under pressure. You can be the life of the party another time. Your friends will understand.

Chapter 5

Taking Supplemental Steps on the Road to Baby

*Y*ou're feeling tired. You've charted your ovulation, timed your sex life, and possibly even tried a few of the more basic fertility medicines. Nothing has worked so far, and your doctor may be suggesting stepping up the pace, as if the present pace isn't hard enough. His advice may involve injecting medications made from such odd ingredients as powdered Chinese hamster ovaries (actually found in some forms of hCG, or human chorionic gonadotropin). "Wait a minute!" you cry out. "Isn't there another way?"

Yes, there are other ways, and you may already have tried one of them. In the first stages of trying to conceive, you may have been met with the well-intended, but unasked for, opinions of those who tell you to just relax and you'll get pregnant. Sometimes, this directive may actually work, but more often it doesn't. Now, as you prepare to move to the next level, the middle-tech road to baby, you'll more than likely hear of (and from!) others who swear by other, nontraditional ways of conceiving.

In this chapter, we talk about those "other" ways to become pregnant, alternative measures from basic to beyond, and help you decide which ones are worth trying and which ones may just result in expensive urination.

Eating for Two? Sampling a Fertility Diet

Eat meat if you want to get pregnant with a boy, and eat sugar if you want a girl, an old wives' tale states. But what if you just want to have a baby — of *any* kind? When I (coauthor Jackie) first ventured online to learn more about this road that had become a little longer than I had first anticipated, I found an entire civilization of people trying to conceive by using a variety of dietary means, claiming that diet changes put them in tiptop reproductive shape. These women (and men) had purged their diets of red meat, dairy products, white flour, sugar, and a host of other staples that I viewed as necessary. I was terrified. Their list of don'ts was my diet in a nutshell.

Some people swore by omega-3 fatty acids, found most commonly in salmon and other fish, as the magic potion for improving and/or restoring fertility. The only fish I consumed were Goldfish (those popular snack crackers, that is). I thought I was in big trouble. The prospect of shots, whatever they were made of, seemed more attractive to me than a complete overhaul of my diet, but I didn't want to skip what could be a crucial step. But is your diet a factor when trying to get pregnant? Here's a brief look at some foods and our recommendations:

- ✔ **Red meat:** Studies show that red meat can neither help nor hurt your chances of getting pregnant. Trim all visible fat and cook the meat thoroughly.

- ✔ **Dairy:** Many women trying to conceive cut dairy products from their diet, but there's no conclusive medical or scientific data that supports the notion that dairy foods compromise fertility. Use organic products if possible. If you're lactose intolerant, dairy products can create havoc on your system, so be aware of your personal dietary needs.

- ✔ **White flour and processed sugar:** No studies have proven that refined sugar or processed flour decreases fertility. We recommend limiting their intake.

- ✔ **Artificial additives:** Despite hot debate, no definitive studies prove that additives such as aspartame and MSG are harmful. Limit or eliminate these additives from your diet if the controversy worries you.

- ✔ **Omega-3 fatty oils:** Studies are underway to evaluate the use of omega-3 oils in male infertility and in women with endometriosis. Omega-3 oils, present in fish, soybeans, flaxseed oil, canola oil, wheat germ, and walnuts, have been shown to reduce heart disease. We recommend that you avoid fresh tuna, swordfish, and shark in favor of salmon, whitefish, or mahi mahi, and limit canned tuna to two servings a week.

 Do not eat raw or undercooked fish, meat, or poultry when trying to get pregnant or during pregnancy. These products have a higher than normal chance of carrying listeria, a bacteria that may make a mom somewhat ill but wreak havoc on an unborn child's nervous system. Listeria has also been linked to an increased rate of spontaneous abortion.

✔ **Soy:** Some studies have shown that a very high soy intake may decrease fertility, and soy may disturb thyroid function, decreasing fertility. The recommendation: Skip the soy or limit it severely.

Soy is a source of phytoestrogens, weak estrogens that can enhance or suppress natural estrogen production. Knowing whether you produce enough, or too much, estrogen on your own is a part of the diagnostic process in your fertility treatment. Confusing the matter with outside sources of estrogen will do just that — confuse the matter. Keep it simple.

Good nutrition is something that you should *not* ignore. Consider it common sense, as well as medical sense, that the healthier your body is, the healthier all its systems, including the reproductive system, are. Nutrition is part of the bigger picture that also includes such basics as getting enough sleep, exercising, and nourishing your body as well as your mind. Although good nutrition is rarely the sole factor that brings about a baby, it does help to better preserve your overall health so that you may enjoy your future child as well, and as long, as possible.

If you choose to opt for a complete nutritional overhaul, realize that this is a long-term commitment and is unlikely to produce a quick fix for your fertility issues. Books such as *The Infertility Diet: Get Pregnant and Prevent Miscarriage*, by Fern Reiss (Peanut Butter and Jelly Press), can provide you with a menu plan of fertility foods if you want to try a complete dietary overhaul. For most people, this is a major lifestyle change and may lead to better overall health. On the fertility front, however, keep your expectations in check; diet changes alone are unlikely to get you pregnant.

For those looking to take the more moderate road, consider planning your diet around the major food groups that we discuss in Chapter 2. You may also choose to consult a nutritionist to make sure that you get the proper balance of vitamins and minerals. A good diet is a good idea whether you're trying to conceive or not.

Looking at Supplements — Vitamins, Minerals, Herbs, and More

Dietary supplements are very popular; one survey shows that over 40 percent of all Americans use some form of supplement. Dietary supplements include herbs, vitamins, minerals, amino acids, enzymes, and extracts. Because they're considered a dietary product rather than a medicinal product, they aren't regulated by the U.S. Food and Drug Administration the way prescription medications are. This lack of regulation means that the ingredient amount may vary from one pill to the next. Supplements have also been found to be contaminated with animal parts and toxic molds in some cases.

Because they're sold over the counter, without a prescription, supplements are often viewed as harmless. Studies have shown that many supplements are far from harmless. Some supplements, such as ephedra, have been implicated in causing death, and others, such as comfrey, can cause severe liver damage.

Yet many naturopaths, who believe that the body will heal itself if kept in proper balance, and herbalists tout supplements as a way to help get (and stay) pregnant. Internet sites abound with happy moms claiming that supplements were responsible for their pregnancies. So who do you believe, and are there any supplements that you absolutely should not take?

Herbs

Although herbs have been used for centuries, studies on their safety and benefits have been few. That's beginning to change, with the National Institutes of Health (NIH) now studying many herbs and other alternative medications. Herbs aren't benign, and someone with some knowledge of their interactions should oversee their use. Practitioners in this area may include chiropractors, osteopaths, nutritionists, and naturopaths (those who employ a drugless approach to keep the body in balance).

Here's a look at some of the more popular herbs used in the treatment of infertility. This list represents a small sample of herbs that can be used and represents herbs that are both Western in origin as well as Chinese.

- **Black cohosh:** An herb with estrogenic qualities, black cohosh is often used to relieve the discomfort associated with menopause (hot flashes, for example). Studies have been mixed on whether black cohosh is effective. Black cohosh is also recommended to boost estrogen production, although there's no proof that this works. Side effects of black cohosh are dizziness, nausea, low pulse rate, and increased perspiration.

- **Dong quai:** Dubbed the "ultimate herb" for women, dong quai is used for everything from restoring menstrual regularity to treating menopausal symptoms. Dong quai is a blood thinner and should not be taken during an IVF cycle or by women who have very heavy periods.

- **False unicorn root:** Native Americans used this herb to improve menstrual irregularities and to alleviate problems associated with menopause and problems with infertility due to irregular follicular formation.

- **Nettle leaves:** This herb is considered to be an overall uterine tonic that better prepares the uterus for implantation of the embryo.

- **Primrose oil:** A fatty acid, primrose oil may increase cervical mucus to make it easier for sperm to get to the egg. An unwanted side effect of primrose oil may be thinning of the uterine lining, making implantation more difficult.

- **Red clover:** This herb is often used to boost estrogen in a women's body. This exogenous, or outside the body, form of estrogen may raise your estrogen levels artificially; raising your estrogen levels artificially is meaningless if the rise isn't caused by the production of a mature egg.

- **Red raspberry leaves:** Another uterine toner, this herb reportedly increases the uterine lining thickness (in order to make the uterus more receptive to the embryo). Red raspberry causes uterine contractions and absolutely should not be used in early pregnancy.

- **Vitex:** Also known as chaste tree berry, this herb has been used by herbalists for many years to help regulate women's hormones. Some use Vitex to increase luteinizing hormone levels and help an egg release. According to others, Vitex can also increase progesterone levels and should be used only after you ovulate — not before. If taken earlier, it may keep you from releasing an egg. If taken in the luteal phase, after you ovulate, it may regulate and lengthen your cycle to give the embryo a chance to implant. Vitex is slow acting, so it may take several months for any effect to occur.

- **Wild yam:** In large doses, wild yam is used as a contraceptive; in smaller doses, it may promote progesterone production. Don't take wild yam until after ovulation occurs.

The following herbs stimulate the uterus so you absolutely should not take them after you get pregnant:

- Black cohosh
- Dong quai
- False unicorn root
- Feverfew
- Golden seal
- Pennyroyal

In addition, avoid these drugs if you get pregnant:

- Blue cohosh: May cause fetal heart defects
- Mugwort: May cause fetal abnormalities

Herbal treatment of infertility is not a do-it-yourself approach! Let all your doctors know whether you're taking any kinds of herbs, whether they're the over-the-counter variety or prescribed to you by another source. Undesirable reactions may occur between one herb preparation and another. In addition, they may all cross-react with the drugs your reproductive endocrinologist is giving you. Deciding what to take on your own is complicated, because the same herb may be described as useful for two entirely opposing actions.

Vitameatavegamin and all that jazz

A good multivitamin has the correct amounts of the vitamins you need, so rarely do you need to supplement with additional vitamins. Your body takes in only what it needs from water soluble vitamins (generally the maximum recommended daily dose found in most multivitamins) and urinates out the rest (talk about good money down the drain!). In addition, overdoing it on some vitamins can cause adverse reactions in your system. Excess amounts of fat soluble vitamins, such as vitamin A, are stored in your body instead of being excreted. Although adequate levels of vitamin A help to preserve your vision and immune system, an excess of vitamin A can result in liver disease and birth defects when taken by pregnant women. So, yes, you can really have too much of a good thing.

Overdosing on vitamins *through foods alone* is highly unlikely. Because most foods contain small amounts of any individual vitamin or nutrient, you would have to eat bushels of bananas, oranges, or spinach to get too much. Overdosage of any particular vitamin, mineral, or nutrient is generally only a danger if you consume it in a concentrated form, such as vitamin pills or powders.

Is taking a prenatal vitamin when trying to conceive premature? Not really. The primary difference between multivitamins and prenatal vitamins is the greater concentration of folic acid and iron in a prenatal vitamin. Folic acid is crucial in pregnancy to help prevent spinal and neural tube defects, while iron is often needed as a supplement for the loss of iron due to pregnancy. An excess of iron *can* result in constipation, which can be remedied through the introduction of additional fibers, fruits, and vegetables in your diet, a good thing no matter where you are on the baby-making quest.

Lydia Pinkham's tonic

For half a century, Lydia Pinkham's Vegetable Compound was a best-selling "medicinal" used by women for a variety of female complaints, including problems with menstruation and symptoms of menopause. Whether the drug was so beloved because of its high black cohosh content or the 36-proof alcohol in the bottle is something we'll never know. But if you have an old bottle of this sitting around somewhere (it's still manufactured, but with different ingredients), don't dump it — antique collectors will be glad to take it off your hands!

Over-the-counter (OTC) prenatal vitamins may boast that they contain even higher levels of the necessary vitamins and nutrients. In order to achieve this, however, the OTC brand may require dosages up to three times a day while prescription prenatal vitamins pack their punch in one dose per day. If you're feeling childlike, even though you're not with child yet, you can also get the same ingredients of a prenatal vitamin by taking three Flintstones Complete vitamins per day.

If you're taking a standard multivitamin rather than prenatal vitamins while pregnant, make sure that it doesn't contain extra ingredients such as herbs. Many health food stores sell blends that contain herbs. Don't take these types of vitamins during pregnancy.

Are certain vitamins, taken in greater (or lesser) quantity, more likely to result in increased fertility? At the time of this writing, no direct evidence supports this. We advise you to stick with a standard multivitamin or prenatal vitamin. Your local pharmacist can recommend a good OTC brand, and your doctor can steer you toward a good prescription choice.

Some studies have shown that liquid prenatal vitamins are better absorbed than pills. They may also be less likely to make you nauseated after you become pregnant.

All the vitamins in the world won't get you pregnant, but they will help you keep your body in the best nutritional shape possible, along with proper diet, exercise, and general care. This balanced state is the best place for babies to come from!

Folic acid

Folic acid, a B vitamin, is essential when trying to get pregnant. Many studies have shown that 0.4 mg of folic acid a day cuts the chance of having a baby with neural tube defects by 50 percent. Neural tube defects occur in 6 of 10,000 births in the United States and include problems with the spine and brain. Neural tube defects develop very early in pregnancy, in the first four weeks, so taking a good multivitamin containing this amount while trying to get pregnant is essential. Many foods, including leafy green vegetables, fortified cereals, orange juice, and lean beef, contain folic acid, but overcooking can destroy folic acid, so take a vitamin even if you eat well.

Wheatgrass

For me (Jackie), it was a litmus test. When I dropped a wheatgrass pill on the floor, my basset hound (also known as the canine garbage disposal) raced toward it. Before I could grab it, he had it in his mouth. Then, to my disbelief, the dog, who has been known to view dead squirrel as a delicacy, dropped the wheatgrass pill and scurried away. It was not a testament to taste.

Despite my dog's opinion, many others claim that taking regular shots of wheatgrass (meaning a liquid taken in a shot *glass,* not through injection) or a daily handful of pills has lowered their FSH (follicle-stimulating hormone) levels, allowing for better egg production and/or egg quality.

What is wheatgrass anyway? Wheatgrass is a dark, leafy, green vegetable that can be harvested, dried, and bottled in pill form. Some people attest that the homegrown or fresh grown variety is better and raise their own wheatgrass from seed, later shaving off the grass and blending it into a questionable-looking green froth. Many health food stores do this blending for you; however, *you* still must drink the stuff. In all honesty, wheatgrass juice is fairly flavorless, with a slightly sweet taste and an aroma similar to, well, freshly cut grass! You probably won't find a wheatgrass-flavored Blizzard at Dairy Queen anytime soon, however. Many people follow up a wheatgrass shot with a "chaser" of fresh vegetable juice.

Wheatgrass is an antioxidant, meaning that it can cleanse your body of impurities and toxins. It's also used to build hemoglobin (iron stores) in the blood, reduce blood pressure, and keep your hair from going gray.

Regarding the claims that wheatgrass lowers FSH levels and thus improves the number and/or quality of eggs, remember that you're born with a limited number of eggs that only decrease over time. There is virtually no way to increase that number or to change a bad egg into a good one. FSH is merely a measurement of ovarian reserve and is generally checked to determine the probable response to stimulation via fertility medicines.

The question in this area is, if you artificially lower FSH levels (through wheatgrass, herbs, or exogenous estrogen), are you actually changing anything to do with your egg quality or quantity? The confusion lies in the fact that FSH numbers can often vary from normal to high (signifying diminished ovarian reserve) during *perimenopause* (the period preceding menopause). Doctors are still in discussion as to which reading to believe, the high or the low. Many doctors claim that after an FSH value is returned high, any other reading, even a normal one, is insignificant. In other words, the egg stash is dwindling.

Other doctors look at any month's specific FSH value (typically taken on cycle day three) as predictive of that month's egg supply. If you opt for the latter train of thought, then methods that may help lower your FSH levels could be beneficial for future cycles. However, at this writing, no available evidence shows that wheatgrass can lower your FSH levels.

Ann Wigmore, the mother of wheatgrass

Wheatgrass as a way to good health was popularized by Ann Wigmore (1909–1994), who immigrated to the United States at a young age from Eastern Europe. She believed that wheatgrass cured the insanity of King Nebuchadnezzar in the Old Testament after he was forced to live on grasses for seven years while wandering the fields. She also believed that the fact that animals ate grass when they were ill showed the value of eating various grasses. Her ideas became well known through her many books on the subject of raw diet and through her Hippocratic Health Institute. She was sued several times for claiming her elixir could cure AIDS or prevent cancer. Her institute is still active as the Wigmore Foundation. "Dr. Ann," as she was known, had no medical degree and was a self-taught naturopath. (Naturopaths believe that the body will heal itself if balance is maintained.)

L-arginine

L-arginine is another example of a product that has received cult status over the past few years for treating everything from immune disorders to sexual problems. L-arginine is a nonessential amino acid found in whole wheat, rice, nuts, seeds, corn, soy, grapes, carob, and other foods. Nonmedical individuals in the fertility community have used L-arginine (also known as arginine) in concentrated pill form during fertility cycles in efforts to improve egg quality. Some studies also show increased blood flow to the uterus. In males, some studies (but not all) have shown increased sperm motility and production when taking L-arginine.

A study published by the professional journal *Human Reproduction* pointed out a negative effect of L-arginine if you're taking fertility medications. The study showed that in a small test group, the use of L-arginine supplementation was detrimental to embryo quality and pregnancy rate during a sample cycle when the test also used fertility medicines.

If you're prone to cold sores, L-arginine may exacerbate them. Use with caution.

Like many supplements, L-arginine can cause adverse reactions at higher doses when taken in pill form as a supplement. It is virtually impossible to overdose on the amount of L-arginine found in foods, as even foods that contain it have it only in trace amounts. However, L-arginine can reach less than desirable levels when taken in more concentrated forms, such as pills. Pregnant women are advised not to use L-arginine.

Natural doesn't necessarily mean safe. If your fertility doctor prescribes any medication for you, let him or her know of any other herbs, pills, or treatments that you're already taking, in order to prevent a possible harmful drug interaction.

Supplements for better sperm production

Fertility is not just a female issue. In fact, 40 percent of the time, male factor is responsible for a couple's failure to conceive.

So women aren't the only ones who may venture onto an alternative path for treating medical problems related to infertility. Keep in mind that studies have been mixed as to the efficacy of taking supplements. Also remember that in male problems where surgery is deemed necessary (to fix a varicocele or any other structural issue), diet and/or supplements won't do the trick. These tips, however, can benefit overall health, which can contribute to better reproductive health. A man produces new sperm every three months, so what you do today can affect conception down the line. The following supplements have been shown to benefit sperm count and motility in some studies:

- **Zinc:** May increase sperm motility and sperm count
- **Vitamin B12:** May increase sperm count
- **Vitamin C:** May increase sperm count
- **Vitamin E:** May increase sperm motility
- **Selenium:** May increase sperm motility
- **L-Carnitine:** May increase sperm motility and sperm count
- **L-arginine:** May increase sperm motility and sperm count
- **Folic acid:** May increase sperm motility and sperm count
- **CoQ10:** May increase sperm motility and sperm count

A good multivitamin should contain an adequate amount of all of the preceding.

Visiting a Traditional Chinese Medicine Practitioner

Traditional Chinese medicine (TCM), often referred to as Eastern medicine, works on a different set of principles and beliefs than Western medicine (that which is practiced in the United States and many other parts of the world).

Traditional Chinese medicine views the individual as an integral mind/body organism and, in essence, believes that a delicate balance, the yin and yang, is necessary for optimal health and well-being. TCM divides the body into various *meridians,* or pathways, along which *qi,* or energy, flows. For example, fertility problems might be explained by liver qi stagnation, that is, congestion in the liver meridian. Primary treatment in TCM includes the administration of herbal formulas and acupuncture to clear the body passageways and restore normal function.

Although traditional Chinese medicine has been practiced since 204 B.C., only during the past two decades has it been recognized in the United States and other parts of the world. According to Western medicine, anecdotal evidence, as demonstrated in TCM, awaits confirmation in randomized clinical trials. Currently, however, the National Institutes of Health (NIH) has set up a division to further investigate alternative medicines and treatment. More definitive findings probably will become available in the coming years.

Despite this lack of scientific evidence, many patients, suffering from diseases ranging from cancer to chronic fatigue to infertility, have found a haven in the TCM community, which many times is warmer and fuzzier than the classic Western doctor/hospital setting. Some who have given up on Western medicine (or on whom Western medicine has given up) have found palliative relief, remission, and results under the guidance of a traditional Chinese medicine doctor.

Before you jump on the TCM bandwagon, check the credentials of the practitioner whom you select. TCM doctors must complete training, just as they do in Western medicine, and should be licensed or certified (if your state offers this). In addition, they should be nationally certified through the National Certification Commission for Acupuncture and Oriental Medicine. To confirm certification, visit the commission's Web site at www.nccaom.org.

Help from herbal formulas

Your TCM practitioner may prescribe an herbal formula containing up to ten different herbs. The combination of herbs to create a formula is one of the main differences between the Western and Eastern views. TCM relies on this ability to modify formulas in order to customize an individual approach based on a patient's needs. TCM herbal formulas are also available in pills that can be purchased from your TCM practitioner; however, they're considered to be less effective due to the extraction process necessary to convert them into this form.

Because there are over 6,000 herbs to choose from, this formulation is a science in and of itself and, unlike the single-ingredient, Western herb approach, can't be self-administered.

Most TCM practitioners also use *moxibustion,* in which small mounds of herbs are burned over certain areas of the body, in the treatment of infertility. TCM practitioners also treat male infertility issues, so feel free to go as a couple.

Don't view traditional Chinese medicine as a shortcut. Nothing in medicine ever is. The treatments require consistency and commitment, but they may provide you with a more palatable process than Western treatments.

We also recommend that you "pick your poison," for lack of a better term. Whether your treatment is traditional Chinese medicine or Western medicine, don't try to combine the two. Many herbs, when taken with fertility medicines, can cause adverse reactions. Particularly when combined with treatments that involve surgical procedures, such as in vitro fertilization, the ingestion of herbs or other tonics can cause more severe problems, such as bleeding, or simply complicate matters. As a result, both your TCM doctor and your Western doctor may find it impossible to accurately define and treat your condition.

If you choose to try both TCM and Western medicine simultaneously (despite our suggestions to the contrary), make sure that all of your practitioners, doctors, and nurses, are aware of your protocol. Not revealing this information is an ideal way to confuse the people whose goals are to help you conceive.

On pins and needles — acupuncture for infertility

Perhaps one area of traditional Chinese medicine that has benefited the most from the recent interest on behalf of Western medicines is acupuncture. Acupuncture is based on the belief that a person's health is determined by a balanced flow of energy (qi) in the body. This 5,000-year-old practice is most often used to relieve chronic pain by inserting needles into a variety of pressure points on the head and body. Acupuncture also is used for treatments for everything from the common cold to drug addiction.

In April 2002, the prestigious medical journal *Fertility and Sterility* cited evidence that acupuncture, when used in conjunction with in vitro fertilization, notably improved pregnancy rates. In the study involving 160 patients, acupuncture was performed just prior to the transfer of embryos into the uterus and again after the transfer took place. Needles were inserted along the spleen and stomach meridians, as well as other sites, in an effort to stimulate blood flow to the uterus. Forty-two percent of the acupuncture group got pregnant, compared to 26 percent of the non-acupuncture group. The sedative effect of acupuncture is also believed to assist in relaxing a woman, quieting her uterus, and making it more receptive to embryos.

Although this study will require additional follow-up to make sure that the previous results were not psychosomatic and are indeed repeatable, the findings were certainly of great interest to those in the fertility community.

Acupuncture has long been a popular alternative form of treatment for infertility. Many woman have used this treatment in hopes of increasing blood flow to the uterus, thus helping to thicken the uterine lining. Other women have found that acupuncture has been crucial in helping them relax through the trials and tribulations of fertility treatment.

Whether its effects are actually physiological or not, acupuncture is an excellent adjunct to a fertility regimen. However, be sure that those performing the treatment are certified. Many fertility clinics work in conjunction with an acupuncturist and/or can recommend someone who specializes in fertility-based treatment.

Many states have their own acupuncture society, and some states have specific requirements that must be met. For example, in Indiana, people need a prescription from a physician in order to be treated by a certified acupuncturist. You can check online for your state's rules and regulations, as well as for acupuncture societies, which may also provide you with specific recommendations.

If you're scared of being stuck with acupuncture needles, take heart! The average acupuncture needle has the thickness of a human hair. You may feel a small prick, but it's far less discomfort than a blood test. But if you're still a bit apprehensive and too needlephobic about the procedure, you may be better off skipping this particular form of treatment. Remember that the goal is to relax.

Bring along a favorite tape or CD to listen to during acupuncture treatment. Most acupuncture treatments require you to lie still with the needles in place for a short period of time, usually 20 minutes or less. This may also be a great time to use your visualization techniques (see "The Eyes Have It: Visualizing Your Baby," later in this chapter).

The Eyes Have It: Visualizing Your Baby

Have you ever come across an individual who appeared to set her mind on something and ultimately achieve it? Some credit this ability to positive thinking, while others say it's dumb luck.

Philosophers through the ages have said that if you change your mind, you change your life. Now, no amount of positive thinking will reverse uterine or tubal scarring that may be preventing conception, but your attitude can certainly help you walk whatever path you're on with greater ease and peace.

A study conducted by the American Society of Reproductive Medicine (ASRM, the medical organization for fertility professionals) saw a marked improvement in the response of in vitro fertilization patients who showed a more positive attitude going into the process. These findings were noted in the number of eggs produced, quality of eggs, and the overall pregnancy rate. Indeed, very few people doubt the negative impact of stress on all areas of your life and your health.

Visualizing your goal, whether it's to move peacefully through the process of fertility or to imagine the feeling of holding your own child, is a wonderful tool for both relaxation and focus. Legions have sworn by the teachings of Shakti Gawain, Deepak Chopra, and others whose books and tapes can lead you through the journey to your goals. Visualization can help you identify the skills (such as persistence, patience, or diligence) that can help you reach your goal and can also help you name and let go of those traits that may stand in your way.

I (coauthor Jackie) found moments of peace, along with the occasional glide into a nap, while listening to Shakti Gawain's *Creative Visualization* tape. I listened to that tape on my personal tape player while waiting in many a fertility doctor's office and found that it helped me escape a difficult or painful situation by refocusing my thoughts. This consistent, positive reinforcement helped me to turn down the volume on the voices of naysayers, including myself.

Saying Om: Meditation and Yoga

For those who need a little more help than self-help, consider the structure of a class such as meditation or yoga. Although they're not cure-alls, these ancient arts can go a long way in easing your body and spirit.

Staying sane through the process is a goal that can carry you through your fertility rites. This goal is something you *can* control, and meditation or yoga can help. Check with your local gyms or wellness centers to see whether they have classes. Or ask your family or fertility doctor to recommend a particular class or instructor. You may be surprised at how many medical folks use the same techniques to bring peace to their own lives.

Both meditation and yoga can carry you through your pregnancy as well. Meditation can help relieve the discomfort and pain of everything from morning sickness to labor, and yoga can keep your gestating (or pregnant!) body fit and focused all the way through.

How do you spell relief? R-e-l-a-x

Medical researchers have known for some time about what's called *relaxation response,* which is defined as a series of physiological changes that occur when a person blocks out intrusive thoughts by repeating a word, a sound, a phrase, or a prayer. Relaxation response can cause a decrease in metabolism, heart rate, rate of breathing, and brain wave activity.

When used in conjunction with nutrition and exercise, relaxation response has been proven to be effective therapy in treating a number of conditions, including cardiac disease, chronic pain, symptoms associated with cancer and HIV/AIDS, anxiety, mild and moderate depression, and the stress brought on by infertility and its treatments.

Some research says that infertile women are twice as likely to experience depressive symptoms as fertile women. No matter how large or small the effect may be, excessive stress and depression can certainly contribute to or exacerbate infertility.

I (coauthor Jackie) participated in a six-week program that applied the techniques of relaxation response and that was conducted by a nurse who worked for a local fertility clinic. Although I was initially skeptical about the benefits, I did find the relaxation techniques, nutritional information, open dialogue, and camaraderie to be helpful. Partners were invited to participate in the last class of the session, where we focused on communication skills to better express our individual problems and fears related to our infertility and treatment. I enjoyed this opportunity immensely, and my husband appreciated the refreshments.

To find out more about workshops in relaxation response in your area, ask your doctor (ideally your Ob/Gyn or a fertility specialist) or contact your local chapter of Resolve by visiting www.resolve.org.

Massaging Away What Ails You

If you're more relaxed with a hands-on approach, consider massage. Although no evidence proves that regular massage improves fertility or increases the likelihood of pregnancy, few people question its ability to relax the body and mind. And although relaxation itself won't get you pregnant, it certainly makes the fertility process a little more tolerable.

Consider massage as a healthy, lowfat, guiltless way to reward yourself as you go through the fertility process (or any other stress-producing activity for that matter!). If the hormones, either naturally produced or artificially added, are getting you down, schedule a Swedish massage. Other, more vigorous forms of massage, such as shiatsu, may be useful in energizing your body. Some people believe that massage helps promote better blood flow.

Although massage can be very beneficial, make sure that your massage therapist knows that you're trying to conceive. Massaging certain areas can be harmful during pregnancy. Your massage therapist should be aware that you could be pregnant during this process, and she should be skilled in what areas to focus on and what areas to avoid.

When choosing a massage therapist, make sure that the therapist has graduated from an accredited school and is a member of the American Massage Therapy Association (www.amtamassage.org) or the Associated Bodywork and Massage Professionals (www.abmp.org). An unskilled massage therapist can sometimes cause more damage than good.

If you can't afford the cost of a professional massage, ask your partner, a friend, or a relative to provide a massage. Scented oils, soft music, and a comfortable surface can help even the most rank amateur produce soothing results.

If you think that you may be pregnant, consider skipping the massage treatment from anyone other than an accredited professional familiar with massage during pregnancy.

A few clinics nationwide claim high success rates with the practice of deep muscle massage and internal massage to reduce or eliminate scar tissue such as endometriosis and other types of structural anomalies that might prevent pregnancy. Little proof supports these claims, as no one has shown that massaging away excess or scar tissue is possible. Take great care if pursuing this type of treatment. Internal massage can be detrimental, if not just painful, expensive, and altogether unnecessary.

Seeking Help from On High

When you're caught up in the minutiae of fertility management (and there's plenty of minutiae!), you may have trouble seeing your daily struggles as part of a larger plan designed by a power greater than yourself. Whatever your faith, solace and relief are available to you.

Coauthor Jackie has witnessed many women online and in person walking through the fertility process with confidence as they placed their fears and worries in the hands of their God, a special saint, or an icon. Many chat rooms started their own prayer group. And although many people claim to be disbelievers, the old adage "there are no atheists in foxholes" seemed to be true. Online prayer groups grew at a lightning pace, bearing the names of those who were pious by nature, as well as those who just figured prayer couldn't hurt. And it can't.

Through the ages, certain groups have turned to the power of prayer for healing the sick and giving sight to the blind. A study was released in the United States in early 2002 that claimed that patients in a test group who were prayed for by outside individuals made a quicker and better recovery than those who weren't. Some physicians scoff at this notion. However, many people find credence in the idea that prayer helps patients relax and, in doing so, helps them to release whatever stranglehold they may have on their condition and to stop trying to force results. This type of help may make whatever road you travel a little less bumpy.

Individuals and couples may also benefit from the moderation of a third party, such as a priest, rabbi, or other religious figure. These professionals often act as counselors to help an individual or couple work through problems resulting from outside stressors, such as fertility. Religious leaders also respect your privacy and maintain confidences just as a therapist or doctor does. Their consideration of all things spiritual may also help to reveal another point of view or option. If nothing else, your local clergy can provide additional support, something that you can never get enough of, regardless of your situation.

Exercising without Overdoing It

I (coauthor Jackie) found that one of the most difficult parts of infertility and its treatments was the loss of certain aspects of my life (for example, free time that I used to have was now spent running from one doctor appointment to another). As an avid runner, I questioned my exercise routine and wondered whether the constant jarring might be preventing me from getting pregnant. I asked my doctor, who recommended moderate exercise. I'm not the type of person who understands the word *moderate,* regardless of its context. I decided not to take any chances and replaced running with a workout on a stair-climbing machine. After a few more months of failed attempts at pregnancy, I reevaluated the stair-climbing workout as well. And so it went until I was reduced to walking, which also became a personal no-no during the two-week wait after the time of ovulation. As the fertility bar seemed to get higher and higher, my stress management tools, such as exercise, had diminished to almost nothing. It was not a pretty sight.

Regular exercise is a good thing when trying to conceive, just as it is at almost any time in your life (except maybe when you're in traction). The key is to participate in moderate (there's that word again) activity that's consistent with your past routines. For example, if your previous exercise plan consisted of wind sprints to the refrigerator and back, training for your first marathon while trying to conceive isn't a wise idea. Some doctors recommend keeping your heart rate to a maximum of 140 beats per minute. You can use this as a guide to help build your exercise plan. When it comes to nonaerobic activity, the sky is (virtually) the limit. Again, use common sense when making your choices. Full-contact boxing may be a bit more precarious during this time (actually during any time!), but kickboxing for fitness could be a good compromise.

If you're someone who overexercises as a means to lose weight, your behavior could affect your fertility. Check with your doctor to make sure that you're within the proper weight limits. Carrying too little weight can affect your menstrual cycle as well as your hormones, therefore compromising your ability to conceive.

Above all, no matter what exercise you engage in, stay well hydrated at all times. Doing so is especially important when trying to conceive and even more so while pregnant. Wear comfortable clothing and be aware of how you feel at all times. Exercise shouldn't be painful — ever! If it is, stop, rest, and consult a trainer or exercise physiologist before resuming your routine.

Ironically, after tiring of my lack of exercise and treating my body as though it was spun glass, I (coauthor Jackie again) began running again during my third year of trying to conceive. After one month of resuming my former exercise routine, I found out I was pregnant. Go figure.

Counseling: Separately, Together, Both

Everybody needs a shoulder to cry on from time to time. Those of you going through fertility treatments may need more than one person's shoulders.

In this chapter, we discuss finding alternative ways to deal with the stress, depression, and anxiety that often accompany infertility. Understanding that these are normal reactions to the diagnosis and to the process is crucial in moving through and past this point. Yoga, meditation, exercise, and prayer are often just what the doctor ordered to pull you out of the dumps. But at other times, the hole feels a little too deep, and you may need further professional intervention.

Whether the problem feels like yours, your partner's, or the guy's next door, an outside source is sometimes the best thing for helping you find your way. Don't minimize the stress you're under. By acknowledging how difficult this may be for you, realizing that it may not be that difficult for your partner, and recognizing all points in between, you can define your starting point, a necessary step in determining your direction.

Although many of the more complex decisions in fertility treatment require medical guidance, you may find yourself getting stuck in areas that seem far simpler. Perhaps you're overwhelmed, a natural response when the path in front of you seems confusing. Talking about your options with your doctor is certainly one way to get clarity. A therapist, however, can help prevent you from getting bogged down with the small stuff and often help you to realize what's behind it all. Perhaps you're feeling the weight of the world on your shoulders in trying to conceive. Your partner's admonishment to "take it easy" may seem insensitive and unaware. It probably is.

Couples counseling is a great place to have your thoughts and feelings translated into a language that your partner may better understand. Do you find yourself snapping at every mail carrier and store clerk in town? Therapy may be a good place to unburden your frustrations before people scatter at the sight of you. Are you resentful of your or your partner's fertility problems? Telling one another over dinner may exacerbate the problem, but the helpful mediation of a therapist can allow you to acknowledge your feelings and your partner's and move on.

There's an old saying that what doesn't kill you makes you stronger. Therapy is a good place to develop the mental muscle you need to succeed.

Evaluating the Good and the Bad of Antidepressants

Few conditions seem to warrant the use of an antidepressant more than infertility. The insecurity brought on by the inability to conceive, the physical and psychological stress associated with treatment, and the repeated disappointments seem to be the perfect setup for creating a person in need of a little more help. Indeed, infertile women are twice as likely to experience depression as fertile women.

As with all things medical, refrain from diagnosing yourself. No matter how much your symptoms fit the latest commercial for Paxil, Prozac, or Zoloft, you still need to be evaluated by a psychiatrist (the only *mental health* professional who can prescribe medication).

Your fertility doctor can, and may, offer to put you on antidepressants to help you over the hump. Some doctors aren't sure of the long-term effects and may prefer to avoid them. Still other physicians use antidepressants as part of their fertility treatments (particularly when addressing immune issues). Be aware, however: Antidepressants aren't benign medications, and you shouldn't take them as such. You're better off being evaluated by a doctor who specializes in this area. Your fertility doctor, general practitioner, or therapist can certainly refer you to an appropriate specialist. You also can ask for recommendations from friends or family if you feel comfortable doing so, or you can contact your local mental health center and keep your request anonymous. Don't start taking your sister's or your best friend's antidepressant prescription. These drugs are individually dosed, based on a person's needs, size, and medical history.

No significant long-term studies have been done on the effects of antidepressants on fertility. The jury is still out on these relatively new medications (which have been on the market 20 years or less), and no conclusive results of the effect of these medications on fertility may be available for many years.

Antidepressants, however, do have some side effects that may affect fertility. Decreased sexual desire is among the possible reactions, possibly opening the door to other reproductive interaction. Antidepressants can also dry up cervical mucus, which is crucial in transporting the sperm to the egg and in helping to build up the uterine lining. You and your fertility doctor are the best judge as to whether you're experiencing these side effects.

Ultimately, as with most medications, you must weigh the pros and cons when deciding whether to take antidepressants. Depression can be consuming and can affect your health, work, relationships, and, consequently, your fertility. If you're suffering through this, the uncertain risks of antidepressants may be far outweighed by your need for relief.

Fertility Consultants: More Dollars than Sense?

Wouldn't it be wonderful if someone could take all the decisions of fertility, including what doctor to see and what treatment to follow, off your hands? Tempting, isn't it? Today, there is such a certain someone. With the increase in fertility treatments and patients, a new vocation has emerged: the fertility consultant.

These practitioners, some of whom have gone through fertility treatments themselves, work on an hourly or daily basis. Although their duties may vary depending on the individual providing the service, you can expect your fertility consultant to assist you with the following:

- Picking a doctor and clinic
- Getting the first appointment available
- Assisting you with special needs (such as locating an egg or sperm donor agency)
- Providing moral support and a bit of direction as you decide which way to go

Some fertility consultants are attorneys and thus more skilled in helping you negotiate a donor agreement or other type of contract. Others may have worked in a health profession and can help you decipher some of the information you receive, including test results, a diagnosis, or protocols. Still others may possess a background in social work and provide you with a consistent support network as you go through the process.

Proceed carefully when considering whether to use a fertility consultant. They don't come cheap and are generally not covered by any type of insurance that we're aware of. Considering the high costs of fertility treatment in general, you may be better off taking a little extra time to research information yourself, using organizations such as Resolve, online bulletin boards, Internet search engines, friends, and family. As tempted as you may be to have someone else do the work, ultimately *you* are the one who must make the decisions related to your treatment. As far as a consultant's ability to help you book appointments with those hard-to-get physicians and clinics, you can often achieve the same results yourself with a good dose of persistence, coupled with daily phone calls to check for cancellations.

If you have far more money than time, however, you can locate a fertility consultant through a Web search. If you want a little more information, contact Resolve or the American Society of Reproductive Medicine (ASRM) via its Web site at www.asrm.org to ask for a referral. If you already have a fertility doctor or clinic, you can start there. And finally, if you decide to use a fertility consultant, consider negotiating the price and make sure that you get your money's worth. Fertility consulting is a relatively small field, and the resources available to the average individual in this highly technological world make fertility consulting a tough sell. Use this to your advantage. Whether your road to baby is short, medium, or long, you'll have plenty of opportunities to spend your savings later!

Taking a Break from Your Fertility "Job" — You Deserve It

When all else fails to help you relax, consider taking off, whether that's a break from your efforts or a real vacation!

Fertility often becomes a job with no benefits and dismal working conditions. Just like any job, time off is necessary in order to clean your mind, refresh your spirit, and come back to greet another day with your best efforts.

Many individuals and couples take anywhere from a few weeks to a few years off from the process of trying to conceive. This doesn't mean adhering to a celibate lifestyle. Instead, it's a reintroduction to sex sans schedule, trying to conceive a baby the old-fashioned way. Obviously, your age and condition are critical in determining just how much time away from fertility treatment you can spare, but a short respite probably will do nothing *but* refresh you. Try to avoid feeling guilty for needing the break. Actually, in giving your mind and body the time and space they need, you're taking the best possible care of yourself. And don't minimize your partner's need for a break either. He may need a respite from "performing" on demand, undergoing batteries of tests, or just providing you with the support you need, but he may not feel comfortable suggesting it.

Getting away from the daily grind also helps you to gain a better perspective and make decisions that best suit you, your partner, and your living style. Some people can do this by taking a fertility-free weekend that includes no discussion of anything to do with physicians, fertility, treatments, or future plans. Others find it necessary to truly get away from home. You'll be amazed by the perspective and peace that you can gain from a well-needed vacation. And although we don't advise planning a vacation with the hidden agenda of making this getaway the one that does the trick, perhaps it will! In the meantime, throw caution and your medical records to the wind and relax. Your baby will wait for you.

Chapter 6

When the Beginning Is the End: Early Pregnancy Loss

As upsetting as it is not to get pregnant, getting pregnant and having the pregnancy end in loss is even more devastating. Why do so many pregnancies end early, and what does it mean for future pregnancies? And how can you avoid personal feelings of failure when a loss occurs? In this chapter, we discuss how and why pregnancies are lost in the first 12 weeks, and we offer advice on how to pick yourself up and try again if this happens to you.

Getting "a Little Bit" Pregnant — It's Possible

Most of you have heard that there's no such thing as "a little bit" pregnant. This statement is true in one sense, but at times, you do feel that you're "almost" pregnant . . . and you may be right.

More than 50 percent of all embryos stop developing before they develop a heartbeat. Most of these, up to 30 percent, are lost before the time when you would notice any signs of pregnancy. If this happens, you may have no pregnancy symptoms at all, not even a missed period. Or you may have very early pregnancy signs, such as breast tenderness, which suddenly disappear. These signs may be followed by a slightly late, heavier-than-normal period, which is actually the passing of a very early pregnancy. You may pass more clots than normal (for you), or you may feel "crampier" than usual. You probably wouldn't even realize that you had been pregnant unless you did a sensitive early pregnancy test, such as a blood test.

If you're under treatment by a fertility doctor, you may be asked to do a blood pregnancy test, called a BSU (beta sub unit, or "beta" for short), about two weeks after ovulation or embryo transfer. Your beta number may be positive (anything over 5 is considered positive) but very low when first tested, and it may be negative a few days later, at the second test. Your doctor may say that you had a *chemical pregnancy* if this happens.

At least 50 percent of the time, chemical pregnancies are caused by the implantation of a chromosomally abnormal embryo, but other factors can also cause very early miscarriage. Your doctor may do tests, such as checking your progesterone level, to see whether there are other reasons why the embryo isn't "sticking." In a normal pregnancy, the *corpus luteum,* or leftover "shell" of the ovulated egg, produces a hormone called *progesterone.* Progesterone is necessary for the implantation and growth of the early embryo. If your progesterone is lower than normal, the embryo may not be able to grow properly.

A simple blood test or an endometrial biopsy can check your progesterone levels. In a biopsy, your doctor takes a tiny scraping of your uterine lining and sends it to a lab to have the amount of progesterone in the tissue measured. If the tissue sample shows less than normal progesterone, your doctor can recommend supplementing progesterone in the form of shots, pills, or vaginal suppositories. A biopsy can be done after a negative pregnancy test; it needs to be done within a day or so of the test because it will not be accurate if your period has started.

So even though people may say that you can't be a "little bit" pregnant, the truth is that a pregnancy can start to implant and then stop before you even miss a period. You may not realize this is happening to you without a very early blood pregnancy test. If your doctor suspects that you're having chemical pregnancies, he or she will order further testing to see whether an easy fix, such as adding progesterone supplements, can solve the problem.

Suffering a Miscarriage

A *miscarriage* is a pregnancy loss that occurs after you know you're pregnant but before the fetus is *viable,* or able to live on its own.

Miscarriages are very common: One in four women has a miscarriage during her reproductive years. But knowing that miscarriages are common events and not likely to recur doesn't make them any easier to deal with.

Eighty percent of miscarriages occur in the first 12 weeks of pregnancy. Based on this fact, many couples decide not to shout the news to friends and relatives before this time has passed.

The first sign of possible miscarriage is usually spotting. But because spotting is common in pregnancy (occurring in one in five women), doctors don't always take it as a dire sign. If spotting and cramping stop quickly, the chances are excellent that the pregnancy will carry to term. Most doctors restrict sex and heavy exercise if some spotting has occurred. Your doctor may call cramping and spotting a *threatened abortion.* Bleeding can be caused by implantation of the embryo or by the sloughing off of the lining around the area where implantation has occurred. An internal exam will show whether your cervix has started to open. An ultrasound done around six weeks will show whether a fetus is in the uterus and may show a heartbeat. A heartbeat *should* be seen by seven and a half weeks.

If your cervix has started to open, or *dilate,* and you're bleeding, you'll almost certainly miscarry. Your doctor may call these symptoms an *inevitable abortion.* An ultrasound may show no fetal heartbeat. Your doctor will want you to watch for signs of infection, such as a temperature over 100 degrees or a foul-smelling discharge. Hospitalization isn't necessary in most cases of miscarriage. Save any tissue that you pass so that your doctor can send it to a pathologist, who can evaluate it for chromosomal abnormalities. You'll probably continue bleeding for seven to ten days.

A *missed abortion* occurs when the pregnancy stops progressing but there are no signs of miscarriage, such as bleeding or cramping. Your pregnancy blood levels may be lower than expected, and the ultrasound shows no fetal activity. A missed abortion may require a dilation and curettage, a minor surgery, to remove the tissue.

Will you need a D&C?

You need a D&C, or *dilation and curettage,* if you don't pass all the pregnancy tissue on your own. This procedure involves opening the cervix and scraping the uterus with a blunt instrument called a curette, or with a suction vacuum, to make sure that no tissue is left, because leftover tissue can cause an infection. This surgery is done under light sedation, usually as an outpatient procedure. Your doctor may tell you not to take tub baths, use hot tubs, douche, or have sex for several weeks. You may be asked to return for a follow-up visit to make sure that you're healing normally. There won't be any stitches to remove after a D&C.

Don't be upset if your doctor calls your miscarriage a *spontaneous abortion,* or SAB. This is the medical term for a miscarriage.

Playing the blame game

Are you feeling guilty about your miscarriage because you once sneaked a cigarette, had a glass of champagne at a wedding, had sex, or went skydiving during your pregnancy? Maybe you've been depressed or had an abortion when you were 17. Whatever, now you blame yourself and your careless ways for the miscarriage. Don't. Although some of these actions may not have been the best decisions, the truth is that almost certainly *none* of them caused this miscarriage.

More than 50 percent of miscarriages are due to chromosomal abnormalities. In these cases, no amount of rest, or anything else that you do — or don't do — will prevent them. Other common causes of miscarriage, such as abnormalities of the uterus, lack of progesterone support after ovulation, or vaginal infection, can be evaluated before you try to get pregnant again.

You should know, though, that regular cigarette smoking can increase the rate of miscarriage by 30 to 50 percent, so cutting down drastically or stopping smoking is a good idea if you want a successful pregnancy.

Playing the guessing game: Why did things start off so well?

Miscarriage has a number of causes, some of which may not be easy to pinpoint. More than 50 percent are related to chromosomal abnormalities.

In trying to understand chromosomal abnormalities, you can compare a growing fetus to a house being built. If a builder orders a lot of lumber but no roofing materials, a house's walls can be built, but only up to the point where the roofing materials are needed. If the genes needed for the baby to develop are processed wrong at the time of conception, the baby will develop to the point where it needs those genes to keep growing. Without those genes, the fetus can't continue to develop. Its "walls" will be built, but without the "roof," it can't continue to grow.

Blighted ovum

A blighted ovum is a variation of chromosomal error. *Blighted ovum* occurs when the placenta and amniotic sac develop and put out pregnancy hormones but the fetus itself doesn't develop. So you may test pregnant, but there is no fetus. You and your doctor may discover this fact when you start spotting and the doctor tests for fetal activity and finds no fetus.

Molar pregnancy

Another, somewhat rare type of chromosomal anomaly is called a molar pregnancy. Molar pregnancies occur in one in a thousand conceptions in the United States; it is more officially called a "hydatidiform mole." *Molar pregnancies* result when the egg is abnormal; it has no chromosomal content to pass on, so there is no fetus, only a placenta. The placenta usually grows very quickly; you may show signs of pregnancy very early and have unusually high beta levels. Molar pregnancies are treated with methotrexate, a chemotherapy drug, to stop the abnormally fast cell division. A D&C will probably be done as well; in fact, you may need more than one. Molar cells can spread very quickly into other areas, similar to a cancer, and you may need very aggressive treatment to avoid serious complications. You may be advised to avoid another pregnancy for 6 to 12 months after a molar pregnancy to be sure that no abnormal cells remain in the body.

PERSONAL STORY

How it feels to miscarry — Sharon's story

I had three small boys, ages 2, 4, and 6, when I had a miscarriage. I was young, 26, and it never occurred to me that this could happen. I had cramping and spotting, so my doctor put me on bed rest. I followed his orders because I figured that whatever was happening would stop if I did what the doctor told me. (Obviously, I wasn't a nurse at the time.) While lying on the couch, I went through a bargaining stage where I told God that I wouldn't care if the baby were born with a defect, just so long as I could sustain the pregnancy. When the bleeding increased and I realized I was passing tissue, I went into full denial: "Good. This must be what's causing all the bleeding, and now everything will be all right." I was mentally unable to process what was happening until I went to the doctor, who confirmed that I was having a miscarriage. I went to the hospital for a dilation and curettage (D&C), which is sometimes required to remove all the tissue in miscarriages. The nurse who admitted me, obviously trying to make me feel better, asked if I had any children. "Three, but that doesn't matter," I said. "I wanted *this* one."

Oh, was I angry! I couldn't even explain my anger in a rational way. I had three other children and knew I could carry a pregnancy, but that was irrelevant at the time. I was angry with everyone and everything. I didn't want to discuss it with anyone, and I didn't want to be talked out of my anger by being told that "it was for the best," "the baby wouldn't have been normal," or "you already have three children." I can't imagine how much harder I would have taken the miscarriage if I hadn't already had children.

My husband is a pretty compassionate guy, but he had no idea how to deal with me during the period following my miscarriage. When I (angrily, of course!) asked him if he wasn't upset by the miscarriage, he said, "I appreciate the kids we have more," which, of course, made me angrier because it didn't validate my feelings of loss.

I never expected the anger and depression to last as long as they did. What snapped me out of that mood was deciding to adopt a little girl, something we had been talking about for years. Once I had another child to focus on, I slowly became my normal self again. My hormones, of course, were all over the place during this period of adjustment, and I went from happy to sad, and back again, in a matter of minutes. Then came a completely unexpected event — I got pregnant! This pregnancy was unplanned and happened in the month after my D&C. My fourth son was born eight months later, and we put off the adoption for three years (eventually adopting a beautiful little girl from Korea).

Playing the age game

As in most fertility issues, age is a definite factor in miscarriage rates. Consider these numbers:

- If you're under 35, the miscarriage rate is about 6 percent.
- If you're pushing 40, the miscarriage rate increases to 14 percent.
- If you're over 40, your chance of miscarriage is 23 percent.
- If you're around 43, the rate goes up to nearly 50 percent.
- After age 45, 87 percent of all women are infertile, so pregnancy is rare, making miscarriage rates more difficult to gather. Also, periods are more irregular, so what appears to be a late period could be a miscarriage.

These statistics reflect the increased number of chromosomally abnormal eggs still left as you get older; your "best eggs" have already been ovulated. We discuss age-related fertility issues more in Chapter 1.

Suffering the insensitive remarks of family and friends

What's worse after a miscarriage than friends who become pregnant? Or friends who continue to be pregnant when you're not? How about relatives who try to "jolly" you out of depression with stories of how miscarriage was probably a blessing and that you should be thankful for the children you have? Or what about women who regale you with stories of their own miscarriages?

Everyone has her own way of dealing with people you can't avoid. Some women politely ask that it not be discussed. Other women not so politely ask the offender to please shut up. Yet other women agree and pretend that they're feeling better. Try to remember that people are feeling awkward and don't know what to say, but they're trying to make you feel better because they care about you. Spouses may be having an equally difficult time, because few men discuss miscarriage with their friends; if they do, they may find little sympathy for an early loss. They may also feel out of the loop and uninformed about exactly what happened, and may not want to question you for fear of upsetting you more. If you can bring yourself to talk about it, a little conversation goes a long way toward making your partner feel more like a partner and less like a hindrance during this difficult time.

Ectopic Pregnancy: When the Embryo Is Developing in the Wrong Place

An ectopic pregnancy is a different type of miscarriage. In an *ectopic pregnancy,* the embryo may be developing normally, but it's growing in the wrong place, usually in the fallopian tube. Like a miscarriage, an ectopic pregnancy ends your hopes for a baby *this time,* but it can cause other problems as well.

Ectopic pregnancies aren't rare — 1 out of 100 pregnancies is ectopic — and the percentage has been rising over the last 30 years. With an ectopic pregnancy, the fetus may be normal but attaches to tissue outside the uterus, usually in the fallopian tube, and begins to grow there. (Figure 6-1 shows where ectopic pregnancies can occur.) The fallopian tube is much smaller than the uterus, and the baby can't grow beyond a certain point, usually around seven weeks, before rupturing the tube, causing severe complications. Ectopic pregnancy is the leading cause of maternal death in the first trimester of pregnancy.

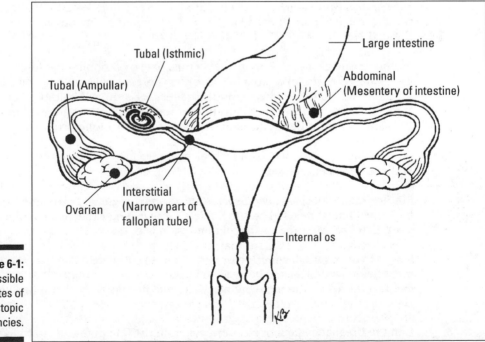

Figure 6-1: Possible sites of ectopic pregnancies.

What to do if you suspect an ectopic pregnancy

Any time you have severe one-sided pain, severe shoulder pain, or a feeling of lightheadedness and weakness a few weeks after missing a period, you *must* go to the emergency room to make sure that you don't have an ectopic pregnancy. A positive pregnancy test and an ultrasound showing no fetus in the uterus can confirm an ectopic pregnancy. If you have no physical symptoms, an ectopic pregnancy may be suspected if the BSU is lower than it should be; rarely, the pregnancy test can also be negative. An ultrasound will show nothing in the uterus — no sac, placenta, or fetus.

What your doctor will do

Treating an ectopic pregnancy involves either dissolving the developing pregnancy with a drug called methotrexate, the same drug used for molar pregnancies (see the section "Molar pregnancy," earlier in this chapter), or removing the pregnancy through surgery. Surgical removal of an ectopic pregnancy can also cause more infertility problems; the fallopian tube may need to be removed, and adhesions or scar tissue may develop after the surgery. An ectopic pregnancy can be a life-threatening event. If the fetus gets too big, the fallopian tube will burst, and you could be in danger of bleeding to death.

Methotrexate causes the pregnancy to dissolve by stopping the rapid cell division necessary for a fetus to grow. Four percent of women taking methotrexate have diarrhea, mouth soreness, or stomach irritation because these cells are also fast-growing and affected by the disturbance in cell division. Serious side effects, such as liver toxicity or lung problems, are rare.

Stop taking folic acid while on methotrexate because it may interfere with the action of the methotrexate.

Methotrexate successfully dissolves an ectopic pregnancy 90 percent of the time, but it must be used before the fetus grows larger than 3.5 cm (a little over an inch). After that, surgical removal is necessary.

If surgery is required, your doctor may try to save the fallopian tube if possible. If the fallopian tube has to be removed, you can still get pregnant. An egg can even be released from the right ovary and find its way to the left tube if the right tube is gone.

Can the pregnancy be moved somehow from the fallopian tube to the uterus? Because the placenta and the tissues involved with growth are "dug in" to the tube, removing the fetus from the tube and reattaching it to the uterus are impossible at this time.

Understanding why ectopic pregnancies happen

Although anyone can have an ectopic pregnancy, ectopic pregnancies are more likely in women who have any of the following risk factors:

- If you have a swollen, dilated fallopian tube, called a *hydrosalpinx,* you're six to ten times more likely to have an ectopic pregnancy. Hydrosalpinx is frequently caused by pelvic inflammatory disease (PID), often associated with a chlamydia infection. (See Chapter 2 for more on chlamydia.)

- If you smoke, you're one and a half to four times more likely to have an ectopic pregnancy.

- Have you had a previous tubal ligation reattached? You have a 15 percent chance for an ectopic pregnancy.

- Previous use of an IUD slightly increases the chance of an ectopic pregnancy.

- Current use of progestin-only birth control pills also increases the chance of an ectopic pregnancy.

- If you've had a previous ectopic pregnancy, your chance for another is 7 to 10 percent.

- If you douche regularly, at least three times a week, you're more likely to have an ectopic pregnancy.

Other origins of ectopic pregnancies

Some infertility treatments, such as in vitro fertilization, are associated with a higher rate of ectopic pregnancies. Twin, triplet, and other multiple pregnancies are also associated with ectopic pregnancies; in some cases, one fetus may implant in the uterus and another in a tube, a condition called a *heterotopic pregnancy.*

Recurring Miscarriage: Why It Happens

Two percent of all couples suffer *recurrent miscarriage,* which is the loss of three or more early pregnancies. After three losses, the chance of a fourth loss increases to 45 to 50 percent. What causes this repeated heartbreak?

- Uterine problems, such as fibroids that intrude into the uterine cavity, scar tissue in the uterine cavity (Asherman's syndrome), or malformations of the uterine cavity shape, can result in a miscarriage. If your mom took DES, a drug to prevent miscarriage, in the 1950s and 1960s, you may have an unusually shaped uterine cavity. Between 15 and 20 percent of recurrent miscarriages are caused by uterine problems. (We discuss this topic in depth in Chapter 7.)

✔ An incompetent cervix is responsible for 5 percent of all recurrent miscarriages. An *incompetent cervix* is a cervix too weak to stay closed during pregnancy. The cervix dilates painlessly, resulting in the loss of the pregnancy; this usually occurs after 12 weeks, when the growing fetus puts more weight on the cervix. An incompetent cervix can be diagnosed on ultrasound; the cervical length will measure less than 20 mm. An incompetent cervix can be caused by DES exposure before you were born, trauma to the cervix (such as a cone biopsy done to diagnose possible cervical cancer), or congenital deformities. Pregnancy loss can be prevented in most cases by placing a stitch, called a *cerclage,* through your cervix to keep it from opening too soon. This is usually done after 12 weeks.

✔ Chromosomal abnormalities in either you or your partner cause 5 percent of recurrent miscarriages. Chromosomal karyotyping, performed as a blood test, on you and your partner can be used to diagnose chromosomal abnormalities.

✔ Immune problems, including diseases such as lupus, may be a factor in a miscarriage. Antibodies called antiphospholipid antibodies, which cause clotting problems, and many other possible immune deficiencies are currently a hot topic in fertility workups. (See Chapter 7 for more information about immune issues.)

Pregnancy loss is an issue of biology, not morality. Fertility problems are not a punishment for anything; they're the result of biology gone awry.

Picking Yourself Up after a Loss

As if you haven't heard it enough, your body needs to heal after a miscarriage. Your doctor may recommend waiting up to three months before trying to conceive again. This time period gives your system time to completely recover from the stress of a miscarriage. If a D&C is required, remember that this is a surgical procedure (albeit minor) that needs time to heal. Do *not* rush this process.

Any type of vaginal bleeding (which is normal following a miscarriage or D&C) can interfere with the formation of a good uterine lining. If you try and get pregnant again too soon, the embryo may not have a good place to implant.

Time truly does heal, or at least dulls the pain. Each passing day will help to make your next pregnancy a joyous experience completely its own, not a shadow of the fear and doubt of your early pregnancy loss.

Even the most optimistic of you will experience those times when your hope button is stuck on "off." This phase is a temporary, albeit painful, condition. Rebooting your emotions can go a long way toward resetting your physical condition as well.

What to do while you're waiting

Just like your body needs to repair itself, your spirit needs some help as well. As you count the days until you can begin trying again, consider using this time to help your future child in another way. Here's your to-do list:

- ✔ If you have already been blessed with a child or children, take a moment to appreciate them. A hug from your precious one can right many of the world's wrongs.

- ✔ Allow yourself the time to grieve. Trying to pretend that you're back to normal when you're not may make you feel temporarily better. In the long run, however, covering up grief rather than expressing it and working through it will cause it to resurface again, possibly during your next pregnancy, in the form of resentment or guilt. Take the time to heal.

- ✔ Do something wonderful for yourself. Whether it's a special purchase, a dinner out with your partner, or an ice cream sundae, indulge a whim.

- ✔ Do consider professional help if your sadness is debilitating or lasts longer than three months. A counselor can help guide you through the minefield of emotions that you're facing.

You and your partner are allies, not enemies, no matter how differently you process the stress and grief of your loss. Helping your partner deal with his own emotions will help you come to terms with your own feelings as well. This experience can make you a stronger team if you work together.

What not to do

Taking care of yourself during this time and allowing others to care for you should be your first priority, if not your only one. Part of this task, which may seem daunting enough, is to keep in touch with your own feelings and stay in touch with those who care about you. To help accomplish this, here's our list of things to avoid:

- ✔ Don't force yourself to do anything that you don't feel up to. You may need to decline an invitation to a friend's baby shower, christening, or family gathering, and that's okay. This time is about getting better, emotionally and physically. Don't do anything to compromise your recovery.

✔ Don't go into hiding. You'll want to skip some events, but don't completely isolate yourself. Your community of friends and family can help you heal. Although pain is unavoidable, suffering, particularly alone, is optional.

✔ Don't redecorate the nursery or wander through baby stores. These types of behaviors are similar to picking at a scab. The temptation to do these things is great, and you can talk yourself into believing that these actions will be cathartic. In actuality, they'll most likely cause you more pain and prolong your healing process.

An early pregnancy loss does have somewhat of a silver lining. It confirms that you can conceive, which often can be more than half the battle.

Part III

Medium-Tech Baby Making: Finding the Problem

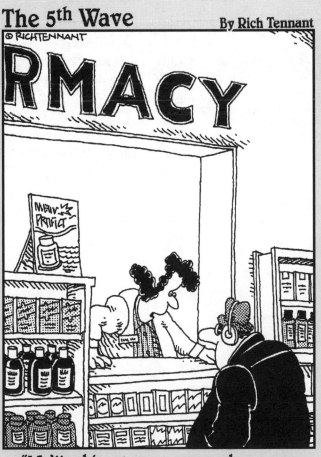

The 5th Wave · By Rich Tennant

© RICHTENNANT

RMACY

MBUY PRFFICT

"We'll whisper your name when your sperm-boosting kit is ready."

In this part . . .

When pregnancy doesn't come easily, you may find yourself in your doctor's waiting room, hoping he or she can help. In this part, we explain the most common tests done in a fertility workup and tell you what the results mean. We also help you pick out a doctor who can best help you through medium-tech treatment such as intrauterine insemination and gonadotropin injections.

Chapter 7

Finding the Problem: Testing 1, 2, 3

In This Chapter

▶ Poking and prodding: blood tests and more

▶ Dealing with male-related problems

▶ Looking to the woman for the cause

▶ Performing reversals of sterilization procedures

▶ Getting pregnant after cancer

*I*f you haven't gotten pregnant after several months to a year, it may be time to start doing some tests. Your doctor may suggest these tests to you, or you may suggest them to him, if you feel that time is slipping away and you want to find out why you haven't gotten pregnant yet, or why you can't stay pregnant.

In this chapter, we give you a rundown of the tests that fertility doctors do most frequently, why they do them, and what you can expect to learn from the tests.

For about 30 percent of couples trying to get pregnant, several problems contribute to infertility. This fact is especially important to remember if one of you has a known factor, such as previous tubal surgery or a known sperm problem. Many couples come to a clinic and tell the staff, "I don't need to do any testing — we already know the problem is him (or her)." You may think that you already know the problem, but keep in mind that for 30 percent of you, tests will reveal another problem, and pregnancy won't occur until both problems are addressed.

Cataloging the Common Tests: ABCD HSG

Many factors can contribute to infertility, and determining what your fertility issue is can take some time and involve some testing. Some tests, such as blood tests, are fairly simple, while others, such as laparoscopic surgery, are more invasive.

Your doctor may start with the most basic tests or go right to the more invasive tests if he or she suspects that your fertility issue involves uterine or tubal factors. The tests we list are the ones most likely to be suggested by your doctor, but you may not need all the tests listed.

Forty percent of infertility is related to sperm problems, so don't forget to have your partner tested, too!

Baseline blood tests

"Let's get some baseline bloods," your doctor may say when you first start looking for an answer to the "why am I not pregnant" question. This test is one of the simplest tests you can have done. You simply wait until your period starts, go to the lab on day two or day three of your period, and have blood drawn. Within a day or two, you usually receive the results, which give you quite a bit of information about your fertility. Here's what the tests reveal:

- **Estradiol:** Estradiol on day two or three of your period is normally greater than 10 but less than 50. An estradiol level that is very low, less than 10, may indicate that your ovaries are suppressed and may not respond well to stimulation to make a normal egg. An estradiol level that is over 50pg/ml may indicate ovarian cysts.

- **Progesterone:** On day two or three of your period, your progesterone levels should be low, less than 2. Progesterone levels go up in the second half of your cycle, after you ovulate, and should be over 12 after you release an egg. Progesterone comes from the *corpus luteum,* the left-over shell of the follicle after you ovulate, and is necessary to help the embryo implant.

- **Luteinizing hormone (LH):** The LH level is usually about 5 on day two or three; women with polycystic ovaries (we discuss this in the section "Polycystic ovary syndrome (PCOS)," later in this chapter) may have an LH level that is significantly higher than their follicle-stimulating hormone level on day two. LH levels rise later in the cycle, usually going over 40 when you're almost ready to ovulate.

- **Follicle-stimulating hormone (FSH):** Your FSH level should be less than 10 or 11, depending on your lab, on day two or day three. A higher than normal FSH level may indicate that you're going into perimenopause, the period a few years before menopause; you may also not be making eggs every month. We discuss FSH in more detail in the section "FSH and Inhibin B," later in this chapter.

Your partner's hormone levels, especially LH, FSH, and testosterone, also need to be normal for good sperm production. Most doctors don't test the levels unless your partner's semen analysis is abnormal, because a good semen analysis means his hormone levels are normal.

HSG (don't even try to spell out the word)

An HSG, or *hysterosalpingogram,* is an X-ray that outlines your uterus and fallopian tubes to make it easy to see where abnormalities may be keeping you from getting pregnant. (See Figure 7-1.) Dye is injected through your cervix to make the uterus and tubes easy to see on an X-ray.

HSGs can be uncomfortable, causing mild to severe cramping, but they're a valuable tool in diagnosing fertility problems you can't see. Some of the problems that can be diagnosed with an HSG are fibroids in the uterus, large polyps in the uterus, an unusually shaped uterine cavity, a septum (a piece of tissue dividing your cavity), or adhesions (scar tissue) in the uterus. If you know that you have fibroids, an HSG can show whether they're intruding into the inside of the uterus, where they may prevent implantation of an embryo.

The dye also outlines the fallopian tubes, so your doctor can see whether your tubes are normally shaped and, most importantly, whether your tubes are open, which your doctor can tell by noticing whether the dye passes through the tubes and flows into the pelvis. The HSG is an important test because it lets you know that if your tubes are blocked in any way, or if they're very swollen, an egg or embryo won't be able to get through to the uterus. If dye does pass through easily, your HSG report will say that the fallopian tubes "filled and spilled," meaning that the dye easily passed up from the uterus, all the way up the tubes, and out the end of the tube into the pelvis.

How uncomfortable is an HSG? That depends on your own pain tolerance and whether your tubes are open. If the tubes are slightly blocked with debris, your doctor may need to push the dye more forcefully to clear the block, which may increase cramping. Most doctors tell you to take ibuprofen or a similar pain medication an hour or so before your test.

Schedule your test for the early part of your menstrual cycle, usually before day 12 (before you ovulate), because both the dye and the pelvic X-rays can be harmful if you're pregnant.

Many doctors also do cervical cultures for gonorrhea and chlamydia before doing an HSG because pushing dye through the uterus and fallopian tubes can spread the infection and cause serious complications. Your doctor may also prescribe antibiotics for you to take starting a few days before your HSG because between 1 and 3 percent of women experience some type of infection after the procedure.

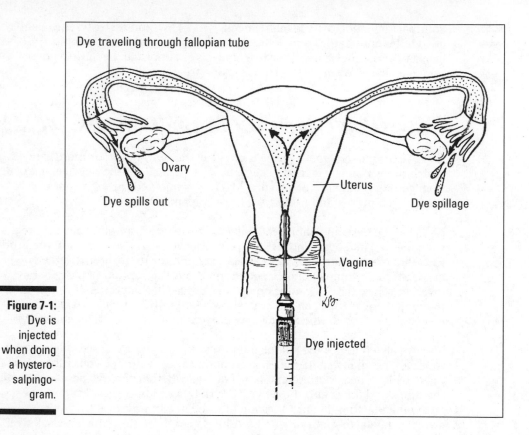

Dye traveling through fallopian tube

Ovary

Dye spills out

Uterus

Dye spillage

Vagina

Dye injected

Figure 7-1:
Dye is injected when doing a hystero-salpingo-gram.

If you're allergic to contrast dye or shellfish, you may not be able to have the test done. Contrast dye and shellfish both contain iodine, and some doctors believe an allergy to shellfish means you have a higher chance of having an allergic reaction to the dye.

After the test, a small amount of bleeding is normal; you'll also leak a small amount of dye (which is clear, not colored) over the next day or so. You may be crampy for a few hours after the procedure as well. Take someone with you so that you don't have to drive yourself home.

Hysteroscopy

Sometimes smaller polyps and fibroids are hard to see on an HSG. For a close-up look at the inside of the uterus, your doctor may want to do a hysteroscopy.

A *hysteroscopy,* often done in the doctor's office, is a procedure in which a small tube is guided through the cervix into the uterus. The uterus is distended, usually with carbon dioxide, so that your doctor can clearly see the entire area, including any small polyps, adhesions, or fibroids. You may be given local anesthesia, such as a cervical block, or mild sedation, such as Valium, for the procedure.

If the procedure detects polyps, scar tissue, or small fibroids in the uterus, your doctor may do an *operative hysteroscopy*. In this procedure, the doctor inserts small instruments through the scope to remove the abnormal tissue. Your doctor may perform this procedure in his office, or in the hospital if more extensive work needs to be done. You may have a nerve block, such as an epidural, or general anesthesia for an operative hysteroscopy done in the hospital.

Laparoscopy

A *laparoscopy* involves placing lighted telescopes and other instruments through the abdomen, as shown in Figure 7-2. The incisions made are very small, about ½ inch or less, and the procedure usually involves one to three incisions. Endometriosis and scar tissue can be removed during a laparoscopy. Fallopian tubes that are infected and dilated also can be removed this way.

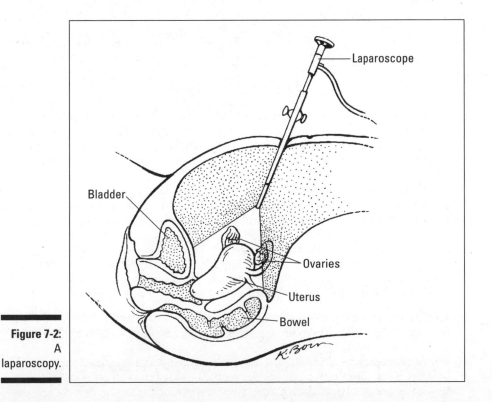

Figure 7-2:
A
laparoscopy.

A laparoscopy is usually done as an outpatient procedure in a hospital or surgical center. The most common problems after the surgery are pain (usually minimal) from the incisions and pain in the right shoulder from the carbon dioxide used to inflate the abdomen. The recovery period is usually short, less than a week.

Postcoital tests

Postcoital testing, also known as the Huhner test, is done around the time of ovulation. Timing of this test is very important to correctly evaluate the results. Your doctor will want you to have sex around the time of your LH surge (determined by blood levels or ovulation predictor kits) and come into the office the next morning, anywhere from 4 to 12 hours later; different doctors seem to have different opinions on the exact timing.

The doctor or a nurse takes a sample of mucus from your cervix for the test, so don't take a bath, douche, or use lubricants, such as KY Jelly, for sex. The doctor puts the mucus on a slide and looks at it under a high-powered microscope. You hope that the doctor sees six to ten sperm moving forward per high-powered field. You *don't* want to see a few inert sluggards or a bunch of sperm seemingly stuck together; stuck-together sperm may mean that antisperm antibodies are present. (See the sections "Semen analysis" and "Testing for immune disorders," later in this chapter, for more information about antisperm antibodies.)

In addition to checking out "the boys," your doctor also examines the mucus itself, which should be clear in color; make a leaflike, fern pattern under the microscope; and be very stretchy, a quality known as *spinnbarkeit*. Good ovulation-time mucus can be stretched about 4 inches, but nobody will blame you if you don't want to check this out yourself! All these qualities are required for sperm to swim rapidly through the vagina without being mired down or destroyed.

Sometimes the mucus seen doesn't live up to all these great qualities; here are a few possible reasons why it may not:

- You may not be ovulating. If your predictor kit says that you're having a ssurge but your mucus is thick, your kit may be wrong. Your LH level could be high in conjunction with a high FSH level; this is common in premature ovarian failure or perimenopause.

- You may have a cervical infection. With cervicitis, normal cells are destroyed, and the squamous cells that grow in their place don't make good cervical mucus.

- If you're taking Clomid (a fertility drug), it may be affecting your mucus. (See the section "The clomiphene citrate challenge test," later in this chapter, for more on Clomid.)

> ✔ If you've had any procedures done on your cervix for abnormal Pap smears, your mucus-producing cells may have been destroyed. Such procedures include cone biopsy, in which a wedge-shaped piece of cervix is cut out and sent to be tested for cancerous cells; loop electro-surgical excision procedure (LEEP), in which a piece of cervix is removed by using a fine wire; laser; and freezing.

Semen analysis

You may find your partner acting a little funny when it's time to "check out the boys," but because male factor infertility accounts for about 40 percent of infertility, semen analysis is a necessary step.

He'll be asked to step into a room, usually complete with videos but maybe just the Victoria's Secret catalog, to "produce." You can help him if you want, but no saliva or lubricants, please. If you want to bring a semen sample from home, you must bring it in within a half hour and use a sterile cup for collection.

If you're bringing in a semen sample, keep it at next-to-body temperature — holding it under your armpit is ideal. Make sure that the lid's on tight!

Sperm are extremely small, but under the microscope, you can see how complicated they really are. A normal sperm (see Figure 7-3) has three sections: a head, a midpiece, and a tail. All three parts need to be normal for a sperm to be considered normal according to the strict Kruger morphology, a system for grading only perfect sperm as normal that was developed in Africa.

> ✔ **Head:** Contains all the genetic material, so a sperm with an abnormal head — either a round head, pinhead, large head, or double head —isn't capable of fertilizing an egg.
>
> ✔ **Midpiece:** Contains fructose, the energy the sperm needs to move rapidly.
>
> ✔ **Tail:** Needed for propulsion. Sperm with no tail, two tails, or coiled tails are all considered abnormal.

The World Health Organization has set standard parameters for a normal semen specimen, so this is what your sperm should have to be graded A+:

> ✔ **Volume:** Should be 1.5 to 5 ml, or approximately a teaspoon.
>
> ✔ **Concentration:** Should be greater than 20 million sperm/ml, or a total of greater than 40 million per ejaculate.
>
> ✔ **Motility:** More than 60 percent of the sperm should be motile, or moving.
>
> ✔ **Morphology:** More than 30 percent should be normally shaped.

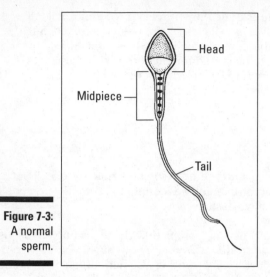

Figure 7-3:
A normal sperm.

(Head, Midpiece, Tail)

- ✔ **Forward progression:** On a scale of 1 to 4, at least 2+ means a good number of sperm moving forward.

- ✔ **White blood cells:** Should be no more than 0 to 5 per high-power field. More could indicate infection.

- ✔ **Hyperviscosity:** Should gel promptly but liquefy within 30 minutes after ejaculation.

- ✔ **Ph:** Should be alkaline, to protect sperm from the acidic environment of the vagina.

- ✔ **HOS, or hypo-osmotic swelling:** Greater than 50 percent of the sperm tails should swell when exposed to a hypo-osmotic solution; this swelling is a sign of normal functioning.

- ✔ **Antisperm antibodies:** A normal semen sample contains no antisperm antibodies. Antibodies cause problems if they're attached to the sperm tail, because they interfere with movement, or to the head, where they may make it difficult for the sperm to penetrate the egg.

- ✔ **Zona-free hamster-egg penetrating test:** A normal human sperm can penetrate a hamster egg after the *zona,* or outside layer of the egg, is removed. Makes you wonder who ever thought this one up!

- ✔ **Acrosome reaction test:** The tip of the sperm is the *acrosome*. It contains enzymes that allow the sperm to penetrate the egg. If the proper enzymes aren't present, the sperm can't get through the egg's *zona,* or shell.

It takes three months for sperm to properly develop, so if your partner was sick, taking medication, or had anything else unusual going on three months ago, his specimen may be abnormal. Check a second specimen in a few weeks to see whether anything has changed.

Sonohysterogram

A *sonohysterogram* is very similar to a hysterosalpingogram, except that a saline solution, rather than a dye, is injected, and ultrasound, rather than an X-ray, is used to show uterine abnormalities such as polyps or fibroids. The test can be done in the doctor's office and requires no medication in most cases.

A sonohysterogram is very effective for evaluating your uterus but not as effective as an HSG for looking at the fallopian tubes.

Thyroid tests

The best state to be in with your thyroid is *euthyroid,* which means that your thyroid is in balance. Thyroid problems are very common, with one out of eight women diagnosed with a thyroid problem at some point in their lives; men can also have thyroid disorders, but women are five to eight times more likely to be affected. Your thyroid can be either overactive (hyper) or under-active (hypo). Both hyper- and hypothyroid conditions can cause infertility problems in men and women.

A thyroid that is hypoactive usually causes fatigue, dry skin, and weight gain. A hyperactive thyroid causes a rapid heart rate, anxiousness, sweating, and weight loss.

In men, thyroid problems can cause a low sperm count and decreased sperm motility. Women may experience an increased rate of miscarriage, lack of ovulation, or irregular periods. Hypothyroidism can cause an increase in *prolactin,* the hormone responsible for maintaining breast milk production in pregnancy. High prolactin can cause a decrease in fertility.

Thyroid imbalances can be treated by daily medication, radiation, or, in severe cases, surgery. Your thyroid medication may need to be adjusted if you become pregnant.

FSH and Inhibin B

Follicle-stimulating hormone is necessary for the production of an egg each month, but, like other things in life, sometimes too much of a good thing is a problem. FSH rises above normal levels when the ovaries stop producing estrogen; similar to what happens in many other parts of the human body, this is a feedback loop reaction. FSH is cranked out in larger quantities, trying to "get" the ovary to understand and put out estrogen, reflected as a higher blood level of FSH. Because the estrogen stays low, no egg is matured. Your doctor may say that you're in *perimenopause,* which is the time from two to ten years before menopause.

Many doctors feel that a single high FSH reading, meaning anything over 10 or 11mIU/ml — the exact number varies with your lab — means that you have diminished ovarian reserve. If you're under 40 years of age, you may be diagnosed with premature ovarian failure (POF). If you're over 40, your doctor may consider this rise in FSH as a normal reaction to aging ovaries.

You may wonder why normal ranges for FSH vary from lab to lab. The reason is that many labs establish their own norms based on their specific patient population. The instruments used in the lab can also cause variations from one lab to another.

Other doctors feel that high FSH levels can be brought down by "fooling" the ovary into thinking that the estrogen is rising. This is done by giving a type of synthetic estrogen. The ovary reduces the amount of FSH produced because it "sees" the estrogen rising, which may give your ovary a chance to start producing an egg, either on its own or with the help of medication.

An Inhibin B blood test is done on day three of your period and may give an idea of how your ovaries are functioning. A low level of Inhibin B may indicate that your ovarian function is decreased.

The clomiphene citrate challenge test

The CCCT, often called the clomiphene citrate challenge test, is a measurement of estradiol and FSH taken on day two or three of your period and then measured again after you take a medication called clomiphene citrate for five days. This drug has the brand names Clomid or Serophene, fertility medications that stimulate egg production. You then recheck your estradiol and FSH levels. Your estradiol level should rise by the fifth day, but if your FSH level is elevated on either day two or after five days, you'll be told that you had a failed CCCT. Your doctor may feel that a failed CCCT means that you have a decreased ovarian reserve, which decreases your chance of getting pregnant with your own eggs.

Interpreting Your Partner's Test Results

With some of the test results back, you may be even more confused than you were before. If your partner's semen analysis comes back with some results askew, he may be too embarrassed to ask what the results mean. Sometimes it's easier to look up the problems in a book, so here you are!

Where's the sperm? Looking for "the real George"

Semen samples can vary from month to month, or even day to day. That's because it takes about 72 days for sperm to develop. Unlike eggs, which are present from your embryonic days, sperm are replenished all the time.

Because men are constantly producing new sperm, one "bad" semen analysis should be followed up to make sure that you're seeing the "real George" (or Tom, Harry, or Bob). An illness, injury, or medication or drug use a few months before may make one sample not so superior, but checking again a month later may show an improvement.

Sometimes a semen analysis shows a very low number of sperm, less than 20 million, a condition called *oligospermia.* If no sperm are seen, it's called *azoospermia.* Between 5 and 10 percent of the male population have either azoospermia or oligospermia.

You can get pregnant without fertility treatments if your partner has oligospermia, but your chances of pregnancy are higher if you do one of the following:

- **Intrauterine insemination (IUI) or intracervical insemination (ICI):** The sperm will be concentrated and "washed" so that the best sperm are used for insemination. (See Chapter 9 for more on IUI and ICI.)

- **In vitro fertilization (IVF):** This treatment utilizes intracytoplasmic sperm injection (ICSI), the insertion of a sperm directly into an egg. The procedure is done by an embryologist under a high-powered microscope. (See Chapter 13 for more information on ICSI.)

If your partner has azoospermia, you won't be able to get pregnant conventionally. Different factors can cause azoospermia; either the production of the sperm or the delivery of the sperm can be at fault.

Sperm production problems can be caused by the following:

- **Sertoli cell only syndrome:** In this condition, the germ cells that produce sperm in the testes are absent. There is no way for a person with this syndrome to father a child.

- **Anabolic steroids:** Their use may cause a possibly reversible shutdown of the sperm production.

- **Abnormal hormone levels:** Low levels of LH, FSH, or testosterone can cause low sperm production. This problem can be treated with hormone injections, pills, or transdermal patches.

If you need a sperm aspiration

Sperm can be aspirated from either the epididymis, which sits on top of the testes, or from the testes themselves. There are four different types of procedures, each with advantages and disadvantages:

✔ **MESA (microsurgical epididymal sperm aspiration):** This procedure can be done only for obstructive azoospermia, because men with nonobstructive azoospermia rarely have sperm in the epididymis. A small incision is made in the scrotum, and then a dilated tubule in the epididymis is cut open and examined through a lighted microscope. Fluid is collected from the tubule and examined for sperm. This procedure can be done in the doctor's office. You may be given a spermatic cord block and sedation during the procedure. You can generally return to work the following day.

✔ **PESA (percutaneous epididymal sperm aspiration):** This procedure is done in the office. A blind needle stick into the epididymis is used to extract sperm. Local anesthesia and sedation may be given.

✔ **TESE (testicular sperm extraction):** A small incision is made, and a piece of testicular tissue is removed. Testicular sperm doesn't freeze or thaw as well as epididymal sperm but may be the only sperm found in men with nonobstructive azoospermia.

✔ **TESA (testicular sperm aspiration):** This procedure is done in the office, using a blind needle aspiration of the testicle.

All four techniques can cause bleeding and *hematoma* (a collection of blood that can be painful). A biopsy usually requires only a one-day recovery and can be done under local anesthesia or mild sedation.

If the problem is obstruction, your partner needs a testicular sperm aspiration (discussed in the sidebar "If you need a sperm aspiration," later in this chapter). This procedure must be done in conjunction with IVF because the sperm need to be injected directly into the egg. Obstructive problems include the following:

✔ Absence of the *vas deferens,* the tube that delivers sperm to the urethra

✔ Previous vasectomy

Mechanical problems with getting the sperm where they need to be include the following:

✔ Retrograde ejaculation, in which the majority of the sperm go into the bladder

✔ Spinal cord injury that prevents ejaculation

✔ Previous injury from trauma

> ✔ Previous injury from surgery, such as hernia surgery
>
> ✔ A disease such as diabetes

Congenital absence of the *vas deferens,* the duct that leads to the urethra, is associated with cystic fibrosis in men. Genetic testing will most likely be suggested if this problem is found. One way to diagnose absence of the vas deferens is to test for a sugar called fructose that's usually found in semen; it won't be found if the duct is missing.

Swimming in circles, or not at all

Sometimes plenty of sperm are seen in the ejaculate, but the sperm themselves are abnormal. Sperm are very complicated little creatures. Despite their small size, they contain three distinct sections, and a problem with any section can cause infertility.

The head of the sperm contains the DNA, or genetic material. If the head is abnormally shaped, the sperm is probably incapable of fertilizing an egg because its genetic material is abnormal.

The midpiece of the sperm contains the energy necessary to propel it to the egg. Sperm need a tremendous amount of energy to get to an egg. If they lack this energy, they're not going to make it the whole distance.

The tail of the sperm makes the sperm move rapidly; if the sperm sample has a lot of coiled, rather than whiplike, tails, or no tails at all, those sperm may go in the wrong direction or may go nowhere at all — they may just twitch a bit. Again, these sperm aren't going to be able to get where they need to be.

Two syndromes that affect male fertility

Kleinfelter's syndrome and Kallman's syndrome are two syndromes that affect male fertility.

Kleinfelter's syndrome is far more common than most people realize. One out of 500 to 1,000 males are affected. Symptoms of Kleinfelter's are delayed puberty, decreased facial and body hair, small firm testes, and long legs. Blood tests show an increase in LH and FSH levels and a decrease in serum testosterone levels.

Chromosome tests will show an XXY karyotype. Treatment is testosterone.

Kallman's syndrome is less common but may be familial. Symptoms are loss of smell, delayed puberty, osteoporosis, red-green color blindness, and possibly cleft palate and urogenital abnormalities. Blood tests show high LH and FSH levels and low testosterone levels. Treatment is with hormones such as HCG or FSH and testosterone.

Considering ejaculation issues: A sensitive topic

Abnormal sperm may be a problem you both can deal with. Problems with ejaculation or the ability to sustain an erection, however, may be so difficult to address that you may have a hard time bringing it out into the open. Yet it's a common problem: Ten percent of men between the ages of 18 and 59 have experienced erectile problems in the last year, and 10 percent of men between the ages of 40 and 70 have complete erectile failure.

Plenty of medical-related conditions can cause problems with erection and ejaculation. The following list gives examples of what can cause such problems:

- ✔ **Medications**
  - Antidepressants
  - Antiulcer medications
  - Certain blood pressure medications
  - Cholesterol-lowering medications
- ✔ **Diseases:**
  - Diabetes
  - Heart attack (myocardial infarction)
  - Hypertension or other vascular disease
  - Hypothyroidism or hyperthyroidism
  - Leukemia
  - Liver cirrhosis
  - Renal failure
  - Sickle cell anemia
- ✔ **Surgeries**
  - Abdominal perineal resection
  - Proctocolectomy
  - Radical prostatectomy
  - Transurethral resection of prostate

Radiation, trauma, heavy alcohol use, and neurological damage from surgery, stroke, epilepsy, or multiple sclerosis can all cause erectile dysfunction.

Erectile dysfunction may also result from psychosexual problems better addressed by therapy. Whatever the reason, the first step in dealing with the problem is being able to discuss it, especially with an outsider such as a doctor or nurse.

Handling the emotional effect of male problems on both of you

A few decades ago, failure to produce a baby was always considered to be the woman's fault. In many cultures, a man could obtain a no-questions-asked divorce from any woman who didn't give him a child. With the advent of microscopes high powered enough to look closely at sperm, it became obvious that male factors are as important for reproduction as female factors.

Intellectually it shouldn't matter which one of you has a problem, but intellect and emotion are two different matters. Women tend to approach medical problems with a "let's just fix it" attitude, while many men approach medical issues with a "let's just bury our head in the sand" approach. For whatever reason, more men than women have an ego issue when it comes to their reproductive parts. Their sense of personal failure may be more pronounced than yours, and they may also be less willing to face the problem and do what it takes to fix it.

If it turns out that he's the problem, you may have to tread very gently around the issue, especially if you're the one more interested in having a child. He may consider the whole subject closed if he's the problem — no sperm, no child, okay, end of discussion. Not all men feel so closely tied to their semen analysis, but if your partner does, be prepared for some tense moments.

Understanding Female Infertility Problems

Men's infertility issues seem simple at first because the problem all comes down to sperm: Are they produced, can they get out, and how do they look when they get there? Women's infertility issues can be more complex because so many different systems can be at fault. Is the problem uterine, tubal, hormonal, age related, or ovarian? Any one of these problems can cause enough trouble to prevent you from becoming and staying pregnant.

Looking in the uterus

Maybe you had an HSG to evaluate your fallopian tubes and uterus, which we discuss in the section "HSG (don't even try to spell out the word)," earlier in this chapter, or maybe you had a laparoscopic surgery for an even closer look into the uterus. Looking at the uterus is an integral part of any fertility workup, because the uterus nourishes and holds a baby for nine months.

Fibroids, or benign tumors, are commonly found inside or on the outside of the uterus. They're extremely common, with 40 percent of women between the ages of 35 and 55 having at least one. Fibroids are even more common in African American women, with 50 percent having at least one.

Fibroids can cause bowel or bladder problems, very heavy bleeding, or pain. Fibroids can be either inside or outside the uterine cavity; their location determines whether they cause a problem with your ability to get or stay pregnant. Fibroids completely outside the uterus, such as pedunculated fibroids, which are attached to the uterus by a stem, don't usually cause a problem with infertility.

Subserosal fibroids are located in the outer wall of the uterus and generally don't impinge on the cavity. *Intramural fibroids,* those within the wall of the uterus, can push the uterus in if they grow large enough. *Submucosal fibroids* grow through the lining of the inside wall and can make the cavity too small for a baby to gestate for nine months. In fact, 40 percent of pregnancies will miscarry if submucosal fibroids are present.

Fibroids can be surgically removed, a process called a *myomectomy.* You may need to deliver by cesarean section after a myomectomy.

Checking out the fallopian tubes

Most women have two fallopian tubes, one on each side of the uterus, next to the ovaries. Because these tubes are the transport path from the ovary to the uterus, a problem with one or both tubes can have a big impact on your baby-making ability.

Sometimes a tube is surgically removed after an ectopic pregnancy, a pregnancy that starts to grow in the tube rather than in the uterus. If this pregnancy is found early enough, it may be possible to dissolve the pregnancy with a chemotherapy agent called methotrexate. However, if the fetus grows large enough undetected in the tube, the tube can burst, causing life-threatening bleeding (we discuss this in Chapter 6). The only way to stop the bleeding is to remove the tube.

You can get pregnant with only one tube, but you must be aware that having one ectopic pregnancy leaves you at a higher risk to have another.

TECHNICAL STUFF

Women who have only the left ovary and the right fallopian tube have gotten pregnant because the egg can "float" to the remaining tube. Of course, this also applies to women who have the left tube and the right ovary.

Sometimes fallopian tubes are seen to be enlarged on ultrasound or during an HSG. If the tubes are very swollen and dye doesn't flow through them, you may have a *hydrosalpinx,* the medical term for a chronically infected tube (see Figure 7-4). If both tubes are dilated, the condition is known as *hydrosalpinges.*

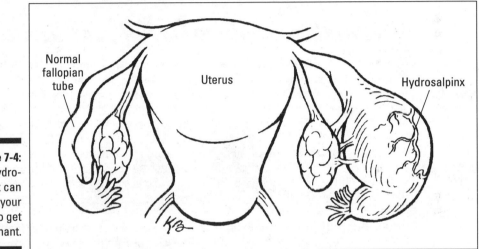

Normal fallopian tube

Uterus

Hydrosalpinx

Figure 7-4:
A hydro-
salpinx can
affect your
ability to get
pregnant.

A hydrosalpinx interferes with pregnancy in two ways:

- The egg may not be able to find its way through the tube because the tube is so large and the passage may be blocked with infected debris.
- The embryo, if it makes it to the uterus, may not be able to survive because the infected material from the tube drips down into the uterus, making an inhospitable environment for the embryo to grow.

The treatment for a hydrosalpinx sounds drastic. The tube or tubes must be removed, and you need to have in vitro fertilization (IVF) to get pregnant because your eggs can no longer float down to the uterus. This diagnosis is a hard thing for many women to accept because it definitely ends any chance that they'll be able to get pregnant on their own.

Women can be born without any fallopian tubes; often the tubes are missing as part of a syndrome in which the external sex organs look normal, but the vagina, uterus, and fallopian tubes are missing. Of course, if you've had two ectopic pregnancies, you may have had both tubes surgically removed also.

Sometimes fallopian tubes look fine on an X-ray or ultrasound, but for some reason, they're blocked so that the egg can't get down to the uterus. *Endometriosis,* tissue growths found anywhere in the pelvis, can grow in or around the fallopian tubes and block the fallopian tubes.

Because the fallopian tubes play such a large role in getting pregnant, you'll probably need intervention, such as IVF, to get pregnant if a problem is discovered with them. Removal or absence of the tubes, or a blockage that can't be removed, makes IVF inevitable if you're trying to get pregnant.

Seeing the complications of scar tissue

In my years as a labor and delivery nurse, I (coauthor Sharon) saw firsthand how scar tissue, or adhesions (as shown in Figure 7-5), can create problems in your reproductive system. Many women having a second or third cesarean section delivery had scar tissue throughout the pelvis that needed to be cut away before the delivery team could get to the uterus.

Adhesions form when blood and plasma from trauma such as surgery form fibrin deposits, which are threadlike strands that can bind one organ to another. They can be removed, but surgery to correct adhesions may result in — you guessed it — more adhesions.

Adhesions in the pelvis are common after a surgery such as a cesarean section, an appendectomy, tubal removal for an ectopic pregnancy, or fibroid removal. Between 60 and 90 percent of surgeries leave adhesions behind. Adhesions often cause pelvic pain; 30 to 40 percent of women with chronic pelvis pain have adhesions, and one out of seven women has chronic pelvic pain.

Your chances of getting pregnant after adhesion removal are highest in the first six months after surgery, before extensive adhesions form again. Some adhesions can't be removed without damaging the tubes or ovaries, and you may need in vitro fertilization to get pregnant.

If you have adhesions in the uterus itself, you may be diagnosed with Asherman's syndrome, also called uterine synechiae. With Asherman's, the adhesions crisscross the entire cavity and make it difficult, if not impossible, for a pregnancy to implant. Asherman's can follow a dilation and curettage (D&C), an abortion, or a uterine infection. It can be diagnosed during an HSG but is best diagnosed with a hysteroscopy, where the inside of the uterus can be visualized. Asherman's also is suspected if you have scant or no menstrual flow or recurrent miscarriages following uterine trauma. If the mild to moderate adhesions are removed surgically, you have a good chance, probably 75 percent or better, of becoming pregnant and carrying to term. Severe adhesions may destroy nearly all the normal uterine lining, and pregnancy may not be possible.

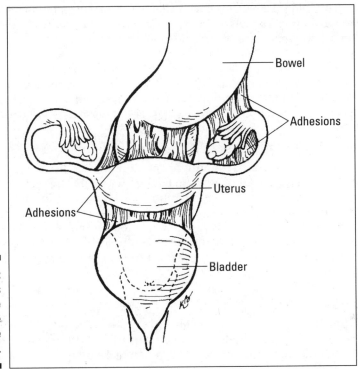

Figure 7-5:
Adhesions
in the
female
reproductive
system.

Testing for immune disorders

Immune testing in infertility is simple. In most cases, only a blood sample is required. Interpretation of the results isn't always simple, however, and different doctors have different opinions of the importance of immune testing in infertility. Some tests are widely done and the results almost universally accepted. Other tests are done only by doctors specializing in immune disorders, and not all doctors believe the results are important. Here are some of the most common immune tests, with information on what the tests mean and how you're treated if the tests are abnormal.

Antisperm antibody (ASA)

Many fertility centers do antisperm antibody (ASA) tests on all their patients. Both you and your partner may be positive for ASA. Women are tested through a blood test, and men are tested through a semen specimen.

Antisperm antibodies in either partner cause problems with fertilization. Males with ASA may need to do IVF with ICSI (intracytoplasmic sperm injection, or the injection of one sperm into an egg) if they have more than 20 percent antibodies, because the antibodies cause the sperm to clump together instead of moving forward. (We discuss ICSI in more detail in Chapter 13.)

About 70 percent of men who have had a vasectomy reversal have antisperm antibodies; they're also common in men who have had injury or insult to the testicle. Ten percent or so of infertile men have ASA.

Antisperm antibodies are less common in women; less than 5 percent of infertile women have antisperm antibodies. They're found in the cervical mucus as well as the blood. The antibodies attach to the head of the sperm and make it hard for the sperm to penetrate an egg. The treatment is IVF with ICSI.

Antiphospholipid antibodies (APA)

You'll most likely be tested for antiphospholipid antibodies (APA) if you've had multiple miscarriages or repeated failure with IVF. The test for APA actually tests for a number of different antibodies; a moderate or high reaction to two or more antibodies is considered a positive reaction. Treatment is either baby aspirin, heparin (an anticoagulant, or blood thinner), or a combination of the two. Antiphospholipid antibodies can interfere with the embryo implanting or can cause miscarriage; they disrupt the normal clotting of blood and the adhesion of the embryo to the uterus.

Antinuclear antibodies (ANA)

A high positive antinuclear antibodies (ANA) test can mean that you have a disease called systemic lupus erythematosus (SLE). At lower positive levels, especially if the pattern is speckled, ANA can increase your risk of miscarriage. A positive ANA level may be treated with low-dose steroids.

Antithyroglobulin (ATA)

Antithyroglobulin antibodies (ATA) can cause problems with your thyroid function. Because the thyroid is so important in maintaining your hormone levels, antibodies that interfere with the thyroid's functioning can cause problems with egg production. A high ATA level may be treated with steroids.

Antiovarian antibodies (AOA)

If you're in premature ovarian failure or early menopause, you may be tested for antiovarian antibodies (AOA).

Leukocyte antibody detection (LAD)

Foreign bodies are usually rejected because they're attacked by antibodies; this would be true of a fetus if it didn't have the protection of *blocking antibodies,* which you make in response to the genetic material from your partner that is present in the embryo. If you and your partner have DNA that is too similar, those antibodies won't be activated, and the fetus will be rejected. A positive leukocyte antibody detection (LAD) test is good; it means the antibodies are present. If the test is negative, you may need to do leukocyte immunization (LI) therapy, which injects white blood cells from your partner into you by using a small intradermal needle, similar to a tuberculin test. At present, LI therapy has been stopped by the U.S. Food and Drug Administration, but approval is being sought to restart this therapy. A newer and simpler therapy being tested is the use of capsules that are inserted into the vagina and contain *seminal plasma,* which is the 90 percent of the ejaculate that is not sperm.

Natural killer (NK) cells

NK cells are part of white blood cells that attack and destroy anything they see as a foreign substance in the body. They're an important part of keeping cancer cells from spreading. A normal NK cell range is about 2 percent; if the count is higher, the cells may be too aggressive and attack a growing embryo. Treatment for high NK cells is intravenous immunoglobulin therapy (IVIG), which is also used in cancer therapy. IVIG is quite expensive (over $1,000 per treatment), quite controversial among infertility specialists, and often not covered by insurance. (We talk more about IVIG therapy in Chapter 16.)

Enbrel, a drug created for treatment of rheumatoid arthritis, can also be used to treat NK cells.

Considering the possibility of endometriosis

More than 5 million American women have endometriosis, a common, complicated condition that affects 30 to 40 percent of all infertility patients. Despite its prevalence, it's often underdiagnosed and undertreated.

Endometriosis is the presence of endometrial tissue, which lines the inside of your uterus, in places it has no business being. Endometriosis can be found throughout the pelvis — around the fallopian tubes and ovaries — but it has also been found in the lungs, skin, and brain. No one is quite sure how endometriosis travels so far, but theories are that it travels through the circulatory system or the lymphatic system.

Because endometriosis is endometrial tissue, it reacts to hormone changes the same way your uterine lining does. So when you get your period or have midcycle spotting, endometriosis tissue also bleeds. Because this tissue doesn't have a handy exit point the way your uterine lining does, the blood stagnates, causing inflammation, irritation, and eventually scar tissue.

You might suspect that you have endometriosis if you have any of the following symptoms:

- ✔ Chronic or recurring pelvic pain
- ✔ History of ectopic pregnancy or miscarriage
- ✔ Backache or leg pain

- Nausea, vomiting, diarrhea, or constipation
- Rectal bleeding or bloody stools
- Blood in urine
- Urinary urgency or frequency
- Chest pain or coughing up blood, especially at the time of your period
- High blood pressure

Because the symptoms are so broad and sometimes nonspecific, endometriosis may be confused with the following:

- Appendicitis
- Irritable bowel syndrome
- Bowel obstruction
- Ovarian cysts
- Pelvic inflammatory disease

Endometriosis affects fertility in many ways. It may cause adhesions, tubal blockage, and problems with ovulation. The problems may include luteinized unruptured follicle (LUF) syndrome, in which a mature follicle develops but the egg inside doesn't release. Women with endometriosis may also have a lower estradiol level at the time of ovulation or a blunted LH surge, so that the follicle may not properly mature.

No cure is yet available for endometriosis, nor is there clear-cut evidence why some women develop endometriosis, although a familial link appears to be a possibility.

Endometriosis is progressive: It starts with clear lesions at the site of the endometrial tissue implant, and these lesions turn red and then black over seven to ten years.

The amount of endometriosis present doesn't determine the degree of difficulty conceiving. You can have severe pain and infertility problems with a small amount of endometriosis, and less pain and fewer problems with a larger amount of endometriosis.

Endometriosis can be surgically removed, although the tissue will most likely grow back eventually. The only way to positively identify endometriosis is through surgery, when the implants can be removed at the same time. Other methods of treatment, such as the use of birth control pills or Lupron Depot to prevent ovulation and decrease the amount of menstrual flow, aren't always helpful.

Amenorrhea — not getting your period at all

Amenorrhea is the absence of menstrual periods. If you've never had a period, undoubtedly you've been evaluated sometime during your teenage years to see whether a structural problem, such as absence of the uterus, malformation of the vagina, or undeveloped ovaries, is the cause. However, many women have periods at one time and then quit having them. This may happen if you have Asherman's syndrome (discussed earlier in this chapter in the section "Seeing the complications of scar tissue") because little normal tissue is left and the exit path from the uterus may be blocked with scar tissue, or maybe you aren't ovulating any longer. If you've had periods previously and no longer do, have a checkup to see whether anovulation (failing to ovulate) is the problem.

Failing to ovulate

If you're not getting your period at all, or if you're having irregular periods, you may not be ovulating, a condition known as *anovulation*. Many factors, including emotional factors and stress, can cause anovulation.

One cause of anovulation is weight gain or loss. Of course, most women don't want to look at their weight. But even a slight deviation — about 15 percent — either up or down may create menstrual irregularities and subtle infertility issues. After your weight falls into normal limits, your chance of getting pregnant without any other therapy may increase.

In today's culture, where thin is in and "you can't be too thin" is a widely accepted standard, overweight women are far more likely to consider their weight a problem than the underweight. The fact is, however, that being underweight is equally as damaging as being overweight if you're having fertility problems.

Frequent, strenuous exercise can also cause anovulation if it causes the body fat percentage to drop to less than 22 percent, the amount needed to keep menstruation occurring.

You may wonder about the role stress plays in anovulation. Stress can alter your body functions, which can affect your menstrual cycle. Lowering stress levels is easier said than done, but if you're under severe stress, you may want to consider therapies such as biofeedback to decrease negative response to stress.

Reducing stress and maintaining normal weight may help correct some cases of anovulation, but not all.

Polycystic ovary syndrome (PCOS)

Between 3 and 5 percent of women have a condition called polycystic ovary syndrome (PCOS). Many of these women have difficulty getting pregnant because many women with PCOS ovulate irregularly or not at all.

Often your doctor will test for PCOS if you're overweight (50 percent of all PCOS patients are obese) and are hairy where you shouldn't be, a condition that may be caused by an overabundance of male hormones called *androgens*.

If your doctor suspects that you have PCOS, he may do a pelvic ultrasound. Women with PCOS have lots of small follicles on their ovaries that are visible on ultrasound. Your doctor probably will check your hormone levels as well; PCOS patients often have a baseline blood LH:FSH ratio that is higher than normal. The high LH levels can cause abnormalities in eggs and also increase miscarriage rates. Insulin levels are often high as well, but these can be treated by taking oral diabetic medications such as Glucophage. PCOS patients have a higher chance of developing adult onset diabetes.

Many women with PCOS respond well and begin ovulating if treated with Clomid or with injectable gonadotropins to induce ovulation. In resistant cases of anovulation, your doctor may suggest laparoscopic laser ovarian drilling, a procedure in which your doctor makes small punctures in your ovary during laparoscopic surgery. Between 70 and 90 percent of women start ovulating after this procedure, although the effect may be temporary. Risks of the surgery are infection and scar tissue formation.

Hyperprolactinemia, or high prolactin

Although less than 1 percent of women have high prolactin levels, high *prolactin* (the hormone responsible for maintaining breast milk production) levels are found in 10 to 40 percent of premenopausal women who have stopped menstruating due to anovulation.

Women who are pregnant or breast-feeding should have high levels of prolactin. If yours is elevated at any other time, it may suppress ovulation. A tumor is found on the pituitary gland in about 30 percent of women with high prolactin levels; these are almost always benign. Many drugs can cause high prolactin levels, including antidepressants and antihypertensives.

A pill called Parlodel can be given to lower your prolactin levels so that you'll start ovulating again.

Reversing Tubal Ligation and Vasectomy

Nearly 50 percent of the American population of childbearing age have been surgically sterilized. Unfortunately, at least 10 percent regret their decision down the road. Can surgical sterilization be reversed? The answer is yes, no, and maybe, depending on when the surgery was done and what kind of surgery it was.

Turning around a tubal ligation: How successful is it?

Surgical sterilization is very common in the United States. A 1995 study showed that 41 percent of ever-married women ages 15 to 44 were surgically sterile. About 1 million women have their tubes tied, a procedure known as *tubal ligation,* each year. Human nature being what it is, at least 10,000 of these women regret their decision and want to have another baby.

A *tubal reanastomosis,* or tubal reversal, has several drawbacks. For one thing, it's expensive — about $10,000 — and insurance usually doesn't cover the cost. For another, the success rate depends on how long ago your tubes were tied and how they were tied.

Before you decide to have your tubal ligation reversed, consider these factors:

- ✔ **Your age:** Are you in your late thirties or younger? If you're over 40, you may have other fertility problems related to age, and in vitro fertilization (IVF) may be a better option for you.

- ✔ **Your partner:** If your partner has sperm problems, you may also be better off doing IVF rather than reversing your tubal ligation.

- ✔ **How your tubes were tied:** If your tubes were blocked off or clamped with clips or rings instead of being cauterized or having a large section removed, your chance of success is higher. Some doctors say that you need about an inch of healthy tube to successfully reconnect the tubes.

If you want a tubal reversal, look for a surgeon skilled in microsurgery. Depending on the surgeon and type of surgery done, your surgery can take up to six hours to perform and require several weeks of recovery.

Risks after surgery include scar tissue formation, infection, and increased risk of ectopic pregnancy. If the fimbriated end of the tube (the part that the egg enters from the ovary) is intact and your doctor believes that you have enough tube left to reconnect, your pregnancy chances after reanastomosis can be as high as IVF success rates.

Undoing a vasectomy: Is it worth the pain?

About 500,000 vasectomies are performed each year. As with tubal ligation, many men regret their decision and decide to have the surgery reversed. Vasectomy reversal surgery is often successful in that sperm will be found in the ejaculate in the majority of cases, but the number of sperm may be too small to make pregnancy likely, or antibodies attached to the sperm may make it nearly impossible for the sperm to swim properly or fertilize an egg.

Antibodies are found in 50 percent of men after vasectomy reversal; men with antibodies generally need IVF for their partner to become pregnant.

As with tubal ligation, vasectomy reversal success depends on what type of surgery was done. The reversal success rate is higher if the surgery was done on a straight section of the vas deferens, the pieces to be joined together are of equal size, and the reversal is done within ten years of the original surgery.

Your chance of pregnancy after sterilization reversal depends on several factors. Consider carefully whether reversal will be more cost effective and offer a better chance of success than IVF, in which tied tubes can be bypassed or sperm can be removed directly from the testicles via sperm aspiration.

A recently reported study showed that there was less pain and less time lost from work with sperm aspirations as opposed to vasectomy reversals.

Understanding Diseases That Affect Fertility

Just a few generations ago, systemic diseases such as diabetes or lupus ruled out the possibility of having a baby. Now, pregnancies in patients with systemic disease are commonplace, and obstetricians or perinatologists who specialize in high-risk patients guide women with a history of cancer, kidney problems, heart problems, or just about any other health condition through successful pregnancies. Discuss the potential problems of pregnancy with your doctor beforehand so that you can be prepared for the problems you may face getting pregnant or carrying a pregnancy to term.

Diabetes: More than a "sugar" problem

Diabetes affects about 17 million Americans, or approximately 6 percent of the population. There are actually several different types of diabetes, including the following:

- ✔ **Type 1 diabetes,** which used to be called juvenile diabetes, usually develops before puberty but can develop at any age. Five to ten percent of diabetics have Type 1 diabetes, which is an autoimmune disease. In Type 1 diabetes, the beta cells of the pancreas stop making insulin altogether, so people with this problem must take injections of insulin every day.

- ✔ **Type 2 diabetes** usually develops in people over 40, but it can develop earlier. It is often associated with being overweight; 80 percent of Type 2 diabetics are overweight. It develops more slowly than Type 1 and possibly can be controlled with diet and pills rather than injections.

Men with diabetes often have problems with erection and ejaculation; about 40 percent of male diabetics have retrograde ejaculation, a condition in which sperm back up into the bladder.

Women with diabetes need to have well-controlled blood sugar during pregnancy. Even with good control, the rate of birth defects in women with diabetes is two to three times the normal rate. Women with polycystic ovary syndrome may develop Type 2 diabetes later in life.

Diabetics tend to have large babies, which can create problems at the time of delivery.

Lupus: Not just a rash

Systemic lupus erythematosus, commonly called lupus, is primarily a disease of women, although a small percentage of men also develop it. One of the outward symptoms of lupus is a facial rash, but lupus can affect every organ in your body. A few generations ago, women with lupus were advised not to have children, because it was felt that pregnancy worsens the disease. More recent studies have shown this belief not to be true, although one-third of pregnant lupus patients have "flares," or increases in disease activity. About 10 percent of pregnant lupus patients find that their symptoms actually improve.

Fifty percent of women with lupus have normal pregnancies and normal deliveries; about 25 percent deliver prematurely, and another 25 percent experience miscarriage or stillbirth.

Miscarriage may be related to antibodies called antiphospholipid antibodies (discussed earlier in this chapter) found in some lupus patients. These antibodies cause clotting and interfere with the growth of the placenta. Baby aspirin and/or heparin may be given in pregnancy to help blood flow to the placenta.

About 20 percent of lupus patients develop *toxemia,* a condition that results in high blood pressure, liver and kidney malfunctions, and premature delivery and can lead to eclampsia, which can cause maternal seizures and death.

Men with lupus often have antisperm antibodies, so fertilization may not occur without IVF and ICSI.

If you have lupus, you need to be followed carefully by an obstetrician who specializes in high-risk patients.

Cancer and Fertility: The News Is Cautiously Optimistic

Just a few years ago, having cancer meant that you would probably not be able to conceive and carry a child. Surgery, radiation, and chemotherapy, the mainstay treatments of most cancers, could destroy ovaries and sperm cells as well as your hope of having a child.

Today, however, new advances have made it possible for cancer survivors to become parents, and the really good new is that more advances are being made all the time. The information of today may be obsolete soon, and the chances for parenthood will hopefully be better than ever.

For women . . .

Breast cancer survivors are now being told that pregnancy after treatment is possible, as long as their ovaries are intact and haven't been irradiated. Many doctors encourage patients to wait two years after treatment before trying to get pregnant. Pregnancy doesn't increase the chance of cancer recurrence, according to most recent studies, but doctors want to make sure that the cancer doesn't recur on its own.

If you do have a recurrence of cancer while pregnant and require chemotherapy, you need to be aware that chemo in the first trimester may cause fetal malformation, while waiting till the second or third trimester may result in preterm labor or fetal loss. If you're taking tamoxifen, you may find that you're no longer ovulating, a side effect for some, but not all, women treated with the drug.

At the time of this writing, a study showed that breast cancer patients trying to get pregnant through in vitro fertilization made more eggs when given tamoxifen.

If you've been treated for ovarian cancer with radiation or ovarian ablation, your ovaries will not be functioning, and you'll need to use donor eggs to become pregnant. If you were treated with multiple-agent chemotherapy, there's a good chance you'll go into premature ovarian failure. One-third of women under age 30 and two-thirds of those over 30 go into POF.

Your baby will not have a higher risk of birth defects or childhood cancer if you become pregnant after cancer treatment.

For men . . .

Although testicular cancer is rare, making up only 1 percent of all cancer, it's the most common cancer found in men between the ages of 20 and 34, with 7,000 new cases diagnosed each year. It is four times more common among Caucasian men than African American men.

If only one testicle is removed surgically, the remaining testicle will produce enough sperm so that fertility won't be damaged. If both testicles need to be removed, several semen samples can be frozen before surgery and used for insemination later on. If only one testicle is affected, the man has a 2 to 5 percent chance of developing cancer in the other testicle.

Some chemotherapy treatment causes temporary loss of fertility, but sperm counts may return to an acceptable level after two to three years. Radiation may also cause temporary infertility, but some men regain adequate sperm counts within a short time.

If certain lymph nodes are removed, the nerves that control ejaculation may be affected, although the sperm count may be normal. This condition may require sperm aspiration with ICSI and IVF to attain a pregnancy.

Chapter 8

Leaving Dr. Basic Behind: Seeing a Specialist

After doing some testing, you may have a better idea of what your fertility problems are, and you may decide that it's time to see a specialist. Or perhaps your testing hasn't shown any specific problems, and Dr. Basic has decided you should move on to a specialist in infertility.

In this chapter, we help you locate a fertility specialist and discuss what a specialist can and can't do for you. We also give you some insight into how an infertility office is run and whom you should get to know well to make your time there (and you will spend a lot of time there!) as pleasant as possible.

Seeking Dr. Perfect: Why Your Ob/Gyn's Golfing Buddy May Not Be the Best Choice

Your family doctor or gynecologist may have already handed you a piece of paper with the name of an infertility specialist scribbled on it. "Go to this guy. He's the best," he may say, and you may do just that, without thinking a whole lot about alternative choices.

Before you set up your first appointment, you may want to ask your doctor *why* he thinks the person he has suggested is the best. Does the specialist have the best pregnancy rates, is he a prolific publisher in journals, or is he just a member of the same health organization?

Even worse, is he your doctor's golfing buddy? Many doctors refer patients to each other, and there's nothing wrong with the practice of referral. That system, however, doesn't ensure that you'll end up with the doctor best suited to you, either.

Although the name that Dr. Basic gives you is a starting point, you should check out other doctors, too, before making a final decision. You may want to turn to Chapter 4 and review the types of doctors doing infertility treatment. At this point, you probably will be looking for a specialist in the field, such as a reproductive endocrinologist.

Start with the phone book. No, you're not going to shut your eyes and blindly poke your finger at a name. You can use the phone book as a starting point, looking under the reproductive endocrinologists listing and accumulating the names of doctors in your area. This approach gives you a basic list to work from and a starting point for some research.

Eliminate clinics that are too far away from you. "Too far away" is a subjective measure; if you work and have a very hectic lifestyle, more than 15 minutes away may be too far, and your options may be limited. If your schedule is more flexible, an hour or even two may seem reasonable. Remember that you may have to go in for blood and ultrasound monitoring several times a month and that some clinics do all their monitoring early in the morning.

Getting Help from Two National Organizations

After you have a core list of infertility clinics near you, you need to check each one out. You can visit each one, hanging around the waiting room and questioning people as they come out the door. Or you can call your local Resolve organization and see whether it has information on any of the offices you're considering. Resolve and INCIID (the InterNational Council on Infertility Information Dissemination) are two large national organizations dedicated to the treatment of infertility.

If you have Internet access, finding your local Resolve organization is easy; the Web site is `www.resolve.org`. Just click on the local chapters hyperlink to find one near you. If you don't have computer access, check your local paper for listings of meetings or call Resolve's HelpLine at 1-888-623-0744.

The Resolve Web site contains clinic success rates published by the Centers for Disease Control (CDC). This information is compiled by the Society for Assisted Reproductive Technology (SART), which you can read more about in Chapter 10. These numbers give you some idea of your clinic's success rates, but keep in mind that these statistics are only for high-tech in vitro fertilization (IVF) treatment, not for medium-tech treatment such as IUI (intrauterine insemination). However, if the clinic you're interested in is listed (remember, it won't be listed if it doesn't do IVF), you can assume that a clinic with good pregnancy rates for IVF probably has good statistics for less high-tech methods also.

Local Resolve meetings will probably connect you with people who can give you the inside scoop on the local clinics, which may help narrow your search or at least give you some ideas about where you *don't* want to go!

The Resolve Web site contains a huge amount of information on insurance coverage for infertility, adoption options, and information on clinical trials and research studies being carried out around the country. (You can find out more about studies in the section "Different Docs = Different Points of View: Sorting Things Out," later in this chapter, and in Chapter 11.) Resolve is very vocal in lobbying for insurance coverage for infertility treatments. The Web site also has bulletin boards, lists of interesting meetings and events around the country, and a host of other information. Check it out!

INCIID's Web address is www.inciid.org. The INCIID site also contains articles, bulletin boards, lists of fertility clinics, a monthly newsletter, and up-to-date information on new treatments in infertility.

Your area may have other groups that meet to help you deal with infertility. Some are informal groups that started out as a few friends meeting to commiserate, and then grew into clubs with monthly meetings. You may also find local psychologists or therapists who have started groups for infertile patients.

All of these are good resources for information on who's good and who's not in your area. Always get more than one person's opinion on a clinic because each person may have a bias one way or the other, depending on her own outcome.

Going Online for More Resources and Information

Resolve and INCIID aren't the only information sources online. In fact, after you start surfing the Net, your sources of information will be limited only by the amount of time you have to spend. Whether you're interested in reading scientific journals, chatting with new friends online, or checking out clinic Web sites, we guarantee that the Internet has enough stuff to keep you occupied until your children leave for college!

Chat rooms and bulletin boards

Perhaps one of the greatest sources of information and strength on the road to baby that I (coauthor Jackie) found came from the countless women I encountered in cyberspace, some of whom became friends in real time as well. I happened upon this wealth of relating and resources right after a failed in vitro fertilization attempt and a subsequent high FSH (follicle-stimulating hormone) reading, which, at the time, seemed a death knell to any future attempts.

After a good cry, I logged on to www.google.com to see what I could find in reference to my new diagnosis of high FSH. Convinced that I was the only one to suffer from this odd disorder (actually a measure of diminished ovarian egg reserve), I was surprised at how quickly Google returned a result listing over 38,000 Web pages on the topic. Okay, so maybe a few others out there had the same problem after all. The first listing, High FSH E-mail Group, connected to me a very lively, upbeat chat room. Through teary eyes, I asked one and all if I was doomed. I logged off in despair and went to work my way through the other 37,999 sites. After visiting two more sites, I went back to the chat room and was amazed to find at least ten responses to my wail. I read each and every one, printed them all (and have saved them to this day), and spent until the wee hours of the morning reading every message of encouragement and every link to more information on high FSH, low FSH, infertility, and the best medical and nonmedical sources for help, including doctors, clinics, acupuncturists, and herbs.

I never left that site through the remaining year of my fertility battle. From it, I garnered hope that I could conceive despite what my doctor had told me. I also found a new (and improved) doctor who (eventually) successfully treated me. I also discovered insights on new treatments and medications and located a 24/7 support network that accompanied me through fertility, pregnancy, and all the stressors in between. I developed a core group of friends from all over the country who were the first ones I called when the pregnancy test came back negative and when it finally came back positive. I can honestly say that my high FSH diagnosis was a blessing, one that led me to a much greater place.

The beauty of the Internet is the availability of libraries full of information right at our fingertips. Bulletin boards help provide links to this information, along with the kinship so helpful in thriving through infertility. Man or woman, whatever problem that ails you, you can be almost certain that the Internet offers a chat room/bulletin board filled with others facing the same struggles.

INCIID, located at www.inciid.org, hosts a vast variety of discussion groups for those with almost every fertility issue imaginable. Sit through the two-week wait with others on a similar site or compare possible pregnancy signs. You also find links to other resources, interactive discussions with doctors, and answers to common, and not so common, questions. If this site doesn't suit you, visit Google at www.google.com or another search engine. Simply type in your issue, disorder, or question and sit back. In today's high-tech age, you're really not alone.

Doctors' Web sites: Separating the glitter from the goods

When I (coauthor Sharon) first started working for an infertility clinic, few infertility clinics had Web sites. Now it seems as if every infertility clinic has a Web site. Some are pretty basic, giving not much more than name, rank, and serial number, and others run a 24-hour-a-day media show, complete with question-and-answer sessions with the doctors, links to published articles, and testimonials from happy clients.

Some sites tell you more about the staff than you really want to know. They have pictures of the staff at work, give everyone's names — right down to the cleaning women — and list everyone's hobbies so you know that the money you spend there is going to good use. I may be exaggerating, but not by much.

Some clinics list their Web site right next to their phone number in the phone book; others direct you to their Web site when you call the office. Some Web sites give detailed and frequently updated pregnancy rates. Other sites either don't supply or don't update statistics.

Here's what *not* to be impressed by when looking at clinic Web sites:

- ✔ **The way the doctor looks:** That picture may have been taken in 1963.
- ✔ **Testimonials from patients:** Unless you know the patients personally and can verify what they say, you have no way of knowing who wrote these glowing reports.

✔ **How many articles the doctor has had published:** What journals? How long ago?

✔ **Great graphics:** Splashy visuals may indicate that the doctor has a son or daughter who knows a lot about Web sites, but those graphics don't reveal anything about a doctor's medical ability.

You can be impressed by the following Web site information:

✔ Clearly written, frequently updated success rates

✔ A list of clinic services, plus how many procedures are performed in a year

✔ The doctors' degrees and the schools they were obtained from

✔ Lab certifications

Manipulating Numbers: What's the (Baby) Bottom Line?

Naturally, you want some idea of how successful infertility treatment is going to be for you. But getting a straight answer to the question "What are my chances?" isn't easy.

Clinics aren't trying to confuse you when they won't give a straightforward answer to the question. Some clinics don't keep really accurate records for their medium-tech treatments, such as IUI. They may keep records only for IVF, so their success rates may be anecdotally based, not based on hard data.

Comparing clinics may also be hard if their statistics compare apples to oranges. For instance, a clinic that bases its pregnancy rates on a single positive pregnancy test is going to have better statistics than one whose statistics are based on live births, because many early pregnancies are miscarried. If a clinic report rates "per patient" rather than "per attempt," its rates will be higher, but you may not be told that each patient did ten IUIs before finally getting pregnant.

Because IUI and other medium-tech methods aren't overseen in the same way that IVF is, there is no national clearinghouse for statistics. However, a clinic that has good statistics for IVF probably also has good statistics for IUI and medium-tech infertility treatments, so you may get some idea of how the clinic you're considering compares.

Different Docs = Different Points of View: Sorting Things Out

Maybe good old Dr. Basic advocated that you try to get pregnant on your own for another six months. He told you he was certain that, in time, you would succeed. Meanwhile, on your first visit to specialist Dr. Perfect, he says that you don't have a minute to spare and that you should proceed immediately to a higher-tech approach. On the other side of town, your best friend, who is the same age as you, is being told that the high-tech method may not be the answer at all and that a more conservative approach is less taxing on the body and produces a healthier pregnancy in less time.

At some point in your fertility treatment, you'll understand that opinions are like noses: Everyone has one, and each one is a little bit different. Although you should adhere to certain accepted protocols and processes when seeking treatment and/or when stepping it up a notch (for example, having basic blood tests, ruling out structural problems via a hysterosalpingogram, and undergoing other such procedures), there are a variety of beliefs and practices on where to go from here.

Some doctors are more conservative in nature and/or prefer treatments involving lesser doses of medications. Other doctors like to be on the cutting edge of technology and use all the options available. Still others have their own theories that they're looking to prove, or disprove, through their extensive work with patients.

But, before you become unhinged at the thought of being a human guinea pig, remember that medicine, particularly fertility, is not an exact science. Many fields of medicine rely on the gold standard for scientific validation, which is proof of performance through randomized and controlled prospective studies. Some people say that the medications and procedures in the field of fertility that can claim this validation can be summarized in one page or less. This opinion doesn't reflect the intelligence or efforts of the physicians in the field. Rather, it is explained by the huge number of variables that can affect the outcome of such research, including age (of both partners), years spent trying to conceive, overall health, egg quality, protocol, and so on.

If your doctor recommends a protocol or treatment that seems off the deep end to you or is vastly different from those you've heard about, read about, or experienced firsthand, ask the doctor whether any research is available to sup-port this method of treatment. Keep in mind that a *retrospective study* (one where data is accumulated *after* the study is complete) is not as thorough as a prospective study. You may also want to look at the size of the group that has undergone this treatment. The higher the number, the more solid the data.

Knowing your rights

Since 1996, the U.S. government has been trying to put together and pass a comprehensive Patient's Bill of Rights. As of this writing, there still is no national Bill of Rights, although more than half the states have passed their own bills. In addition, many clinics and hospitals have written their own Bill of Rights for patients.

Individual states and institutions differ slightly, but most agree that as a patient you have a legal right to expect the following:

- To be treated without discrimination in regard to race, religion, sex, disability, or source of payment

- To receive considerate and respectful care

- To receive full disclosure of your medical condition

- To have the right to refuse procedures or treatments

- To fully participate in decision making about your care

- To receive all information necessary to give informed consent for any procedures

- To refuse to participate in research

- To receive an explanation of any charges

- To have the right to complain without fear of reprisal

- To have your privacy and confidentiality maintained

The rights mean that you, as a patient, have every right to know what is being done to you, why it's being done, and what the possible outcomes are. You also have every right to read your medical chart and to receive a copy of what's in it. Many people in the medical profession still remove your chart from the room when they leave you alone so that you can't read it. The reality is that you have every right to read what's in your chart.

You're also entitled to considerate and respectful care, which means that you have every right to complain if you feel you've been treated badly by any member of the staff, without worrying that someone will decide to take it out on you by treating you badly the next time you're in the office. There are, of course, right and wrong ways to get along with the staff, which we address in the section "Preparing for Your First Visit with Dr. Perfect," elsewhere in this chapter.

These rights are the least that you should expect from your clinic, and any clinic run by a truly caring staff will not be unhappy with you for expecting decent treatment.

If you're a hard-to-treat patient, because of age, egg quality, or other preexisting condition, you might do well with a doctor who is as up to date as possible and offers treatment plans designed to address your particular needs. I (coauthor Jackie) found great solace and hope in working with an out-of-town doctor. His practice consisted greatly of older women (that means over age 35 for those who resent the implication!) and those with high FSH levels, signifying diminishing ovarian reserve. My doctor's methods were off the beaten path just through his willingness to treat me and others like me, patients who may have been turned away by other doctors who look at age and FSH as immovable objects. However, my doctor, whom some people considered a bit out of the mainstream, was actually quite conservative in prescribing medication and treatment, allowing me to save money as well as wear and tear on my body and mind.

Finally, your decision of which doctor and protocol to pick should be influenced by your own history. Try not to compare yourself to others and their treatments. What works for your best friend or colleague may be a poor choice for you. That's not to say that you can't ask your doctor about different approaches, particularly if you've been unsuccessful with your current protocol over a period of time (meaning at least three attempts). However, the mixing-and-matching technique is better left to clothing decisions, not medical ones.

Try to avoid doctor shopping. A second opinion can be helpful, particularly if you feel that the recommended course of action is too aggressive or dramatic or poses risks to your health. However, keeping more than one doc on the clock will only confuse you and probably annoy the team that you have created from your top picks of doctors. Most doctors, whatever the field, have different methods of practicing, if not different approaches or beliefs. The cumulative approach isn't a good one when trying to get the best care possible. Instead, focus on finding the doctor who best suits your needs and let him or her decide which way to go.

Preparing for Your First Visit with Dr. Perfect

It's time to meet Dr. Perfect and friends. Come on into the waiting room, which, if you're lucky, has comfortable chairs and current magazines to read during the inevitably long wait for the doctor. If coffee and cookies are available in the waiting room, that's a nice touch, too, but don't push your luck too much. Even a water cooler is nice. Go on up to the window — it's time to meet the office staff.

Meeting the office staff

Your first contact will most likely be with the front desk receptionists. Start off on the right foot by arriving on time. Call ahead for directions to the office if you aren't familiar with the area, and call if you're going to be late.

You can tell a lot about the way an office is run by the response you get when you first walk up to the window. Does someone greet you right away, or are the receptionists too busy talking about someone's new hair stylist to look over at you? Are they polite, or do they seem frazzled, aggravated, or just plain bored with you?

You can make things easier at your first meeting by having your insurance information handy and being sure that you've brought any referrals needed with you.

If you're lucky, within a few minutes someone will interrupt your magazine reading, and a nurse will get your weight and height, take your blood pressure, and ask some questions before you see the doctor. Smaller offices usually have only one or two nurses, whom you'll get to know well; larger offices may have a cast of, well, not thousands but quite a few nurses. In some offices, the nurse takes your basic history; in other offices, the doctor asks you these questions. Expect to be asked all about your periods, reproductive history, and sex life.

If your partner is with you, he may be sent down the hall to see the andrologist. Andrologists specialize in the study of sperm, and they're responsible for analyzing semen specimens, storing frozen samples, and preparing sperm for use in IVF, IUI, or intracervical insemination (ICI)

While your partner is busy in andrology, you may be sent to the lab to have blood drawn. Not all infertility clinics have on-site labs to draw blood, but many do. The blood lab employees are people you want to be very, very nice to. You'll probably see them pretty frequently — always with a needle in their hand!

After your blood samples are drawn, you may be sent to ultrasound, where specially trained ultrasonographers do your ultrasounds and report their findings to the doctor. In some smaller centers, the doctor or a nurse performs your ultrasounds.

Making friends with everyone

As unfair as it may seem, the doctor's office staff is going to have a powerful influence on how your treatment progresses. Now, no employees are going to deliberately mess up your semen sample or lie about what they see on your ultrasound. Human nature dictates that people are nicest to people they like, however, so you want to be someone the office staff likes. When the front desk people like you, they work extra hard to change your appointment time if you need it, or they put your callback note for the doctor on top of the pile or put you directly through to the nurses instead of sending you to voice mail.

How do you make everyone, from the front desk receptionist to the ultrasound technicians, like you?

✔ Bring them food. Yes, that suggestion is obvious, but it works.

✔ Be nice. Don't sigh, glare at them, stare at the ceiling, make faces, or otherwise act annoyed when you talk to them.

✔ When the inevitable insurance or other conflict arises, be calm. Remember that it's usually not the office staff's fault, and they can only do so much to fix problems with your insurance.

✔ Use your full name when you call the nurses and give a brief overview of your history. The office where I (coauthor Sharon) work receives an unbelievable number of messages from people who leave only their first names. This may work if your name is unusual, but if your name is Sue or Mary, you can assume that there are lots of you in the practice. Leaving your history is also important. For you, it's the only history, but the nurse may have heard a hundred patient histories in the last week alone. As a result, she probably isn't going to remember exactly what the two of you talked about two weeks ago.

Knowing when and how to make waves

Sometimes you just can't be nice. When the staff has been rude, negligent, or otherwise inappropriate, you have to speak up. But there are ways to make waves, and ways not to:

✔ Don't scream, throw a tantrum, or threaten. Even if you fully intend to sue the office for whatever your problem is, don't threaten the staff with a lawsuit. Nothing raises hackles faster in a doctor's office, and your chances of resolving the issue are diminished.

✔ Don't have your partner call to scream, threaten, or throw a tantrum — at least not before you have a chance to tell him all the facts and maybe even sleep on it. Too many times, a partner sees his mate sobbing and immediately decides to do something about it, even if the woman was just going to drop the issue. If you ever want to go back to the office, you'll have a hard time facing everyone after your partner alienates everyone in the office.

✔ Don't complain to the wrong people. Don't complain to the blood lab about the nurses, or to the nurses about the andrologist. People in offices do talk to each other, and you can be sure that the person you told will find a way to let the person you talked about know what you really think about her.

✔ Don't blame the wrong office. For example, in our office (Sharon again), we treat patients literally from all over the world, meaning that our patients get blood tests and ultrasounds done in their area and have the results faxed to us. We're frequently yelled at because we don't have their results, when the problem lies with the office sending the results. Or it may lie with neither office, but with faxing, which sometimes seems to send results to a permanent black hole.

✔ Don't ask the office to do things that are illegal. Don't ask the staff to write prescriptions for you under your sister's name because she has insurance coverage and you don't. Don't ask for a false diagnosis on your insurance reports so your procedures will be covered, and then get mad when the staff won't do it. Doctors can lose their license for this type of fraud.

✔ Do stay calm when problems arise. Remember that it usually takes two people to resolve issues.

✔ Do complain appropriately. Write a letter to your doctor or discuss office problems with him, the office manager, or the head nurse.

✔ Do try not to take things personally. If you don't have an appointment and you come in for an ultrasound, expect that patients with appointments will be scanned before you will, even if they arrive after you did. That's only fair; most likely, no one is trying to punish you by making you wait. Nor is it likely that the nurses *always* lose your blood work or that the blood technician just *loves* to stick you twice.

✔ Do maintain a sense of humor. Funny things happen in a doctor's office, and sometimes they happen to you. If you can laugh along when things go wrong, you'll keep your blood pressure down and maintain your reputation as a great patient, one whom everyone goes out of the way for.

Facing the Stranger in Your Sex Life — Treatment and Your Loss of Privacy

When going through fertility treatment, you open the door to your private life — yes, including your sex life — for all the medical world to see. This loss of privacy is bound to happen and takes some getting used to.

Your doctor (and his staff!) would rather discuss things other than your sex life (like their sex lives for instance!). They will not discuss your private life in their private lives. Their job, however, is to help you conceive a baby, and their inquiries are part of the process. Once again, consider this good training for pregnancy, when your body and your life will be oft-discussed topics with your physicians, your friends, and even your in-laws.

The frequency of intercourse, the quality of your menstrual cycles, and your past history of pregnancies, whether by hit or miss, are crucial bits of information in piecing together your reproductive profile. Offer information gladly because doing so only helps to educate your medical team. Feel free, however, to leave out the details that truly define intimacy. Remember that sexual intercourse is a biological process. Intimacy may occur in or out of the bedroom, and the specifics of that are all your own.

Discussing Dollars with the Doctor

When I (coauthor Jackie) visited Dr. Badadventure for the first time, I was quickly whisked away to meet with Mr. Dollars and Sense, the finance guy. It should have been a warning. Needless to say, my fertility experience with Dr. Badadventure cost considerable dollars and yielded pennies in results.

We're not saying that you should turn tail and flee when the mention of payment comes up. Fertility doctors and clinics are for-profit institutions, so they're permitted and expected to make money from their patients. Most clinics ask for payment upfront for certain procedures, including extensive testing, surgery, and in vitro fertilization. Don't be offended. Because many insurers don't cover fertility, doctors do need to guarantee payment for their time, services, and staff. However, your initial health assessment and plan for treatment should come before you receive a price list for procedures. If you feel like you're getting a hard sell toward high-tech fertility from the finance guy (not the fertility doc), you probably are. If, however, your doctor determines, after careful review of you and your records, that high tech is the way to go, expect the issue of cost and payment to come up. You don't want to be surprised by a bill in the tens of thousands of dollars.

Use your judgment and intuition in deciding whether your fertility doc is too financially motivated for your liking. The financial call should be yours, not your physician's. His or her job is to recommend the best course of action for you, outlining the probabilities for success, the risks, and the costs. It's then up to you, not the finance guy, to decide. For more information on dealing with the costs of fertility treatment, see Chapter 11.

When Dr. Perfect Turns You Down

Imagine yourself sitting on the edge of your chair in Dr. Perfect's office, watching him sift through your paperwork. He looks up, kindly puts one hand over yours, and says, "I'm sorry, but there's nothing we can do for you here."

And you sit, bewildered, wondering what on earth you did to make him issue such a pronouncement. Is it legal to refuse to treat patients? Is it ethical? What did you do wrong?

Doctors can refuse, legally and ethically, to treat a patient if they feel that a patient won't be helped by their treatment. So if you get the "there's the door — don't let it hit you on the way out" speech (and even if the doctor couches it in kindly terms, that's what it will feel like), getting angry at the doctor won't help. He's telling you that, in his honest opinion, he can't help you get pregnant.

So take a deep breath, let the tears come even if the doctor looks embarrassed, and ask why. Is your FSH (follicle-stimulating hormone) level higher than normal? If it is, some doctors feel that your ovarian reserve, or the number of good eggs you have left, is too low for you to get pregnant. Is it your age? If you're over 45, your chances of getting pregnant are very low, but they're not zero. In both of these cases, your doctor may recommend that you use donor eggs.

If you have a problem with your uterus that can't be fixed, then you may need a gestational carrier. If it's a sperm problem, you may need to use donor sperm. If you have Turner syndrome (a chromosomal abnormality that results in small or absent ovaries) or POF (premature ovarian failure), you'll need donor eggs.

The point here is that even if Dr. Perfect says he can't work with you, he may mean that he can't work with you *unless*

✔ You use donor eggs.

✔ You use donor sperm.

✔ You hire a gestational carrier.

✔ You rely on any combination of the above.

In other words, he may not be saying that you'll never have a family. He *may* be saying that you'll have to go a different route (see Chapters 16 and 18) to create a family. And although *he* may not have had any success treating women with your particular history, another doctor may have. It's time to start investigating your options.

Even though you've been turned down by one doctor, other doctors may still be willing to treat you. Some practices specialize in older women or women with high FSH. Now may be the time to revisit the Internet bulletin boards and see whether another doctor out there is available to work with you.

Knowing When to Switch Doctors

So you've tried and tried and tried some more with your initial doctor of choice. Despite your efforts, he or she isn't sensitive to your needs, whether they're physical, emotional, or financial. Perhaps your doctor is stuck in a time warp of sorts, insisting that *eventually* you'll conceive naturally, or with minimal intervention, despite the fact that you've been trying for months or years with no success and a loudly ticking biological clock. Or else your doctor is pushing for expensive, invasive treatment that you don't feel prepared for. Your doctor may be the sort who travels from one office to another, meaning that he or she is virtually inaccessible, except for those occasional appointments.

Any of these reasons, or no particular reason at all, is perfectly understandable in your decision to switch doctors. The personalities of some patients and doctors just clash. For many, this alone can be a reason to run.

Preparing to lose time

Keep in mind that switching doctors results in an inevitable delay in treatment. Sending records to your new physician and giving him or her time to review them take time. Some doctors may choose to repeat tests in their labs to assure accuracy and/or to convert your previous results to their standard levels of measurement. Other doctors may hit the ground running, declining to repeat previous tests and putting you into one of their protocols immediately. Whatever the case, your new doctor needs an adjustment period to become familiar with your body and its response. Fertility is a very individual science, one whose results vary from patient to patient. For that reason, your new physician needs to observe you for a while. Doing so is part of the process.

If you're okay with this slight setback (or if you figure that *anyone* is better than your current doctor), then batten down the hatches and prepare to move on. To avoid unnecessary delays in treatment, meet with your new doctor or potential choices before severing ties with your former doctor. Have a plan in place before moving on. Once your future is secure, you'll want to address your current situation. You don't have to speak directly with your physician regarding your choice and/or your reasons for it. You can request that records be transferred through the front desk staff, or you can sign a release of information in your new doctor's office, which can get the records for you.

If you want to keep the lines of communication open, consider scheduling an appointment with your current doctor to discuss your dissatisfaction and your decision to move on. If your problems with your doctor/staff are due to miscommunication, this tête-à-tête may resolve the situation for you. A less direct approach is to terminate your care in a letter. I (coauthor Jackie) left my first doctor because I felt that he wasn't aggressive enough in his treatment. After a bad experience on the other side of the pendulum, I found myself back in Doctor #1's office, begging him to take me back. Luckily, I had taken the time to write him a very nice Dear John letter before leaving his practice. Instead of blaming him for my infertility, I told him that I wanted to sample a different approach. When I came back with my tail between my legs, he gladly took me in.

Remembering that there are no guarantees

If you switch doctors, remember that doing something different doesn't automatically mean that the results will necessarily follow suit. Many women do get pregnant after switching doctors, but many do not. If you're simply impatient with the process, not the practitioner, you may be better off waiting it out in your current situation. If you're unhappy with the support staff (nurses and front office people) in your doctor's office, remember that you're not guaranteed that a change will solve the problem. Keep in mind that the practice of fertility means long hours for everyone involved. The nurse who seems curt on the phone is probably faced with a huge backlog of patient callbacks. The receptionist who is less than friendly is busy ferrying patients and phone calls and may indeed be a little frazzled.

If you're at a standoff with the nursing staff and/or not receiving correct information, consider discussing the issue with those people and, if necessary, with your physician or the office manager. And remember, as long as the nurses and other staff are providing you with the correct information in a timely matter, the doctor is the one whom you must ultimately like, respect, have confidence in, and feel comfortable with. If that relationship isn't working, then it *is* time to move on.

Understanding What Your Doctor Says

Doctors and nurses aren't *really* trying to confuse you when they spew forth a list of initials or shortcut terms. But when your doctor says something like "Get an HSG and a sono, and then if your APA and FSH come back okay, we'll start the stims," your immediate reaction may be "Huh?"

When I (coauthor Sharon) give a patient instructions, I try to give her terms that are easy to remember. You're more likely to remember that you need an HSG than a hysterosalpingogram (which we discuss in more detail in Chapter 7), a mouthful that even professionals have difficulty saying correctly.

Whenever you don't understand what the doctor or nurse just said, ask the person to stop and explain. Don't write it down, thinking that you'll look it up later, or nod just to look like you know what they're talking about. Of course, you can read Chapter 7 thoroughly before your visit, and then you'll have a pretty good understanding of what's going on. You may even be able to dazzle the staff by interjecting a long, initial-studded sentence of your own!

Verifying exactly what your doctor said

Some of the biggest misunderstandings begin with a simple lack of communication: Someone says one thing, and someone else hears another thing. Don't let this happen with your fertility treatment!

As you move along in your course of action, you may find it important, even necessary, to take notes when your doctor is speaking. Some choose to tape record their conversations with their doctor. In either case, taking notes or using a tape recorder can be a helpful tool in relaying this information to your partner or to your cousin who is a doctor. Always ask your doctor if doing so is okay, particularly when it comes to taping your discussions. Most doctors are glad to accommodate you. However, most _people_ (including doctors) become a bit unhinged if they find out that they were being taped secretly.

You may find it helpful to enlist a second set of ears as well. This can be a perfect spot for your partner to participate! Fertility is an emotional subject. Especially if the doctor is addressing problems that _you_ have, you may be too close to the situation to hear and understand all the options that are available. Your partner or a friend may be a bit more detached and better able to comprehend and communicate the information to you. Many fertility patients view themselves (incorrectly!) in a battle against their doctors. In this case, you may be more open to your partner's interpretation of what the doctor has said. Either way, try to remember that your doctor _is_ on your side. Your doctor is your advocate, and part of that duty involves giving you the complete picture, good and bad.

I (coauthor Jackie) also found my husband's presence to be comforting, both during and after my doctor's appointments. When I was convinced that the doctor was cataloging me as hopeless, my husband would do a good job to reel me in and help me hear the words, rather than try to interpret the feelings (which more often than not would be my own). And while my memory had the potential of rewriting history, my husband kept a second account of the event that I could cling to.

Keeping your own (hit) records

Fertility is certainly a project that can generate a lot of paperwork.

After initially relying on only my doctor's records, I (coauthor Jackie) eventually discovered the need to keep my own records as well. The process was simple, but the organization was not. After every doctor's appointment, monitoring visit, or blood test, I asked for a copy of my records from that day. My records often consisted of nothing more than my notations from the day's blood work results, which I would date and keep in a separate folder. My records proved invaluable during the course of my treatment. Seldom did I have a question that couldn't be answered by reviewing my own information. I was able to compare my results from different cycles to see how I was faring in a historical sense. And, when the time came to switch doctors, I had my own history to present to my new doctor at our first visit.

Keeping your own records certainly provides you with a point of reference as you go through your treatment. Doing so also allows you to double-check doctor's instructions and test results if the communication with your clinic is less than perfect.

As a cautionary note (from one who knows!), try to avoid making your records nighttime reading. If you bring this paperwork to bed with you, you may be becoming a wee bit obsessive about the process. This type of behavior will not help your cause or your sleeping patterns. A lighthearted magazine or book that has nothing to do with fertility is a better sleep aid.

Reviewing your information periodically and having an extra set of records for your files are very helpful to your treatment. Trying to diagnose yourself based on your past performance is a job better left to the pros. Your records are your backup. Your doctors are still the front line.

Deciding Whether to Make Fertility a Full-Time Pursuit

Managing any type of chronic health condition can feel like a full-time activity. Fertility is no exception. Particularly if you're involved in IVF or another high-tech process, you may find that doctor's appointments, ultrasound monitoring, and blood tests chip away at your week rather quickly.

Most fertility doctors offer early office hours (6:30 to 8:00 a.m.) for working patients to monitor their cycles. Others offer after-work hours.

I (coauthor Jackie) found that fertility could take up as little or as much time as I allowed. I could go for daily testing, taking an hour out of my day, and then forget about it. Or I could go for testing, pore over my previous records and results, talk with my husband, log on to chat rooms to compare notes, and anxiously wait by the phone for my next set of instructions. The latter option certainly took up more time than my regular full-time job.

Discipline and time management skills can help keep fertility in its proper perspective. Many fertility patients find that their part- or full-time job can *stop* them from obsessing by requiring them to focus on something else. Your extra time spent worrying won't actually change your results or eventual outcome. If anything, this obsessiveness and worry only hinder your attempts.

You may find that certain processes of fertility treatment may require you to take a few days off here and there. Most of these procedures are on the high-tech side and may include diagnostic surgery, such as a laparoscopy, or in vitro fertilization. Generally, you're given adequate time to prepare for this and to schedule time off if necessary. If you must travel for treatment, you may also need to take time off work. However, in the normal course of events, other than time before or after a surgical procedure, fertility treatment can fit into your regular schedule, albeit making it a little more hectic. Rather than bemoan this stepped-up pace, consider it a blessing. Having unlimited amounts of time to sit around and contemplate your unexpanding navel does you no good.

Chapter 9

A Little Help from Dr. Perfect: Intrauterine Insemination and Fertility Injections

*S*tarting an IUI (intrauterine insemination) cycle or a stimulated medication cycle is a big step up from just trying to figure out when you're ovulating and planning to have sex accordingly. IUI cycles involve monitoring blood and ultrasound results, and often involve injecting potent hormone stimulators called gonadotropins.

In this chapter, we explain how IUI and stimulated cycles work and discuss some of the testing involved and the medications you may be taking. We also help you find those expensive gonadotropins as cheaply as possible, and we give you tips on how to inject them as safely as possible.

Deciding How Much Treatment You Need

There are several roads to travel when seeing a fertility doctor, and which one Dr. Perfect places you on depends on your reason for infertility. If the problem is diagnosed as mild male factor (a slightly lower than normal sperm count or motility), Dr. Perfect will probably suggest doing an IUI.

If your partner's sperm is fine, you may just be monitored with blood work and ultrasounds to be sure that you're making an adequate follicle and releasing an egg every month. Your doctor may do an *intracervical insemination* (ICI), a procedure in which the fresh sperm is inserted into the cervix.

If your partner's sperm count or motility is low, your doctor will probably suggest doing an IUI so that the sperm can be "washed" and concentrated and then placed directly into the uterus.

If you're not producing an egg or not releasing an egg, you may be prescribed stimulating medications to increase egg production. If you're getting your period less than two weeks after you ovulate, your doctor may prescribe progesterone for a suspected luteal phase defect, which we explain in the next section.

If you've gone several months without a positive pregnancy test, you may end up doing all three: IUI, gonadotropins (stimulating medications), and progesterone.

Treating Luteal Phase Defects

Luteal phase, in fertility circles, means the two weeks after you ovulate and before your period starts. You may be diagnosed with *luteal phase defect (LPD)* if your period starts ten or so days after you ovulate, rather than the normal two-week period. If you've been monitoring your BBT (basal body temperature), you may see an early drop in your temperature as well. LPD can be caused by the following problems with the corpus luteum or with the uterine lining.

After you ovulate, the leftover shell of your follicle, now called the *corpus luteum,* starts to produce progesterone. Progesterone stimulates the uterine lining to produce extra blood vessels so that the embryo has a good supply to support its growth if it attaches.

A poorly developed follicle, or one that releases an abnormal egg, won't put out enough progesterone to properly develop the lining. In this case, the treatment is not more progesterone after you ovulate, but stimulating medications to produce a better-quality follicle.

Sometimes you have a follicle that doesn't release the egg inside. This follicle may produce some progesterone, and you may think you've ovulated, but you won't get pregnant, because the egg was never released. An ultrasound before and after your LH surge can help diagnose this syndrome, which is called *luteinized unruptured follicle syndrome* (LUFS).

Some women have a uterine lining that doesn't respond normally to progesterone, and in these cases, progesterone supplements may be helpful. The
best way to evaluate your lining is to have an endometrial biopsy done; an
ultrasound done a week after you ovulate can also show if your lining is
changing to a pattern needed for implantation.

If you get your period less than two weeks after you ovulate, it's important
to have a biopsy done to check your progesterone. An *endometrial biopsy*
involves scraping a little of your uterine lining with a small curette. The
scraping is then checked to see whether the lining contains the proper
amount of progesterone. A biopsy is done in your doctor's office, usually
the day of a negative pregnancy test before your period starts.

"Artificial" Insemination? No, It's Real!

Artificial insemination may sound like it's a fake procedure, but it's the real
thing. *Artificial insemination* (another term for intrauterine insemination or
intracervical insemination) means simply that sperm is placed into either the
cervix or uterus to give it a "leg up" on getting where it needs to go, which is
to your egg.

You may or may not be taking stimulating medications to create more eggs
during an IUI or ICI cycle. Some doctors start with Clomid, a pill given to
increase your egg output, and move up after a few months to stimulation
with gonadotropins. Others may simply monitor your normal cycle and
inseminate, hoping to fertilize the one or possibly two follicles you produce
each month.

Measuring your chance for success

Many doctors say that artificial insemination will not increase your chances
over timed intercourse, if you have a normal semen analysis and normal postcoital test (see Chapter 7 for more about both). Neither IUI nor ICI will be effective if the problem is severe male factor (a very low sperm count or antisperm
antibodies) or blocked tubes.

Although statistics reported for IUI seem to vary widely, most clinics claim
about a 10 to 15 percent per month success rate for women under age 35,
with decreasing success as your age goes up. Producing more than one follicle a month by using Clomid or gonadotropins also increases your chances
of pregnancy per month. Many experts believe that your chance of getting
pregnant after six failed IUIs is slim unless you do in vitro fertilization.

Collecting sperm

When your partner is directed to produce a semen sample in a cup, you may have a mental picture of a little paper drinking cup. Of course, no clinics use paper cups to collect sperm — at least, we hope they're not. Clinics give the guys a plastic sterile container for this purpose.

Semen collection and concentration are a big part of IUI. Several methods are used both to collect and to concentrate the sperm:

- ✔ **Clean container collection:** A sterile container is used to collect the sample obtained through masturbation.

- ✔ **Condom collection:** A special condom containing no lubricants or spermicides is used if the semen sample has to be collected during intercourse. This method is useful for those whose religious beliefs prohibit masturbation.

- ✔ **Split ejaculate:** This method of collecting uses a two-part container; the first "squirt" of ejaculate goes into one part, and the rest goes into the second part. Obviously, this method requires some coordination. The advantage to this collection is that the first bit has the highest concentration of sperm, so using it for insemination results in a higher sperm concentration.

Don't be insulted if the andrologist (the person who deals with sperm) asks whether there was any spillage. This isn't a comment on your general clumsiness or the look of your sample! The first part of the semen has the highest concentration of sperm, so if any was lost, your semen sample may not be as good as it should be.

Sperm need to be "washed" before they're ready for IUI. (ICI sperm aren't washed after collection.) Washing must be done because unwashed sperm contain large amounts of prostaglandins, chemicals that cause smooth muscle contractions. If a large amount of semen — more than 0.2 ml — is injected unwashed into the uterus, the prostaglandins can cause severe cramping at the least and a shocklike, life-threatening reaction at worst.

If you're picturing the washing process being done in a little machine with a spin cycle, you're partially right! Sperm are spun down into a little pellet in a centrifuge before being placed in the uterus. One method spins the sperm in a centrifuge, and another puts the sperm on the bottom of a test tube and allows the best sperm to swim up. Another common method used puts the sperm on top of several layers of washing media; the tube is spun down, and the pellet on the bottom will contain the largest amount of motile, healthy sperm. The sperm pellet is then placed via catheter into the uterus.

The main risks of doing IUI are risk of infection and risk of multiple births if you're taking medication to stimulate growth of more than one follicle.

Checking out your egg

IUI, ICI, and timed intercourse (timed for your ovulation) will work only if the sperm is placed in the right place at the right time — when you have a mature egg. Making sure that you're making a follicle and checking it for maturity before an IUI increase your chances of pregnancy.

Monitoring your hormone level

One way to be sure you're making a good egg is to monitor your hormone levels. As you start to make a mature egg, your estradiol starts to rise. A good egg should produce an estradiol of 150 to 300 pg/ml. About 30 hours before your egg releases, your LH will also start to rise; a good LH surge is usually over 40.

Thar she blows: Ultrasounds before and after ovulation

Many fertility doctors use pelvic ultrasound to monitor the growth of ovarian follicles. Ultrasound works by bouncing high-frequency sound waves off internal organs. Unlike X-rays, ultrasounds don't expose you to radiation. There are two types of pelvic ultrasound:

- **Transvaginal ultrasound:** This procedure uses a long, wandlike probe that can be embarrassing if you're very modest. In addition, the moving probe can cause uncomfortable pressure. This method, which can be done with an empty bladder, gives better images than abdominal ultrasounds in most cases.

  For a transvaginal ultrasound, you undress from the waist down, cover yourself with a sheet, and lie flat on your back with your legs in typical exam table stirrups. The ultrasound technician or your doctor inserts the vaginal probe after covering the tip with transducing jelly and placing a condom over it. The tip of the wand is smaller than a vaginal speculum. Some centers ask you to insert the probe yourself. The technician moves the wand from side to side to record good pictures of your ovaries and uterus.

- **Abdominal ultrasound:** This procedure requires a full bladder. The images aren't usually as clear as the transvaginal ultrasound.

  For an abdominal ultrasound, you pull your pants down to the pubic hair line. Jelly is placed directly on your stomach, and the technician then moves the transducer (a small hand-held device about the size of your hand) over it. Be aware that, because you have a full bladder, this pressure can be uncomfortable.

A full bladder is needed for abdominal ultrasound for this reason: The uterus and ovaries normally lie behind the intestines, but a full bladder moves the uterus back and pushes the intestine up, so the uterus and ovaries can be seen more clearly. The bladder also provides a fluid contrast that makes the uterus easier to identify.

There are no known side effects from ultrasound. When your ultrasound is finished, you can go home with no special instructions.

If your doctor does ultrasounds during the first two weeks of your cycle, you'll see your follicle growing as your estradiol rises and your LH surges; usually the follicle is about 22 to 25 millimeters at the time of ovulation. Many centers do an ultrasound the day of IUI and the day after, to make sure that the egg has released from the follicle; when this happens, the follicle shrinks on ultrasound. Without a release ultrasound, you may be making a good follicle but not having the egg release. Pregnancy can't occur unless the egg releases.

Moving Up to Controlled Ovarian Hyperstimulation

Clomid is usually the first drug given to start your follicles growing because it can be given orally and has fewer side effects than injections. If Clomid isn't working for you after a few months, your doctor may suggest moving up to the big time: injecting gonadotropins, a technique called *controlled ovarian hyperstimulation,* or COH for short. We talk about gonadotropins in the section "Defining gonadotropins," later in this chapter.

Understanding the need for injections

With COH, the goal is to make more than one or two follicles. The reasoning is that if you make a few more follicles, you have a better chance of getting pregnant each month. The chance of pregnancy with one egg each month is between 5 and 20 percent, depending on your age.

Because pills pass through your intestinal tract and your liver, they're not as well absorbed as injections, and they may not be as effective in making more than one follicle. So the logical next step, if you're not making follicles on Clomid, is to move up to injections.

Obviously, taking injections is a big step. Not only do you have a possibility of making too many follicles when taking injectable stimulating medications, but you also have to deal with the logistics of COH, including going in for frequent blood tests and ultrasounds and finding someone to give you your injections. Some clinics may offer to give the injections, usually for a small fee, but others want your partner or someone else to come in and learn how to give the shots.

Getting injections from your partner

Believe it or not, most partners do very well giving injections — after the first few times, that is. Giving shots is a learning experience, and unfortunately, *you* are the learning tool in this experience.

Your clinic will probably show you and your partner how to give injections, and it may send you home with a video and an informational tearsheet that you'll refer to frequently in the first few days.

Is it really safe to put a needle in the hand of a totally untrained person and tell them to have at it? Statistically speaking, yes. Millions of diabetics inject themselves every day or have someone else do it. The biggest risks are from infection and hitting a nerve. You can prevent infection with a careful sterile technique, and hitting a nerve can happen to anyone, even a professional, because your anatomy may not look like the textbook picture.

If at all possible, insist on doing your first injection in front of someone at your clinic, so a person skilled in this procedure can critique and give pointers. Also, after you and your partner have done it once, your partner is less likely to pass out the first time you do an injection at home.

Giving yourself shots

Sometimes, for whatever reason, you may have to give yourself the shots. Maybe you don't have a partner, maybe your partner is locked in the bathroom refusing to give you a shot, or maybe you travel a lot. You can inject yourself, although it's a bit trickier.

If you know that you'll be doing your own injections, ask your doctor if he can give you subcutaneous gonadotropins. These are injected with a very tiny needle — like a diabetic needle — and can be used in the top of your leg, in your stomach, or in the back of your arm, although this latter site is a hard place to inject yourself. Subcutaneous gonadotropins are *recombinant* — meaning that they're made in the lab from animal, not human, proteins — and they have less impurities than urinary-based gonadotropins, so they can be injected subcutaneously without causing a rash. The medication your doctor orders depends on whether he believes you need the extra LH found in urinary products.

If you end up taking intramuscular injections, such as Pergonal or Humegon, made from human urinary proteins, standing in front of a mirror when you give them may be helpful. Or ask your clinic if you can inject them into the top of your leg.

Your doctor may recommend that you take all medication intramuscularly if your body mass index (BMI) is over 30, so that the medications will be absorbed better.

Defining gonadotropins

Gonadotropins are stimulating medications (see Chapter 21), meaning that they make follicles grow. Each follicle should contain an egg, so making five follicles each month rather than one or two gives you a better shot at getting pregnant.

Gonadotropins contain either all follicle-stimulating hormone (FSH) or a combination of FSH and luteinizing hormone (LH). Pure FSH (also called recombinant FSH) is manufactured in the lab by several manufacturers and is the most expensive — about $60 a vial. Gonadotropins made from human proteins — in this case, urine — contain some LH because filtering all the LH out of urine is hard. Some doctors prefer that you have a little LH because they feel it aids stimulation, while others prefer a pure FSH product. Urinary products are cheaper and most need to be injected intramuscularly; they cost about $35 a vial.

Some doctors have definite preferences about which type and brand of drug you should take. Sometimes the preference is medical, and sometimes it depends on which drug company representative has been in the office most recently.

Exploring the side effects

Because these drugs contain hormones, you can expect to be more hormonal when taking them. The most common side effects are headache, bloating, weight gain, and mood swings. Obviously, the hormone changes are going to be a big part of making a stressful situation worse for some people.

Deciding which medication to use

The choice between recombinant, pure FSH and urine-based LH/FSH combination medications depends on several things:

- Which medication does your doctor feel most comfortable working with? If your doctor has a preference, ask him why. He may have done or read studies that have influenced his opinion that one is better than the other.

✔ Do you have drug coverage? Which medication will it cover? If your prescription plan covers only one type of injectable, that's probably what you'll get. If you have no drug coverage, you may want to go with what's least expensive.

✔ How needlephobic are you? If you're extremely needlephobic, you'll need to go with subcutaneous medications (see the section "Giving yourself shots," earlier in this chapter) or risk being a wreck for two weeks, dreading each shot.

✔ Do you have someone to give you your injections? If you'll be doing most of your shots yourself, you'll probably want to do subcutaneous injections.

✔ Have you taken one or the other in the past? How did you respond? If you've taken stimulating medications before, you have some kind of track record. Did you do well on that medication? If not, you'll probably want to try something different. If you did well, you may want to do the same, because changing to something else may change your results.

Recombinant medications are more expensive — about a third more — because they're produced in the lab. But they're all given subcutaneously.

Urinary LH/FSH products are less expensive, but they need to be intramuscularly injected because the proteins in them can cause skin rashes.

New, nearly pure urinary FSH products can be given subcutaneously and are a little cheaper than recombinant products. Chapter 21 contains the names of all the current stimulating medications and their manufacturers.

Mimicking nature with a minipump

A somewhat newer method of getting your ovaries to respond to hormones and make an egg involves an infusion pump. The pump, which can administer either intravenous or subcutaneous doses of gonadotropin-releasing hormone (GnRH), attempts to mimic nature by releasing a small dose of GnRH every 90 minutes. This stimulates your body to produce LH and FSH.

The benefits of the pump over LH and FSH injections are the following:

✔ It doesn't require daily injections.

✔ Ovarian hyperstimulation syndrome, described in the section "Ensuring proper monitoring throughout your cycle," later in this chapter, is not as common.

✔ You have less chance of a multiple pregnancy.

Disadvantages of the pump are the following:

- ✔ It's expensive.
- ✔ It must be inserted and refilled by a physician.
- ✔ It increases the chance of infection.

Injecting hCG to mature your eggs

The last injection you'll take when doing COH is called hCG, or *human chorionic gonadotropin,* a luteinizing hormone substitute given to mature your eggs and help them release from their follicles. It's usually given a day or two before your IUI.

Not all doctors give hCG. Some doctors prefer to see whether you release your egg on your own. Taking gonadotropins sometimes affects your follicle release. Your LH may rise but may not rise enough to mature and rupture the follicle and release the egg. If this happens, you'll probably be given hCG. If you have an adequate LH surge on your own, you won't need to take hCG.

HCG helps the eggs in the follicles to mature and complete the cell division needed before they can be fertilized. HCG is made by several companies (see Chapter 21) and is usually given intramuscularly; a newer laboratory-created hCG called Ovidrel can be given subcutaneously.

Don't take nonsteroidal anti-inflammatories such as aspirin, Motrin, or ibuprofen during the middle part of your cycle. They may inhibit prostaglandin production, which may keep you from ovulating.

Ensuring proper monitoring throughout your cycle

If you're taking stimulating medications of any kind — injectables or Clomid — your clinic may want to monitor you to make sure that you're not making too many eggs. Some centers will cancel your IUI or insist that you do in vitro fertilization if you're making a lot of eggs, because the risk of hyperstimulation and getting pregnant with triplets — or more — is increased.

Ovarian hyperstimulation syndrome (OHSS) is a serious complication that could land you in the hospital. It starts when you take injectable stimulating medications and make a lot of follicles. If your estradiol rises over 1500, OHSS may occur; it's more common with IVF but can also occur with IUI cycles. Some symptoms of OHSS are the following:

- ✔ Difficulty urinating
- ✔ Difficulty breathing
- ✔ Sudden weight gain of ten pounds or more

If you have OHSS, your clinic may want to monitor your blood count, liver function, weight, and urine output. OHSS may not resolve itself for several weeks, and symptoms may worsen if you're pregnant.

OHSS isn't the only complication of taking gonadotropins or Clomid; multiple pregnancies of five or more babies are usually the result of stimulating medications. These high-order multiples are more often the result of IUI or timed intercourse than IVF because IVF can control the number of embryos put back into the uterus, whereas IUI can't. The number of follicles you have is the number of babies you could end up with!

Boosting Progesterone

Because progesterone is essential to maintain pregnancy, many doctors give progesterone supplements in pill, suppository, or injection form to all their infertility patients on an "it can't hurt and might help" basis. Most doctors want to see a progesterone blood level of at least 10 and preferably 15 ng/ml after ovulation.

Another way to raise progesterone levels is to give HCG "boosters," usually a 2,500 IU injection of hCG every few days. HCG stimulates the corpus luteum so that it puts out more progesterone. The disadvantage to boosters is that your pregnancy test will be positive, even if you're not pregnant, for up to ten days after the last hCG injection.

If you've taken gonadotropins, you may be given both progesterone and estrogen supplements after you ovulate. Your doctor may prescribe them because gonadotropins can affect embryo implantation in several ways.

Gonadotropins can shorten the luteal phase; progesterone is given to make sure the two-week wait actually *is* two weeks, so the embryo has time to implant before the lining starts to break down.

Stimulated cycles usually result in higher than normal estrogen levels. Higher estrogen may cause the lining of your uterus, where the embryo will implant, to develop too quickly. When the embryo arrives in the uterus, the lining may have developed past the point where an embryo can attach to it.

Higher estrogen levels can also affect the movement of the embryo through the fallopian tubes. If the embryo moves too quickly or too slowly through the tubes, the lining won't be ready for it to implant when it arrives in the uterus.

A few recent studies have shown that the ratio of progesterone to estrogen is as important as the actual values of each. Some doctors are now giving both estrogen and progesterone after ovulation to patients who've taken stimulating medications, to keep the estrogen and progesterone in proper balance during the luteal phase.

Getting Your Medications for Less

As any smart shopper knows, it's always best to avoid paying the retail price. Instead, look for outlets, sales, and other bargains that can help you get the same product for less money. In this section, we discuss some of the "deals" available when purchasing fertility medications.

Shopping at mail-order pharmacies

Many doctors suggest that you order your medications from one of the mail-order pharmacies now specializing in fertility medications. (See Chapter 21 for a list of some of the biggest mail-order pharmacies.) These pharmacies carry all fertility medications, can ship quickly, and often offer the best prices. In addition, they may provide 24-hour access to nurses or pharmacists who can answer questions for you and Web sites that address common concerns. Many mail-order pharmacies offer overnight shipping at no additional cost with a minimum order. Many mail-order pharmacies also provide booklets, tapes, and hotlines to provide you with information any time of the day or night. Another added benefit is virtual anonymity. You won't risk standing next to a nosy neighbor who's certain to share your fertility battle with the neighborhood, if not the world. Mail-order pharmacies are subject to the same Food and Drug Administration (FDA) regulations as your corner drugstore and are completely safe to use.

If you're paying for your medications out of pocket and every penny saved is important, your doctor may be able to order your medications from pharmacies based in Canada or Europe. They provide generic or other name-brand equivalents to the United States prescriptions. For example, Puregon is a gonadotropin that is pure FSH, similar to Follistim, and is commonly distributed in the United Kingdom and throughout Europe. Pergonal is another FSH/LH combo that is more popular in Canada. Although some fertility patients swear by one name brand or the other, most patients find that the drugs are interchangeable, as long as they contain the same amounts of LH and/or FSH.

One advantage to offshore pharmacies is that the costs can be significantly cheaper than those in the United States. Keep in mind that you'll pay more for shipping charges and you can't count on overnight delivery in a pinch. In addition, beware of recent holdups at customs for drugs being shipped to the United States from Europe. The FDA can, and will, occasionally hold an order and/or stop delivery of overseas prescriptions if it believes that its standards aren't being met by the provider. Pressure from local drug companies to avoid being undercut by foreign competitors is also a contributing factor. Although this has occurred with orders from Europe, it's not often the case for Canadian-based facilities.

Before completing your order, ask whether the pharmacy has had any problems with United States delivery. Your medications, even those bought at a good price, will do you no good if they're stuck in customs!

Making a quick trip over the border

If the mountain won't come to you, maybe it's time to venture to the mountain! For those adventurous types who would rather use the drive-through to get low-cost medications, consider a trip over the border. Mexico and Canada are both sources for lower-cost medications, and for some people, they're only a car ride away. Do remember, however, that the standard in the United States, set by the FDA, is quite rigid, and you have no guarantee that other countries will employ the same quality controls. The more Westernized a country, the more likely it is to maintain standards similar to those of the United States. But if you want the security of homegrown products, the only option is to stay home!

When we speak of going over the border to buy medications, we're not referring to scoring fertility drugs from the guy on the corner. Your only source should be the local pharmacy. Some individuals and couples join forces and elect a representative to travel across the border and fill prescriptions for the group.

Turning to drug studies or "leftover" drugs

Another option for low-cost or no-cost medications is to get involved in a drug or protocol study, which is generally run by larger institutions or drug companies. Ask your doctor if he is aware of any existing studies for which you may qualify. Internet bulletin boards also have this information, and other fertility patients often pass along information on studies that their doctors or others are conducting. Studies usually provide only free medications. You would still be required to pay for any procedures, such as IUI or IVF.

You will also find that many doctors are the recipients of medications that have been donated from former patients. Generally, this reserve is used for emergencies (for example, when you break your last vial, and the pharmacy is out). However, some physicians help out a patient whose protocol has run a little longer, and a little more expensive, than planned. It never hurts to ask!

Deciding How Long to Keep Trying

The odds have it. As with most fertility procedures, the numbers help to give you an indication of how likely you are to conceive and (for some) how long conception might take. You may find that a lot of data is available regarding in vitro fertilization, but much less data is available for some of the medium-tech methods, such as IUI. You may also notice that every doctor has a different take on your odds for success. Although most doctors quote you numbers that reflect their *own* success with any given process, they may also alter them a bit to better reflect your age or your response to treatment so far.

Many doctors use the "three strikes and you're out" rule. In other words, they have you try a particular method three times and then move on to something else if that approach doesn't work. Others point out that if a particular protocol hasn't worked by (for example) the fourth try, the odds of success are greatly diminished.

Speaking on my own behalf, my husband and I (coauthor Jackie)were beyond my doctor's statistics, which showed that 87 percent of his patients became pregnant by IUI #4, if at all. In fact, it was the baker's dozen, the lucky stimulated cycle #13 (IUI #7), that finally stuck!

But, regardless if you're on IUI #1, 4, or 40, after a while, it *all* becomes a bit too much.

Growing sick of getting stuck

Perhaps you grew sick of waiting when the first home pregnancy test read negative. But even if you're more patient, what if a month, or two or three, of nightly injections of hormones is just about all you can handle?

First off, be assured that your impatience and irritability aren't a reflection of your winning personality, but more likely the side effects of the drugs you're taking. Most women find that acknowledging that their moods or mood swings are largely chemical in nature does lessen the burden. If you haven't confided in a friend about your fertility struggles, perhaps now is as good a time as any. You'll find that friends or relatives in the know will treat you with kid gloves right about the time that you're ready to pull out the boxing gloves.

One woman talked about looking at fertility, the shots, ultrasounds, and doctor visits as a project or a job that she didn't particularly like but had to get through. She then viewed each test or treatment as a task to be completed, much like cleaning the house. This detachment helped her get through 22 assisted reproductive cycles (in two and a half years) before achieving success!

Another thing to remember is the numbers game that is human reproduction. One of our favorite stories is that of a professional basketball player who smiled and clapped every time he missed a free throw. When asked about this odd behavior, he responded, "With every miss, I'm one shot closer to success." Consider *your* shots the same way.

Being sensitive to your partner's feelings

Just as you may find the fertility rituals to be all consuming, your partner may be sharing your views, more than you know. The partner being treated may feel that he or she is undergoing the lion's share of discomfort and disappointment. But remember, even if your partner isn't experiencing every needle stick or test result, that person is watching you go through it. "Big deal!" you scoff. Well, it can be. Watching another person experience pain or sadness can be as difficult as going through it yourself. The silent partner also must suffer with feelings of inadequacy and powerlessness in being unable to relieve your discomfort. Partners of terminally ill patients often need their own support networks as well. And, as a recent study reveals, fertility patients, due to the sometimes long nature of their treatment, share some of the same issues faced by the chronically and terminally ill.

Encourage your partner to share his or her feeling with friends, family, or a professional. Although you may feel as though you're losing your sanity, your partner may feel as though he's losing you.

Coping when you're both sick of everything, including each other

Many say that the rigors of fertility are an opportunity for couples to grow closer. We say that this is generally *not* the case. With chemically induced moods raging, money being spent at warp speed, and disappointment doled out in monthly doses, it takes a lot for couples to remain civil and calm with one another.

Trying to maintain this level playing field is a good goal for your relationship when going through the fertility rites. My husband and I (coauthor Jackie) tried to make our visits to our out-of-town fertility doctor a chance to unwind. Ironically, our favorite fertility times were those when we actually traveled the farthest from home (1,000 miles each way) and were entirely inconvenienced. On each visit to Philadelphia, we planned day trips to local museums, the nearby shore, and Atlantic City in order to break up our tightly wound schedules. We found a favorite restaurant that made each trip something to look forward to, and we made a point to treat ourselves as much as we could afford.

The seriousness of fertility treatments actually allowed us to put aside trivial arguments more easily. No matter how angry we were at each other over daily issues, we had to reconvene each night for my shot of gonadotropins. Believe me, it's hard (to say nothing of unwise) to harbor a grudge toward someone who's sticking you with a long needle. But seriously, when I watched my husband carefully mixing medicines and grimacing at my every "ouch," it was easy to remember how much I loved this kind man and easier still to forget any past resentments.

Although fertility treatment may not seem to be a bonding experience, it certainly is a time for teamwork. Split up the work, whether it's making doctor appointments, dealing with insurance companies, or paying the bills. Many couples find that the growing experience is more about growing *up*. Yes, fertility requires a lot of time and effort, but so do most worthwhile things in life. This reality is a good one for an immature partner to grasp, particularly *before* you welcome a baby, a responsibility that makes fertility treatment pale by comparison.

If you and your partner are unable to deal with anything, including each other, you may want to consider counseling and/or a break from your fertility routine. Don't forget the importance of your relationship. Couples who do may find themselves miles apart, whether or not they conceive. Remember, your goal is to make a family, not break one up.

Part IV
The High-Tech Highway: Moving Up to In Vitro Fertilization

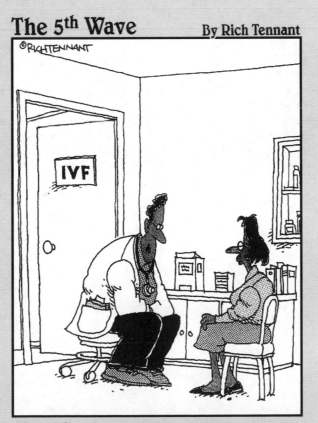

"In brief, we'll stimulate your ovaries with daily medications or hormones, perform an oocyte retrieval at the hospital, incubate the eggs in a petri dish at the laboratory, and then sit back and let nature take its course."

In this part . . .

When medium-tech fertility approach fails and you find yourself at the door of the in vitro fertilization (IVF) clinic, you'll have lots of questions and concerns. In this part, we explain what IVF is, how it works, and how you should pick your clinic. We also give you some ideas for reducing the cost of high-tech treatment. Then we take you through a typical IVF cycle, from stimulating medications to what happens in the embryology lab.

Chapter 10

Welcome to the Big Time: In Vitro Fertilization

In This Chapter

▶ Moving up to in vitro fertilization

▶ Finding the right doctor

▶ Determining your clinic's personality

▶ Adding up the cost of IVF

In vitro fertilization (IVF) is the top of the high-tech mountain of infertility treatments, so naturally, you may be a bit nervous about moving into an invasive, expensive, no-guarantees treatment.

The term *in vitro fertilization* means fertilization (the joining of egg and sperm) that occurs in a test tube; that's where the term "test tube baby" comes from. Before you get to the fertilization point, you have to make eggs with the help of stimulating medications called gonadotropins and retrieve them from the follicles they grow in during an egg retrieval. Twenty years ago only a handful of clinics performed IVF. Now almost 400 clinics offer this service, and IVF has become a big (and lucrative) business.

In this chapter, we help you evaluate different IVF clinics, decipher the confusing statistics about IVF success rates, and give you some help in deciding whether IVF is the next step for you.

Reaching the Top of the Mountain: What In Vitro Fertilization Means for You

For those of you who just basically need to know when to show up at the clinic, here's the scoop on IVF:

- IVF is expensive.
- IVF is time consuming.
- IVF is unpredictable.
- IVF does not guarantee success.
- IVF involves injections.
- IVF requires frequent ultrasounds and blood work.
- You will scream at the IVF nurses at least once during your treatment.
- You will scream at your partner at least once, and then *he'll* scream at the IVF nurses.

That's all you really need to know — you can pick up the rest along the way. But we thought you'd like some insights.

Perhaps the most intimidating part of IVF is the notion that you're at the end of the technologic line, the top of the fertility treatment mountain in your quest for a biological baby. While part of you may feel enormous excitement anticipating that you've finally found the magic path, the other part may fear what will happen if IVF doesn't work. If it fails, you may find yourself going back to less-technological methods, or you may move forward to other means of creating a family, such as donor egg or adoption. Think of IVF as a beginning and one step closer to your dream, however it may be attained.

Understanding that IVF may not work

Although IVF gets a large share of publicity when it comes to infertility, the fact is that only about 2 percent of infertile couples actually end up doing IVF. Because the techniques used and the ethical issues are so cutting edge, media coverage of IVF far exceeds that of, say, intrauterine insemination. So it may seem that way more people are doing in vitro than really are.

Publicity for every celebrity IVF baby may also make it seem like IVF is a sure-fire success method, when at best, the statistics for live births per IVF cycle are about 35 percent — and that's for women under age 35. The statistics break down this way:

> ✔ **Under age 35:** A 35 percent chance of a live birth per IVF cycle
>
> ✔ **Ages 35 to 37:** Approximately 30 percent chance of taking home a baby per IVF cycle
>
> ✔ **Ages 38 to 40:** A 22 percent chance of a live birth per cycle
>
> ✔ **Over age 40:** A 12 percent chance of a live birth per cycle
>
> ✔ **Over age 45:** Virtually no chance of pregnancy unless you use donor eggs

The cost of one IVF cycle is about $8,000 to $10,000, which may or may not include your medication, blood draws, and ultrasound, all of which may or may not be covered by insurance.

Looking at the preceding success rates, you can see that it may well take two or more cycles to get pregnant with IVF, and the cost equals or exceeds a new car. Plus, you have no guarantees of success. Sounds like a great way to spend money, eh?

On the brighter side, if insurance covers IVF, including medications and ultrasounds, the only thing you have to lose is time.

Managing your expectations

When you're spending a large amount of money on a procedure such as IVF, you have high expectations. And some doctors with large practices (and egos) to support may feed those expectations. As the Romans said, caveat emptor (let the buyer beware).

When I (Jackie) first sat down with the doctor whom a friend later termed Dr. Badadventure (based on my less than glowing praise), he summarily dismissed many of my questions and concerns about this expensive procedure by waving his hand and declaring, "IVF cures everything."

If you hear this comment from any doctor, turn tail and run — and don't forget your wallet. The idea of IVF as a cure-all is a misnomer, carrying with it a slew of great expectations, most of them false. IVF will not take care of all that ails you, particularly if your problems are not structural. IVF is, among other things, a good solution if you suffer from blocked tubes or other structural malformations that require bypassing the ovaries and/or fallopian tubes, or if you have certain types of male factor that require the use of intra-cytoplasmic sperm injection (ICSI).

And although IVF, through the retrieval and examination of eggs and subsequent embryos, can diagnose many issues of egg quality, it can't repair your eggs and hence is *not* a solution for women with "old" or chromosomally poor-quality eggs.

Jackie's personal mountain

"I never thought I'd be at this point," I (coauthor Jackie) lamented to myself, and anyone else who would listen. Married at 34, I had been trying to conceive for two years now to no avail. My local doctor had been convinced, and convincing, that I would get my baby through the low-tech intrauterine insemination (IUI) procedures. "You have stingy ovaries," he would say with a wink. "We'll just push you a little harder and hope you don't end up with more than one."

After three failed attempts and increasingly higher doses, that dialogue began to wear thin. My faith in him and in myself had waned, and I was off to find a new doctor and a more direct line to baby. Now, here I stood contemplating a $10,000-plus, two-month procedure for what I thought would have been accomplished in one night after a bottle of cheap wine. The mountain was indeed much higher than I thought.

Sometimes, regardless of your problem, or lack thereof, your lack of success may simply call for a few more tries, be it IUI or timed intercourse. "I've already tried IUI six times," I whined to my out-of-town doctor during a late-night call." "Then try twelve," he remarked impassively. Need I tell you that the eighth time was the charm? If you have no indication of structural issues or if age or your reproductive history is in your favor, you might consider spending a little more time on the old ways instead of a lot more money on a new one.

Knowing the true nature of your fertility problem, as best you or your doctor can, can help you to best assess whether IVF will provide you with your golden egg, or eggs, or if it will merely drain whatever nest egg you have left.

Just because a procedure is more expensive or more advanced doesn't mean that it's going to work!

Looking at the risks of IVF

Although IVF has become a familiar and accepted way of dealing with infertility, it's not without risk. Some risks are well established, and others are not as clear-cut. Before you decide to move on to IVF, consider these factors.

High rate of twins or triplets

The best documented risk of doing IVF is the high rate of twins or triplets. Because more than one embryo, usually two to four, is placed into the uterus at one time, the risk of getting pregnant with more than one baby is high. In the normal population, twins occur a little over 1 percent of the time, or about 1 in 90 births in the United States. Contrast this with the fact that about 25 percent of IVF births are twins! You may see this as an advantage — two for the price of one — but the price tag on multiple deliveries is high.

About one-half of twins are born prematurely, before 35 weeks gestation, or with a low birth weight. Up to half have a lower than expected birth weight, compared to 10 percent of single babies. One-half or more of twins are delivered by cesarean section, as compared with about 30 percent of the normal population. Mothers of twins are twice as likely to have preeclampsia (high blood pressure and fluid retention, factors that can cause maternal stroke).

Premature infants in general are three to six times more likely than full-term infants to die in the first year of life. Premature babies also have a higher risk of vision problems, cerebral palsy, and learning difficulties.

Increased risk of ectopic pregnancy

Ectopic pregnancies implant somewhere besides the uterus, usually in one of the fallopian tubes. Because space for growth is limited, the pregnancy can't continue past seven or eight weeks. If the tube bursts, the woman faces a serious risk of bleeding to death. Ectopic pregnancies are twice as common in IVF pregnancies, which seems strange when you realize that the embryos are placed directly into the uterus and don't come down the tubes at all. The embryos apparently move out of the uterus and up into the tube to implant.

Ovarian hyperstimulation syndrome

Ovarian hyperstimulation syndrome (OHSS) occurs in 1 to 5 percent of all stimulated cycles in which gonadotropins, medications that stimulate growth of follicles, are taken. OHSS can cause serious maternal illness, including stroke.

Birth defects

Birth defects are a controversial and as yet unproven possibility in IVF. Some studies show an increase in birth defects in IVF pregnancies, while other studies don't support this claim. Much more research will undoubtedly be done in this area as IVF children become older. Techniques such as ICSI and assisted hatching (see Chapter 13 for more on assisted hatching) have been done only in the last ten years, so the children conceived are still young.

Some proof exists that men who need to do ICSI for male factor issues may pass the gene responsible to their sons, who may also need to do ICSI (or whatever the equivalent technique is) 20 or 30 years from now.

Deciding Whether to Stay with Your Current Doctor

The clinic you've been going to for IUI or monitoring may also perform IVF. And if you're comfortable with the staff and the doctors, know the routine, and have all your insurance coverage set up there, you may decide to stay with that clinic.

You should, however, think about it and do some reading before deciding to stay with your current center. Almost 400 U.S. clinics do IVF, and they range from little more than the "weekend dabbler" that does maybe 30 to 40 egg retrievals a year to the megacenters that do more than 1,000 or even 2,000 egg retrievals a year.

Bigger isn't always better, but when it comes to high-tech procedures such as IVF, success rates are highly dependent on the quality of the IVF lab. It stands to reason that a small center doing 30 or 40 retrievals a year may not have the same lab setup as a center doing 1,000 a year.

One way to evaluate centers is to compare their statistics and what they offer via the Society of Assisted Reproductive Technology (SART). SART is the statistic watchdog of IVF. We describe in detail what it monitors and how the statistics are compiled in the section "Sorting through SART statistics," later in this chapter.

Another way to evaluate your current center is to talk to patients who are currently doing IVF there and to your doctor or the nurses. Sometimes the nurses are more candid about whether you should stay or move on, especially if they've gotten to know you, like you, and want what's best for you. If the nurse slips you a little note about another clinic a few towns away, pay attention!

Moving On: Finding Dr. Magic

Sometimes the decision to move on to another clinic is easily made. For example, if your current clinic doesn't take your insurance, you don't like the staff, or its hours aren't convenient for the more intensive monitoring of IVF, you know you need to switch doctors. Or maybe you need or want specialized treatment that your present clinic doesn't do, such as sex selection, preimplantation genetic diagnosis (PGD), or sperm aspiration. Lucky for you, Dr. Magic most likely has a Web site, a good place to start looking for your IVF doctor.

Searching through IVF Web sites

Most medium to large IVF clinics have a Web site. At the very least, the Web site should tell you the following information:

- ✔ How many egg retrievals the clinic does in a year
- ✔ How many embryo transfers the clinic does in a year
- ✔ Pregnancy rates for all age groups, broken down per egg retrieval and per embryo transfer
- ✔ Whether it freezes embryos
- ✔ Whether it does ICSI
- ✔ Whether it transfers three-day embryos or blastocysts (see Chapter 13)
- ✔ How many doctors do IVF
- ✔ The educational level of the doctors and whether the doctors are reproductive endocrinologists
- ✔ Whether the clinic cycles patients through all the time or you have to wait for the next group
- ✔ Whether the clinic has a donor egg or embryo program

You may have other concerns pertaining to your own situation. If you can't find the answer on the Web site, you may be able to call the center and ask to speak to an IVF nurse. Usually they're happy to answer any questions you have about their program, and you won't feel as committed as you might after talking to a doctor. (You don't have to give your real name, either!)

Sorting through SART statistics

The Society of Assisted Reproductive Technology (SART) is an organization affiliated with ASRM (American Society of Reproductive Medicine), the organization for health care professionals involved with reproductive medicine. SART's members are the approximately 370 IVF clinics in the United States that submit the following information to SART for publication each year:

- ✔ The number of cycles they do
- ✔ The types of infertility their patients have
- ✔ The outcome of their cycles
- ✔ Pregnancy rates

✔ Multiple pregnancy rates

✔ Miscarriage rates

✔ Cancellation rates

In short, the clinics provide information on just about anything and everything concerning their patients' IVF cycles.

SART takes the information and compiles a booklet of information about every one of the 370 clinics and distributes it to its members; it also publishes the data on *its* Web site. SART data is also found with other data from the Centers for Disease Control and Prevention (CDC).

Clinics that are members of SART can be audited and their data checked for accuracy. The amount of information required by SART is astounding: Your age, Social Security number, infertility type, and type of cycle are reported to SART for every IVF cycle that you do. In most medium to large clinics, compiling and reporting SART data take a tremendous amount of time.

SART confirms clinic-reported data by visiting about 30 clinics a year and auditing selected patients' charts to make sure that the submitted information is accurate.

SART statistics can be difficult to read because not all clinics report their numbers in the same way. For example, one clinic may report pregnancy rates per retrieval, and another may report per transfer. Try to compare apples to apples when sifting through SART data. Also, SART statistics don't tell you anything about the clinic population but their age. A center dealing with only the crème de la crème of patients, the place everyone else calls the "mecca," certainly has higher pregnancy rates than the center that treats everyone, including patients rejected at the mecca.

Here are a few statistics from SART:

✔ In 1999, approximately 86,000 IVF cycles were done in the United States.

✔ 90 percent of IVF centers offer embryo freezing.

✔ 83 percent of the clinics have a donor egg program.

✔ 67 percent of clinics have labs accredited by a national organization; all SART member labs are accredited.

✔ 20 percent of IVF patients have problems with their fallopian tubes.

✔ 24 percent of IVF patients have male factor issues.

✔ 15 percent of IVF patients have problems with ovulation.

✔ 14 percent of IVF patients have endometriosis.

✔ 8 percent of IVF patients have unexplained infertility.

Looking for a clinic

Although SART statistics make interesting reading and may help you decide which clinic to use, they don't tell the whole story. You'll also need to check into the following information:

- ✔ The clinics that are nearest to you. Long-distance IVF is possible but complicated.

- ✔ The clinics that are accepting new patients.

- ✔ How much clinics charge if you don't have insurance.

- ✔ Whether the clinics take insurance — not all do!

- ✔ Whether the clinics treat patients like you, an important consideration if you're over age 40 or have been turned down by another clinic.

- ✔ The kind of feeling you get from the clinic. For the answer to this question, you'll probably need to make a consultation appointment with a doctor. The clinic usually charges for this appointment.

You don't need to commit to a program at your initial consultation. It never hurts to go home and think everything over before you go any farther. Remember, also, that if you're at one of the big-name clinics, you're also being sized up as a candidate for its program, and you could be turned down for treatment if you don't fit the clinic's criteria. Some centers don't want to give you false hope if they don't believe that they can help you, and others don't want to bring down their statistics.

Whether you need or want to know everything about a clinic before you go there depends on your personality. You may be happy to go wherever it was that your best friend went or to go where your insurance tells you to go, or to the clinic around the corner. There's nothing wrong with trusting your instincts and other people's personal experiences. However, if you're already filling up infertility notebook number three, your family doctor's recommendation that you just go to his golfing buddy probably isn't going to convince you.

Tracking down all the stuff you want to know

The best way to find a lot of information about fertility clinics is to check the Internet. The information will be much more up-to-date than what you find in books or the phone book; most clinics have Web sites that they update fairly often. Just type "IVF clinic" into a search engine such as Google, and you'll get somewhere around 10,000 hits. Some hits will be redundant, but it's a safe bet that the clinic you're considering (remember, there are only about 400) will be listed.

Now you want to check out the centers closest to you. Although IVF can be done outside your home area, it's much simpler to do IVF within a 100-mile radius of where you live. Monitoring needs to be done frequently, and having blood and ultrasound work done in your hometown isn't that easy if you're doing IVF 300 miles away. Your hometown doctor could be understandably a bit peeved at doing the scut work and not getting to do the IVF procedure or make any of the decisions. Here are the only reasons to go outside your part of the country for IVF:

✔ No one in your area will do IVF for you.

✔ No one in your area does IVF cheaply enough for you.

✔ You need extremely sophisticated testing or procedures that are done only at a handful of clinics in the world.

After you have a list of all the clinics in your area, you should do two things:

✔ Ask a doctor you know and trust which clinic he recommends.

✔ Find out where your insurance is accepted.

You shouldn't always go to the clinic that takes your insurance, but knowing what you'll need to pay should certainly be a factor in your decision.

Evaluating a Clinic's Personality

IVF clinics have personalities just like people do. Usually but not always, the head honcho or main doctor at the clinic sets the tone for the whole office. Sometimes instead of one main doctor, a clinic has a team of fairly equal doctors, all of whom leave their impression on the way the clinic functions. Here's a rundown on the most common types of offices and what you may encounter when you enter their doors.

Razzle-dazzle: Where the receptionists wear cheerleading skirts

You may already know the razzle-dazzle offices by name and reputation — they're the meccas of infertility patients. Even if you aren't aware of the office's national reputation when you walk in, you will be by the time you walk out. They're the best, they know it, and they capitalize on it.

The razzle-dazzle is usually apparent the moment you pull into the parking lot. The place is spotless, the flower beds are manicured, and the staff uniforms may be color coordinated, even if they're not actually wearing cheerleading skirts. The doctors are well dressed even for doctors —check out the shoes and the imported silk ties. All kinds of achievement awards and recognition certificates line the walls, and everything is organized. Information is handed out in tidy little packets, and employees make much mention of the clinic's reputation as the first this or the best that. Doctors are referred to as simply "Doctor" by the receptionists, as in "Doctor will see you now," as if there were only one in the world.

These places are selective and often expensive, but you'll probably feel like you're in first class if you go there.

The serious office: Seeing the world through horn-rimmed glasses

Some doctors take everything about life much too seriously, including themselves. Stepping into Dr. Serious's office is like stepping into a museum; it's very quiet, with carpeting on the floor because squeaky shoes make Dr. Serious nervous. Nothing is funny here. Infertility is serious business, and none of the office staff ever seems to get your jokes. If you're a serious type yourself, you'll probably love Dr. Serious, but if you're a kidder, you'll never make it through your first visit because you'll start laughing too loud and they'll throw you out. If you liked Dr. Peter Benton on *ER,* Dr. Serious may be your kind of guy, but if you were a *St. Elsewhere* fan a few years back, Dr. Serious is not for you. Instead, you may prefer the type of clinic we describe in the section "The madhouse: Shouldn't these people be locked up?" later in this chapter.

A variation on Dr. Serious is Dr. Seriously Published. He's written a million journal articles, all of which he tries to explain to you during your one-hour appointment. He also gives you a stack of papers to take home and read over at a later date, which you'll probably decide means like never.

Drs. Doom and Gloom

Just as some doctors feed false expectations, others may choose to starve reasonable ones. Drs. Doom and Gloom can also be known as Drs. Prove It To Me, as in "Prove that you can actually get pregnant." Some women find this attitude to be the challenge they need, not unlike that provided by a high school coach. Others would rather the doctor at least *appear* to be in your corner, fighting for your fertility and your family almost as hard as you are.

Drs. Doom and Gloom are certainly realists. They recognize the innate difficulty associated with human reproduction, to say nothing of how hard it becomes when other factors are thrown in. These doctors will certainly keep your feet firmly planted on the ground. Remember, however, that there *is* another side to the statistics — the successful side, the side Drs. Doom and Gloom do not acknowledge *until* you are successful.

Women who have spent time and money to consult with Drs. Doom and Gloom often walk away with a heavy heart after being handed the diagnosis of a 1 percent chance of success. Listen closely. If a doctor tells you that he has never had a patient with your statistics succeed, translate that into the fact that *he* has no experience in making this happen. Other doctors may routinely work with patients such as yourself and report better odds.

The madhouse: Shouldn't these people be locked up?

The madhouse clinic is easy to spot. You open the front door and are appalled. The waiting room is jam-packed, the phone rings nonstop, the receptionists are throwing charts at each other, and the doctors are yelling over the intercom system.

A normal reaction might be to turn around and walk right back out, but these "madhouse" clinics are some of the biggest and best; they're just incredibly busy and often disorganized. You need to be a strong character to survive at this type of clinic. You need to stay on top of everything, keep duplicate records of all your tests (these places lose your chart at the drop of a hat), and be persistent enough to get good care.

Checking up on your doc

One way to check out your potential doctor's reputation is to ask another doctor, particularly one who lives in the same area. Doctors within a specialty, especially one as small as reproductive endocrinology, usually know one another. Although doctors are usually reluctant to criticize other doctors, you can tell a lot by noticing whether his eyebrows go up and down or whether you detect a notable lack of enthusiasm when you mention the doctor's name.

A negative or neutral reaction doesn't always mean that you should pass on that doctor. Some doctors are less mainstream in their thinking, so the majority of practitioners may frown on their practices. Such a doctor, however, may be exactly the type of person you're looking for.

If you can tolerate the chaos, you may find that you get good care at a reasonable price, plus you get to watch the three-ring circus every time you walk in the door.

Why IVF Costs So Much — Especially without a Free Toaster

No, you won't get a free toaster at your IVF clinic, but you may feel like you should. Why on earth does IVF cost so much? Although supply and demand may have a bearing on costs — in other words, doctors charge what they can — the fact is that IVF costs are high because IVF is a high-tech procedure and high-tech costs money. An IVF lab costs over a million dollars to set up. In addition, your clinic has many other expenses:

- **Salaries:** Employees include doctors, nurses, andrologists, embryologists, ultrasonographers, phlebotomists, file clerks, front desk staff, billing staff, medical assistants, and cleaning people.

- **Supplies:** The nursing side of the clinic where I (coauthor Sharon) work uses the following disposable supplies in a month for 100 or so egg retrievals: 300 bags of IV fluid, 400 drape sheets, 200 patient gowns, 100 Tyvek jumpsuits, 100 retrieval needles, 300 pairs of sterile gloves, and 10 oxygen tanks.

- **Maintenance of equipment:** Clinics need such things as a hemocue machine (to test iron levels), pulse oximeters (to measure oxygen levels in the blood), automatic blood pressure cuffs, a complete crash cart of medications, and ultrasound machines.

- **Embryologists' equipment:** These specialists use expensive culture media to grow and nurture embryos, micromanipulation tools for ICSI and assisted hatching, and expensive microscopes, plus liquid nitrogen tanks to store sperm and embryos.

- **Basic office expenses:** These costs include rent, utility bills, the phone bill (which can be enormous), health benefits for employees, copiers, paper, computers, and so on.

An IVF practice is an expensive practice to run.

Chapter 11

Sticker Shock —
Paying for IVF

*O*ne of the greatest misunderstandings about fertility treatment is that it is a practice reserved for the bored and well to do. And although some women and men who do turn to fertility treatment, whether it's low tech, medium tech, or high tech, are in the position where money is no object, generally speaking, that's not the case.

Yes, infertility treatment in general and in vitro fertilization (IVF) in particular are very expensive — so expensive, in fact, that insurance companies have been reluctant to pay the costs in most cases. This situation is slowly beginning to change as infertility is being treated not as a lifestyle issue but a medical issue.

Many individuals and couples faced with extended periods of fertility treatment and/or some of the more expensive procedures associated with high-tech procedures have found themselves needing to borrow money, refinance a house, sell possessions, or dramatically scale down their lifestyles. Managing your insurance benefits is one way to help bring home a baby.

In this chapter, we look at the current state of insurance coverage and show you ways to work with your employer to improve your coverage. If you're still in a state without mandatory coverage, we give you some ideas for lowering your IVF bill and/or increasing your chance of leaving treatment with a baby in your arms.

Looking at the Insurance Situation

The average IVF cycle costs between $8,000 and $15,000, and more if you don't have insurance coverage for your blood work and ultrasounds. Of that, about $4,000 to $5,000 is spent on medication, and another $4,000 to $10,000 goes to your clinic.

No one can deny that this is a lot of money. In addition, in most clinics the success rate is less than 50 percent per cycle, meaning that one try may well not be enough for you to get pregnant. It's no wonder that insurance companies aren't anxious to cover the cost of IVF.

Unless you're the one in a million infertility patients with unlimited funds, you may already be spending sleepless nights trying to figure out how to pay for this. If you have insurance coverage, you may be breathing a sigh of relief, at least until you read your policy's small print and find out that you're not as home free on costs as you thought you were.

Insurance companies and HMOs have traditionally avoided paying for IVF and other infertility treatments by saying they aren't medically necessary, meaning that you can live without a biological child. In other words, they were equating infertility treatments with a face-lift or liposuction — nice to have, certainly, but not really necessary.

Here are some other arguments that insurance companies give for not covering infertility treatments:

- ✔ The treatments have a low success rate.
- ✔ Success rates vary widely from clinic to clinic.
- ✔ There is a lack of accountability and oversight within the field of reproductive medicine.
- ✔ Very few people actually need the coverage, so it's not fair to make people who don't need it pay for those who do.

The last argument is rather ridiculous. Not everyone needs bypass surgery either, and insurance still covers that cost. And the fact that 10 percent of the population has some type of infertility issue certainly proves a documented need for coverage.

Obviously, this position is arguable, somewhat like saying that infertile people should just accept that they won't have natural-born children and live with it.

Underneath this view seems to be an underlying opinion that infertile people are somehow responsible for their infertility and that infertility is a result of their lifestyle. This opinion is like saying that people injured in car accidents shouldn't get medical attention because they were driving too recklessly.

If all the people writing the laws that govern infertility coverage were suddenly infertile, or their children were, you would see a big change in the insurance laws very quickly. Meanwhile, the laws crawl through the state legislatures, doling out coverage a little piece at a time, one state at a time, leaving thousands of infertile couples crying out for help with the costs.

Studies have shown that the cost of adding infertility treatment coverage to all insurance policies would increase consumer costs by less than $25 a year.

The extent of health insurance coverage largely depends on why you're seeing a doctor. For example, *menstrual dysfunction* is a commonly used term among gynecologists and fertility doctors alike. It can certainly *cause* infertility, but monitoring or treating it doesn't necessarily constitute infertility treatment. Polycystic ovary syndrome (PCOS) is another common cause of infertility, but again, it can, and often must, be treated, whether the woman is trying to conceive or not. The same can be said for polyps, cysts, and endometriosis.

Discovering what your insurance plan really covers

Even if you have insurance coverage, you may be amazed to see how little of your bill is covered. Some insurance plans cover only monitoring, meaning the frequent blood draws and ultrasounds. Because these can run well over $2,000 per cycle, this coverage is a help. Other plans cover only the medications, which is a help, but not by any means relief from the total cost.

Nor is it easy in some cases to decipher your insurance plan. Check out your plan before you start treatment. Even if you live in a state with mandated coverage, your particular employer may find several loopholes to slip through. Finding out you're not covered at the pharmacy the night before your cycle is supposed to begin isn't a good way to start treatment.

Many insurance companies require preauthorization even if you do have coverage. Preauthorization can take several days to complete, so don't leave this step until the last minute!

Insurance 101: The differences between types of insurance

You may be confused over whether your insurance is public or private, group or individual. Public insurance is paid for, at least in part, by the government. Medicaid, for those on public assistance; Medicare, for those over age 62 or disabled in some way; and Champus, for military families, are public insurances. Private insurances are paid for by you, either directly or indirectly. If your employer pays the costs for you as part of a benefits package, you have group insurance. If you pay the entire cost yourself, you have an individual policy, which is usually quite expensive.

You may be covered only if you go to an "approved" clinic. But what if you don't want to go to this clinic? Maybe it doesn't offer treatments you want, or it doesn't have high success rates. In that case, you'll be forced to make an unpleasant choice: Will you go for care that costs you less but may not succeed, or will you pay more for a higher chance of success? These decisions would have had even King Solomon, the master of wise decisions in the Old Testament, in a quandary.

Changing jobs or changing insurance to get infertility coverage

People have been known to change jobs to get better insurance, or to drop insurance at their place of employment and pick up coverage under their spouse's policy, even if it costs more per month.

Is it worth taking a lesser-paying job to cover IVF costs? If the drop in pay isn't too much, it might be. Three or four IVF cycles could certainly cost you more than $40,000 over a year or so.

Consider a part-time job as another means for establishing fertility coverage. Some companies offer insurance to part-time (20 or more hours a week) employees as well — insurance that may cover fertility treatments.

For a listing of major companies that offer infertility coverage (of some sort), visit http://if.freehosting.net/insurance_list.html.

But don't quit your current job yet. You still need to confirm this information with the organization (after you get the job, that is!) to determine the specifics of the plan.

Before you throw away your law career or consider moonlighting, you may want to check out any other insurance your company may offer. Some companies offer a choice of plans. You may pay more for a plan that covers infertility, but the savings may be worth the extra cost.

Some companies allow you to change insurance only at certain times of the year; usually this is called "open season." Check out your choices ahead of time so that you can have your insurance in place before you need to start using it.

Getting coverage from professional associations

So your insurance company won't give an inch, and the option of a new or second job is just not an option at all. Is it over? Maybe not.

That flier inviting you to your industry association dinner may come in handy after all. Many organizations have professional associations that offer open enrollment programs for insurance, meaning that if you're a member (you pay the monthly dues), you can't be turned down for insurance. Because these associations generally boast large memberships, you benefit from group coverage, which may include some of the "ups" and extras not found in smaller companies or individual plans. You can start by checking out associations within your profession.

Long-time resources for the self-employed who often have trouble getting coverage of any kind, professional and trade organizations are a popular way to cover yourself. Associations can be found in almost any field, particularly those that tend toward the self-employed or those underrepresented in business. Examples include the National Writers Union, Graphic Artists Guild, Public Relations Society of America, American Marketing Association, and Women in Communications. Often, you must be a member for a period of time before you can enroll in an insurance program. Sometimes, the insurance policy may have a one-year preexisting condition rider as well.

In either case, proper advance planning can help you meet these requirements if necessary. Not all professional organizations allow "laymen" to join. For example, you can't simply sign up for the American Medical Association or the American Bar Association to avail yourself of their benefits (unless of course you actually are a doctor or a lawyer). Some associations require a minimum of hours worked in the profession or a minimal base salary. Others, however, welcome those who may be practicing a vocation, even if they're doing so in their spare time. Requirements depend on the size of the group and how much they want and/or benefit from membership dues.

States are in charge — for now

No federal mandate for insurance coverage for infertility treatment exists at this time, although a few bills were sent to Congress in 2002. When you consider that the federal government has spent years arguing over general health care coverage for U.S. citizens, one can only imagine how bogged down a specific coverage for infertility treatment would become in Washington.

For now, it's up to individual states to pass and enforce infertility coverage. States can force employers to cover treatment in two different ways:

✔ They can mandate companies to cover infertility treatment.

✔ They can mandate that employers *offer* coverage.

If your employer is only mandated to offer coverage, you'll usually have to pay extra for the coverage, in the form of a *rider,* or extra policy, attached to your main insurance coverage.

Touring the States That Mandate Fertility Coverage

As of this writing, 15 states mandate some sort of reimbursement for in vitro fertilization. No consensus exists between states on how coverage should be applied or who has to offer it. This coverage is still a mixed bag for the average patient; even if your state mandates insurance coverage, your employer may be exempt from offering coverage if he meets certain requirements listed below.

States that currently have some infertility coverage mandates are Arkansas, California, Connecticut, Hawaii, Illinois, Louisiana, Maryland, Massachusetts, Montana, New Jersey, New York, Ohio, Rhode Island, Texas, and West Virginia.

Some states include IVF; some specifically exclude it. Others have a mandate to offer coverage, but the employer isn't required to pay for it; the cost is passed on to the individual buying the insurance. The current state coverage looks like this:

✔ **Arkansas:** Requires coverage for infertility, including IVF up to a lifetime cap of $15,000.

✔ **California:** Employees must make available a policy covering infertility treatment, excluding IVF but covering gamete intrafallopian transfer (GIFT), a much more expensive and invasive procedure.

✔ **Connecticut:** Must offer a policy covering infertility, including IVF.

✔ **Hawaii:** Requires coverage, including one cycle of IVF.

✔ **Illinois:** Requires coverage of diagnosis and treatment of up to six IVF cycles. Employers with fewer than 25 employees are exempt.

✔ **Maryland:** Requires coverage for IVF after certain conditions are met; HMOs and companies with fewer than 50 employees are excluded.

✔ **Massachusetts:** Requires comprehensive coverage.

✔ **Montana:** Requires HMOs to cover infertility as part of "preventive care."

✔ **New Jersey:** Requires coverage, including IVF.

✔ **New York:** Requires coverage of diagnosis and treatment as part of a correctable medical condition.

✔ **Ohio:** Requires HMOs to cover infertility under "preventive care."

✔ **Rhode Island:** Requires comprehensive coverage but allows a 20 percent co-pay for consumers.

✔ **Texas:** Requires certain insurers to offer coverage for IVF only.

✔ **West Virginia:** Requires HMOs to cover infertility costs.

Some states exempt HMOs from mandated coverage. Some states make HMOs cover infertility treatment. Some states cover everything except IVF; others cover IVF but not medications.

After you get past what is and isn't covered, in some states your employer can refuse to pay for infertility treatments if

✔ The company has fewer than 50 employees.

✔ The company doesn't cover maternity care.

✔ You haven't done at least several cycles of intrauterine insemination (IUI) before moving to IVF.

✔ You've had a vasectomy or tubal ligation.

✔ You're over a certain age.

✔ You haven't had two years of documented infertility.

You can find a very specific, detailed list of state coverage with exclusions at www.asrm.org/Patients/insur.html.

Fighting City Hall: Insurance Appeals

Insurance appeals need to attack one of the three basic reasons insurance companies give for not covering infertility treatments:

- Infertility is not an illness.
- Infertility treatments are not medically necessary.
- Infertility treatments are experimental.

You need to address one of these issues to win your claim. In some cases, your doctor may write a letter of "medical necessity" for some of your treatment.

A policy with vague wording may be easier to appeal than coverage that specifically excludes infertility treatment.

When Having Insurance Doesn't Help

You can have the world's greatest infertility insurance that can end up being worth nothing to you if your clinic doesn't accept insurance. Why would a clinic choose not to accept insurance? Because the amount the insurance offers isn't enough in the eyes of the clinic. Clinics that won't take insurance are usually the "mecca" types; they're the best, they know it, and they don't see why they should accept the typically low payment that your insurance offers.

Some clinics take your insurance amount but require you to pay the rest of the bill out of pocket. If a clinic is a preferred provider for that insurance, it's generally required to accept the amount offered as payment in full. If a clinic doesn't want to accept the amount offered, which is usually quite a bit below what most clinics charge for high-tech treatments (such as IVF), it simply refuses to take the insurance at all.

Getting Creative When You're Out of Other Options

If you don't have insurance or if your insurance doesn't pay anything toward IVF treatment, you may need to get creative. There are ways to have your IVF cycle paid for if you meet certain requirements and are in the right place at the right time!

Donating eggs to reduce costs

A few clinics have innovative donor egg programs that let you donate half your eggs to another couple in return for treatment. The recipient of your eggs pays for your medications and your IVF retrieval and transfer. You need to pay for your own pretesting (such as infectious blood work and a hystero-salpingogram), blood and ultrasound testing, and the cost of freezing any excess embryos you have.

You usually must meet certain requirements to be an egg donor. Generally, you must be under 35 years old and have a normal follicle-stimulating hormone (FSH) level. Usually a donor list is sent out every month or so by the clinic, and you need to be picked by a recipient to be able to do a retrieval cycle. The donors and recipients need to be matched ahead of time so that their cycles can be synchronized, thereby ensuring that both the donor and the recipient can have a fresh embryo transfer.

Your chances of getting picked are highest if you meet the following requirements:

- ✔ **You're young, preferably under 30:** The younger you are, the better the chance that you'll make a lot of eggs.

- ✔ **You're of normal weight and height:** Overweight donors aren't usually a first choice. Recipients may worry that obesity is hereditary and also may be concerned that they may have infertility problems, such as poly-cystic ovaries, a condition in which many eggs are made but the egg quality may be lower than normal.

   Very short donors may also not be picked as quickly, because given a choice, more people choose to have a taller donor (and hopefully taller children).

- ✔ **You have proven fertility:** If you have children already, you're more likely to be picked as a donor.

- ✔ **You have a male factor issue:** If your only fertility issue is male factor, you may be picked because you don't have any fertility issues yourself.

- ✔ **You have a good family background:** You have lots of brothers and sisters with lots of children, no genetic diseases, and no mental illnesses. These factors make you a prime candidate.

   Everyone has some problem in her background — after all, our grand-parents had to die of something. So if your grandfather died of cancer at 85, that's not likely to be a deterrent to getting picked. If your mom died at 40 from breast cancer, you may have more problems being selected.

- ✔ **You're a nonsmoker:** Evidence exists that smoking can damage eggs, plus nonsmokers are perceived as healthier people who take better care of themselves.

Egg recipients are often looking for someone whose blood type matches theirs and who has certain physical characteristics or racial background, so you may be selected faster if you have what a lot of people are looking for: a common blood type, or a rare one if someone on the list is looking for that.

Your savings as a donor could equal between $8,000 and $12,000, but you need to be comfortable with the idea that your genetic child could be growing up with another family, or that the recipient could get pregnant with your egg and you may not. Only you can say whether you can accept the emotional repercussions of donating eggs to another couple.

Some women say that they don't feel a genetic connection because their egg isn't being fertilized with their partner's sperm, so the child created isn't the same as the offspring form their own relationship. Other women become very angry when their recipients get pregnant and they don't. This is another one of those times where "know thyself" is of the utmost importance.

Joining a drug study

Some doctors' offices are well connected to certain drug companies and do frequent drug studies for compensation. The compensation may be made to the office as well as the patient. Patients may receive anything from a free cycle of medication to an entire paid IVF cycle, including blood work, ultrasounds, and egg retrieval costs.

Some studies have very specific requirements for age, weight, and infertility problem. Others are less strict with their requirements and let the clinic select patients whom they feel are suitable.

In most studies, a new drug not yet approved by the FDA is being tested. If you sign up for the study, you need to understand that you may get fewer eggs or less fertilization than you would from proven drugs. Most studies require that you sign a document stating this. You may also have to keep a journal of all side effects and have frequent interviews with the person running the study.

Centers selected to run drug studies are usually the larger centers, so you may want to check and see whether the clinics you're considering ever participate in drug studies.

Shopping for "sales" and money-back guarantees

Some clinics try to overcome resistance to the high cost of IVF by offering a money-back guarantee. This offer sounds good, but it does have a few catches.

Some centers call these "shared risk" programs. The specifics vary, but usually you pay an upfront fee, such as $15,000, for three or four IVF cycles. If you get pregnant in any one of the cycles, the clinic keeps all your money. If you don't get pregnant at the end of the last cycle, you get your money back. You must pay extra charges for intracytoplasmic sperm injection (ICSI) or using an egg donor or gestational carrier.

Patients must meet certain requirements for acceptance into the programs; usually you must be under a certain age and have a normal uterine cavity and normal baseline blood test results.

Are these programs a good deal? That depends. Obviously they try and hedge their bets somewhat by selecting patients they feel have a good chance of success. If you get pregnant on the fourth try, you'll have gotten a good price per try. If you get pregnant on the first try, you'll have spent a great deal of money for one cycle, far more than you needed to. But if you get pregnant on the first try, will you care about the cost? Only you know the answer.

If you're able to look at a pregnancy on your first try as an incredible blessing and not count the cost, this program may be for you. After two cycles, the clinic begins to break even on you, so if you get pregnant on the fourth cycle, this is a good deal for you financially.

Other clinics advertise a "twofer" deal, offering two cycles for the price of one for a limited time when they open a new office. As long as the office is a reputable one, you have nothing to lose by signing up for this offer. If the clinic doesn't have a proven track record or a good success rate, you may not be getting a good deal no matter how many free cycles it gives you.

ASRM (the American Society for Reproductive Medicine) has supported shared risk programs as a way to decrease costs to patients if they don't get pregnant. If you do get pregnant on the first try, you're basically subsidizing other people's third and fourth tries.

Ask your doctor whether his or her practice offers this type of quantity discount (or any discount at all for that matter). For specific information on networks of physicians who offer this type of pricing, visit your local search engine on the Internet. One such organization is www.arcfertility.com, but other such networks are available as well.

Chapter 12

Let the IVF Cycle Begin!

*I*n vitro fertilization (IVF) is the highest-tech method of getting pregnant. During an IVF cycle, you take powerful stimulating hormone drugs called gonadotropins so that you'll make more than one or two eggs. Then you go through an egg retrieval, a minor surgery to take the eggs out of the follicles they grow in. After that, the eggs are fertilized in the lab and then put back into your uterus so they can grow.

The treatment sounds complicated, and it is — but not so complicated that you can't understand the basic idea and walk into your clinic confident that you know what to expect.

So, if you've sent in your payment for in vitro after hassling with the billing office a few times, gasped at the hole left in your wallet, spent days on the phone arguing with your insurance company, bought all your medications, and gasped again at the cost, you're ready to start an IVF cycle. In this chapter, we discuss how to get through an IVF cycle with the least amount of frustration, explore what egg retrieval involves, and explain how your best friend's cycle may be completely different from yours and why you shouldn't worry about it.

Starting an IVF Cycle: A Roller Coaster Ride of Emotions

In vitro fertilization is a complicated process. It involves injecting potent medications with possibly serious side effects for several weeks, taking time out of your schedule to have blood work and ultrasounds done, and undergoing surgery, albeit minor, to retrieve your eggs. And that's just the beginning! Every step of the way through IVF is crucial, and every day brings news that will either thrill you or bring you to your knees in despair. Is it any wonder that you're feeling scared?

Even though you're scared to death, you're also excited. You've probably been through a lot to get here, you've spent buckets of money, and you have high hopes that high tech will not fail you.

Behind the excitement may be depression. This is where you've ended up. You've tried all the simpler methods of conception, and they failed. This is your last shot, and it may seem that there's nowhere to go from here. Before you got to IVF, you always knew you had one last thing to try. Now, you're trying IVF, and if it fails, you don't know what you'll do next.

Aggravation is a given in IVF. You're late for work too often because the ultrasound department was backed up. Your lab results are lost again. Your partner isn't giving you the injections right. Your numbers aren't good. You didn't get a callback. Be prepared for all the aggravation, and you won't be quite so upset when it occurs.

Try to reframe your anxiety as excitement. You *are* in the big time and probably closer to your dream of baby than ever before. In vitro will also give you answers that will help your doctors understand exactly what's going on. For the first time, your medical team will see your eggs, determine their quality, see firsthand whether fertilization is occurring, and figure out what kind of embryo you make. You'll know a lot more when all is said and done.

From the emotional side, rely on that support network that you've been building. Many women on chat room sites, in Resolve meetings, and in mind-and-body classes find "cycle buddies," literally other women going through IVF (or any of the lower-tech measures) at the same time. (For more details about Resolve, turn to Chapter 8.) You may find comfort in sharing your experiences, good and bad, with someone else who is going through the same thing at the same time. Remember, though, to share and not compare! You're not in competition with anyone. You're trying to have *your* baby.

And try to get your partner to read this chapter, because he's going to be bewildered by the roller coaster ride. Your partner is experiencing much of the IVF process secondhand (with your "hand" being the first line of defense). You're the one dealing directly with the physical discomfort, the scheduling madness, and the emotional ups and downs, so your partner will likely relate to the experience much differently than you do.

Looking at your protocol

When you first sit across the desk from an in vitro fertilization specialist, you may come to think of him as Dr. Magic. He'll probably gave you a stack of totally incomprehensible papers that you'll promptly file in your fertility notebook — you know, the notebook that every patient seems to carry around with her. One of those undecipherable papers is probably your protocol. A *protocol* is nothing more than a blueprint or schedule of how your cycle will be done. It includes the medications you'll be taking, instructions on how to take them, and the procedures you need to follow throughout the cycle.

Dr. Magic may review your protocol with you, or he may mumble something about the IVF nurses going over the protocol with you. If he reviews it that day, you'll probably be too excited, nervous, or scared to remember exactly what he says. Patients have described to me (coauthor Sharon) protocols that they swear the doctor gave them that resembled no IVF protocol on the face of this earth.

So it's time to take out your protocol. Step Number 1: Read the protocol. You would think this would go without saying, but it doesn't. Read the protocol!

Now, your cousin Mary out in Duluth may be going through IVF too, so you call her up and start comparing your protocols. Even though you're only four months apart in age, and everyone says you're more like sisters than cousins, you have two completely different protocols! How can this be? Has one of your doctors made a mistake?

Relax. Doctors rely on a few standard IVF protocols (we list them in Table 12-1), and most doctors prefer to use one over the other. If you're under 35 and your baseline hormone levels are normal, your doctor could choose to start you on a down regulation cycle, starting leuprolide acetate (which has the brand name Lupron) a few days after you ovulate. This drug shuts down your normal hormone receptors and encourages the growth of many follicles instead of one or two. The drug also keeps you from ovulating before retrieval. You start your hormone-stimulating drugs when your period starts. Some centers call this a "long Lupron" cycle, and others call it a "down regulation" cycle. Lupron is a GnRH (gonadotropin-releasing hormone) agonist; it shuts down your normal growth of one dominant follicle by suppressing your pituitary gland. Instead of stimulating a dominant follicle, like you normally would do, Lupron allows multiple follicles to develop at the same time.

Or your doctor may prefer to use a newer drug called ganirelix, a GnRH antagonist (with the brand name Antagon), or cetrorelix (with the brand name Cetrotide), in conjunction with follicle-stimulating medications; this drug suppresses your LH surge so you won't ovulate before your egg retrieval.

If you're over 35, many centers use a modified Lupron protocol, sometimes called a "stop Lupron" cycle because you take Lupron for just ten days following ovulation and then stop when you start your stimulating medications. This protocol is to decrease the suppressing effects of Lupron, which can be detrimental to those over 35 or women who are known to produce fewer eggs. Or you may be given a "microdose Lupron" protocol, in which Lupron is diluted in normal saline so that only a minute amount is given each day; this protocol is used for women who didn't stimulate well in a previous cycle or those who have an FSH (follicle-stimulating hormone) level above normal (10.5 to 15, depending on your lab's values).

You could also be doing a natural protocol, with no or very little medication. This protocol isn't common, but it's used in women who can't tolerate large doses of stimulating medication due to age or previous illness, such as breast cancer.

In addition, your doctor will prescribe gonadotropins, or follicle-stimulating medications, usually taken twice a day, although some centers give only one daily injection. *Recombinant drugs,* or drugs made completely in the laboratory from nonhuman protein sources, are more expensive but are able to be injected subcutaneously, which means they're given with a very tiny needle. (Follistim and Gonal-F are two such drugs.) Because they're made in the lab, they're nearly pure FSH, without any luteinizing hormone (LH) in them. Older gonadotropins, such as Humegon and Pergonal, are made from purified urine from postmenopausal women; they need to be given intramuscularly, with a longer needle, because they're more likely to cause irritation to the tissues. They're equal parts of LH and FSH, because the LH can't be completely filtered out of urine. They're also considerably cheaper than the recombinant medications. A newer drug called Bravelle, made from highly purified human urine, is nearly as purified as the recombinant medications and is slightly less expensive.

Your doctor will prescribe the protocol and medications he feels most comfortable using for your particular case. Try not to compare what you're getting to what anyone else is using.

Table 12-1	Common IVF Protocols at a Glance		
Protocol	*Used For*	*Average Days on Medication Needed*	*Vials of Medication*
Long Lupron	Women under 35; good responders	21 days total, including 10 on Lupron alone	About 40, plus one 14-day Lupron kit (for one cycle)

Protocol	Used For	Average Days on Medication Needed	Vials of Medication
Antagon or Cetrotide	Women who are oversuppressed on Lupron; patients of any age	10 days on stimulating medications; start ganirelix on day 6 of stimulating medications	About 30 to 40 vials of stimulating medications plus 5 to 6 prefilled syringes of Antagon or Cetrotide
Microdose flare	Poor responders women over 35	10 to 12 days of microdose Lupron and stimulating medications	60 vials of stimulating medications; one bottle of microdose (diluted) Lupron
Short flare	Women oversuppressed on long Lupron	10 days of Lupron; start stimulating medications on day 5 for 5 to 7 days	One 14-day Lupron kit; 24 to 30 vials of stimulating medications
Modified long (also called stop Lupron)	Women over 35; poor responders	10 Lupron days of Lupron: then approximately 10 days of stimulating medications	60 vials stimulating medications; one 14-day Lupron kit

After you've read your protocol over a few times, you're ready to call the doctor's office to discuss it and make sure that you understand it. Some offices have an orientation class for IVF patients to review protocols and policies. Some centers make attendance mandatory for their patients. Other centers schedule injection instruction sessions for you and your partner to review your medications and show you how to inject them. Having your partner inject medications is one of the scariest parts of IVF — for you *and* for your partner. Make sure that you get very clear instructions on how to do this. See Chapter 9 for more discussion on both subcutaneous and intramuscular injections.

If your IVF center is large, nurses probably take care of only IVF patients. If your program is smaller, the nursing staff may take care of both non-IVF and IVF patients. Some programs have only one IVF nurse whom you deal with throughout your cycle; others have so many nurses you can't tell who's who without a scorecard!

Try to figure out how your center works and to whom you should be talking before your cycle starts. In many centers, the IVF nurses draw blood and also do your ultrasounds; larger centers have a separate staff that draws blood and ultrasonographers who do the ultrasounds. Make sure that you talk to the right person when you have a problem or need help.

Dealing with a disappearing doctor

After your initial consult appointment, you may wonder where your doctor went. In smaller centers, doctors may do callbacks with your blood results; some also do their own ultrasounds. In larger centers, you may feel as though your doctor has vanished from the face of the earth because all your instructions come from the nurses. This system of patient communication can be upsetting if you came to a center specifically to deal with a particular doctor. Rest assured that your doctor *is* reviewing your callbacks and instructing the nurses on what you should do next, but in bigger centers, doctors simply don't have the time to do more than 50 callbacks a night. Some centers have even gone to a system where you don't talk to *anybody:* Your instructions are left on a message tape you can access.

If your center has more than one doctor doing IVF procedures, you may also feel like you've lost the doctor you came to see. Many centers rotate doctors through IVF on a one- or two-week cycle; you may never see the doctor you had your consultation with again! Sometimes you can request that a certain doctor do your procedure, but granting that request may not always be possible. Your doctor may be doing outside surgery or seeing patients for new appointments the week of your retrieval.

The doctor you saw on your initial visit to the clinic may not be the doctor who is managing your IVF procedure. Try to find out what your center's policy is for scheduling doctors and whether you can request a doctor of your choice.

Taking your medications without having a nervous breakdown

Suppose that you had your injection class a week ago, and on this beautiful bright Sunday morning, you're ready to begin taking your medications. Your partner, with shaking hands, opens the first vial to mix your first injection. "No, no!" you scream, as he proceeds to draw up the liquid. "That's not how she said to mix it!" He stops, and both of you stare dumbfounded at the boxes, the needles, and each other. In one week you've forgotten every word the nurse said. You look at the film you were given on giving injections again, read the colorful pieces of paper that tell you how to mix and inject, and still feel confused, scared, and totally out of control. And it's a Sunday. What on earth are you going to do?

Being confused: Par for the course

First, take a deep breath. Of course, giving yourself injections is hard to do. Do you think doctors and nurses were born knowing how to mix and inject medications? Most people are scared the first time they give a shot or mix a medication. Your reaction is normal.

Second, call your center. Some centers do IVF procedures on weekends, and if yours does, you may be able to talk to someone who can talk you through the mixing and injection.

If no one is there, you can call the answering service and ask for the doctor on call, who may be annoyed but can at least give you some guidance. Some centers also have nurses who carry beepers so they can answer questions when the office is closed. If you got your medications from a large mail-order pharmacy, it may have a nurse on call who can give you instructions also. Call the main number and ask. Never got to know the doctor or nurse who lives next door? Now might be as good a time as any to strike up an acquaintance! Such a person is likely to be more adept than you at handling a needle and walking you through your first shot.

If you can't get anyone, take a little break, compose yourself, and then go back and try again. The procedure probably won't look quite as overwhelming the second time.

Annoying the nurses: A small price to pay

Yes, you may hear a bit of strain in the nurse's voice when she tells you, for the third time in one day, how to mix your medication. No matter. That's what she's there for, and *every* nurse would rather hear from you three times than get a phone call three days later that says you've been taking your medication wrong, wasted your very expensive medications, and probably messed up your very expensive IVF cycle. Every nurse has stories of couples who took too much, too little, or the wrong medication and had to have their cycles canceled. You'll feel angry and stupid, the nurse will feel guilty (nurses always feel guilty when things go wrong), and you may be out a lot of money. So call the nurse — and don't bother to disguise your voice. She knows who you are!

Monitoring your progress (more poking and prodding)

After a few days of injections, you'll start to feel like a pro, your partner will have his injection techniques down pat, and your protocol will start to make sense to you. It's time to find out how well this is working. It's time to have blood drawn and do an ultrasound.

Most centers monitor you every few days to see how you're responding to the medication. If your follicles are growing nicely and your estradiol is rising, your medications will probably not be changed. If you're stimulating too well, or not stimulating well enough, your medications may be decreased or increased.

Stimulating too well can be another example of too much of a good thing. The goal of IVF is to have a number of follicles grow so that more than one egg can be retrieved. This result will hopefully prevent you from having to do multiple cycles of IVF to get pregnant, because your extra embryos may possibly be frozen and used later if you don't get pregnant on your first try. With some women, especially those who have polycystic ovaries (see Chapter 7 for more about this condition), hyperstimulation can get way out of hand very quickly. If your estradiol rises too fast, or if you make too many follicles — 20 or more — you run a risk of developing OHSS, or ovarian hyperstimulation syndrome. Patients with OHSS can be very ill after egg retrieval, with fluid buildup in the pelvis and around the lungs. Some women become sick enough to require hospitalization, and a few patients have died from severe OHSS, which causes fluid volume shifts through your whole body and can make your blood very thick and prone to clotting.

Because OHSS is so potentially serious, most centers watch patients on stimulating medications quite closely, monitoring their blood and ultrasound results every few days. If your clinic thinks that you're in danger of severe OHSS, you may have to freeze your embryos after retrieval and not do an embryo transfer. OHSS becomes worse if you become pregnant, due to the rising hormone levels from the pregnancy. Some centers may not do egg retrieval at all, because the hCG trigger given before retrieval also makes OHSS worsen.

On the other hand, you may not be stimulating well, and your clinic may be increasing your medication to see whether you can do better. This situation also requires closer monitoring because your medications may require frequent adjustment. See Table 12-2 for a typical IVF stimulation cycle, but remember that your cycle may vary.

As a rough guide, you'll probably be on stimulating hormones ten days before you're given hCG to mature the follicle for your retrieval. During those ten days, you'll probably have blood work and ultrasounds done four times, or maybe more or less depending on your circumstances. Some centers insist that all your blood work and ultrasounds be done at their facility; others allow patients to be monitored at outside facilities closer to their homes. You need to find a place capable of doing same-day reports and willing to fax results to your clinic.

Table 12-2		A Typical IVF Cycle — Yours May Vary	
Day of Cycle	*Monitoring*	*Medication*	*Time Taken*
2	Blood and ultrasound	FSH/hCG (stimulating medications)	2 vials a.m./ 2 vials p.m.
3		Keep taking medications	No change

Day of Cycle	Monitoring	Medication	Time Taken
4		Keep taking medications	No change
5	Blood and ultrasound	Adjust according to monitoring results	Change if clinic tells you to
6		Keep taking medications	No change
7		Add Antagon/Cetrotide	Add Antagon/Cetrotide in a.m.
8	Blood and ultrasound	Keep taking medications	No change
9			
10	Blood and ultrasound	Take morning medications/hCG	Morning medications: no change/hCG at exact time clinic tells you
11	Blood work only	No medications	
12	Egg retrieval		

Waiting for the phone to ring . . . again and again

The phone rings at 4 p.m., and you grab it off the hook. "Hi, this is Nancy Nurse," chirps the voice on the other end. Your whole world stops for a second, as you try to decipher from the tone of her voice whether she has good news or bad news.

Blood and ultrasound callbacks consume a huge part of your life after you start IVF. You find yourself leaving whole volumes of information on how to reach you that day (cell phone, home phone, don't leave a message with the babysitter, partner's number, don't call before 6, don't call after 6, don't leave a message, I really need to talk to you) on your callback sheets, because this call, whether good or bad news, is the highlight of your day.

If your clinic has a lot of staff, try to cultivate a good relationship with one or two nurses you feel comfortable with. It doesn't hurt to ask to speak with that nurse when you call. Most nurses are happy to call you if you personally ask for them. Also, if you get to know one or two people well, you hopefully won't have to explain all the ins and outs of your case every time you call in.

What if the clinic has only one nurse and you just don't get along? Try and make it easier for both of you. Maybe you can ask for the doctor to call you; if your personality really clashes with the nurse's, the doctor may be willing to handle your calls. If you have to get your calls from someone you're not happy with, ask the nurse to leave your instructions on your answering machine so that you don't have to talk to her on the phone. Or you may want to fax in your list of questions so that the nurse can write the answers on it and fax it back. That way, you get the answers you need with a minimum of aggravation.

Sometimes you can just *feel* it — you've become an annoyance to the nurses. You picture the nurses throwing the phone to each other when you call, in a version of patient hot potato. You feel terrible about this. Everyone wants to be liked, and every patient also wants her questions answered without feeling like a pest.

If you're getting bad vibes, you may want to try and clear the air with the staff. Politely explain (not at callback time, when everyone is busy) why you feel things are strained, and encourage some open communication about how you can best work together. Everyone benefits if the communication between you and the staff is good, and unfortunately you're the one who will suffer the most if you don't get along with the rest of the team.

Feeling like everyone in the waiting room is doing better than you

There you are in the waiting room, listening to the person ahead of you brag about how well her cycle is going, how she's got 20 beautiful follicles, how good her partner is at giving shots, how she loves the nurses so much she's making them each a ceramic something to say thank you, how great her veins are, and how happy she is to be alive. You look at your poor black and blue arms and think about how you have only seven follicles on ultrasound, how your partner seems to hit a nerve every other day, how much you hate all the nurses, and how much you hate this whole process.

In some centers, the waiting room is like group therapy in a psychiatrist's office: All the patients pull their chairs together while waiting for their ultrasound appointments and talk about IVF and life in general. This kind of place can provide you with new friends who know exactly what you're going through, but it can also turn into a sort of golf course with chairs — she got pregnant on the first try, she has the most follicles, she's doing better than she did last cycle, she's having twins, she's having triplets.

Stay out of the comparison contests, if you can. Everyone responds differently to medications, and in the end, the person with three follicles may get pregnant, and the person with twenty follicles may not. Remember that the only statistics that matter are your own.

If talking to other people about your problems makes you feel worse, don't join in. Bring a book and headphones and put an unapproachable expression on your face. Arrive as close to the time of your appointment as you can, get engrossed in the TV, or hide in the bathroom!

On the other hand, if you can listen to other women's tales and not compare yourself to them, the waiting room can be a great source of camaraderie and a place to make lasting friendships.

Feeling like you've been on gonadotropins your whole life

Are you setting some sort of record for the most days ever spent taking gonadotropins? It probably feels like it. Gonadotropins can cause mood swings, headaches, and bloating, all side effects that make you anxious to discontinue these drugs as soon as possible. You'll probably be on medications at least eight days if you're doing a standard protocol; slow starters may spend nearly twice that amount of time on medications before their follicles are big enough to go to retrieval (usually about 18 to 20 millimeters). Some doctors believe that staying on these medications too long negatively affects your egg quality. Other doctors don't see a problem with continuing these medications for 15 or 16 days as long as your follicles are growing.

Mood swings are a normal response to high hormone levels. You won't be this emotional forever!

Recognizing when your estradiol level is too high

"My estradiol's over 3,000," the skinny little blonde in the waiting room says proudly. Now, you already know not to make comparisons, but you do wonder, "Isn't that too high?" How high is too high? Most programs consider you to be moderately hyperstimulated when your estradiol is over 2,000, and classify you as severely hyperstimulated when the level reaches 4,000 or 5,000. Your estradiol is usually directly related to the number of follicles you have. Each follicle produces an estradiol of 100 to 200, so if you have ten follicles, your E2 (estradiol) will be between 1,000 and 2,000 when the follicles are mature.

If your E2 is too high, you won't be able to do a fresh embryo transfer, so most centers try to keep your E2 and follicle count to a reasonable number. In an ideal world, every patient would have 15 to 20 follicles and an E2 of between 2,000 and 2,500.

Ovarian hyperstimulation syndrome (OHSS) is a potentially life-threatening complication of taking infertility medications; it's more common in IVF patients because they usually take high doses of stimulating hormones. OHSS causes severe fluid shifts in your circulatory system, with fluid from your blood vessels leaking into your surrounding tissues. Sudden large weight gain, difficulty urinating, and shortness of breath are some signs of OHSS that your center will want you to know.

Why feeling blue is normal

We can't stress enough that mood swings are normal with high hormone levels. You also may experience a letdown feeling when doing an IVF cycle. You've planned for it and fantasized about how things would go, and now it's almost over. It's like Christmas: Sometimes the anticipation surpasses the reality. When you're almost ready for egg retrieval, you can't change things. It's too late to say, "We should have waited another month" or "I should have taken more meds, less meds, or different meds."

Taking a Shot in the Dark: Time for hCG

It's Nancy Nurse on the phone again, and this time you can tell that she's got *really* big news. "It's time for hCG!" she says, and because she sounds so excited, you feel like you should get out the pompoms and do a cheer. If you've read your protocol, you know what hCG (human chorionic gonadotropin) is; if you haven't, here's a refresher course.

Defining the role of hCG

HCG is a crucial part of your IVF cycle. HCG is given about 35 hours before your egg retrieval; its job is to mature your eggs and prepare them to be fertilized. Giving hCG allows the IVF staff to plan egg retrievals for a reasonable time during the day, instead of waiting for your natural LH surge to occur. That's why the timing of your hCG is very important.

Watching the clock: Timing is everything with hCG

The hCG instructions include a specific time to take your injection, and following the directions is absolutely critical because timing really is everything. Your injection may be scheduled for midnight, or even a few hours later, if your center has a lot of egg retrievals to do on one day.

If your injection is scheduled for, say, 2 a.m., you can mix the medication ahead of time and put it on your bedside table; then set your alarm for the time you need to take the hCG. Giving the injection at an odd hour is easier if you don't need to fumble around mixing medications when you're half asleep.

If you normally have a doctor's office, close friend, or neighbor do your injections, you may have a problem getting them to give hCG in the middle of the night. Be aware ahead of time that you need to find someone willing to do this when the time comes.

Going for the Gold: The Egg Retrieval

Almost before you know it, it's time for your egg retrieval. All kinds of emotions are probably churning around inside you and your partner. This is the culmination of several weeks of injections, emotions, and worries. It's your big day! How do you feel?

Reducing the anxiety with medication

Surgery is always a little scary, even when it's surgery for something you want very badly. Most centers give you medication to make you comfortable during the retrieval, and some centers give medications before the retrieval to relax you.

Rescheduling the retrieval

You can count on Murphy's Law occurring at retrieval time. If you have a big event coming up around the time of your egg retrieval, the day of the big event will be the same day your retrieval is scheduled. In most cases, your doctor may be able to do your egg retrieval a day earlier or later if it gets you through a big occasion. Sometimes, however, due to your blood levels indicating that you may ovulate if you wait, your center may not be able to schedule around your event.

If you know ahead of time about an event that may conflict with your egg retrieval, tell your doctor about it *before* you start taking your stimulating hormones. Sometimes an egg retrieval can be held off for a few days if you take Lupron or birth control a few extra days before starting your stimulating medications. After you start stimulating medications, influencing the day of your retrieval is harder.

Looking at retrieval schedules

Some IVF centers do egg retrievals every day of the week. Others do retrievals only Monday through Friday and start their patients' medications all at the same time to avoid the weekends. Still others cycle patients through in batches, doing retrievals only every other month or a few months of the year. You probably won't have much say in what day or what time your retrieval is done.

Signing here . . . and here . . . and here . . .

Some centers have you sign consent forms ahead of time for your egg retrieval, but you may be asked to sign the day of the retrieval. Usually a nurse reviews the consent forms with you. Keep in mind that your anxiety level will be through the roof, and the chances that you'll be able to read and comprehend 18 pages of legalese the morning of your retrieval are slim. If possible, ask for the consent forms ahead of time so that you have time to read and understand what you'll be signing.

Some centers let you make changes in the consent forms as long as they know what the changes are ahead of time and can have a lawyer review your changes. Here are the most common concerns that people have with IVF consent forms:

- ✔ Having pictures taken of themselves, their eggs, sperm, or embryos, for use in any type of publication. Many people have no objection to this, but some do.

- ✔ Allowing medical, nursing, or other students in the room to watch the procedure.

✔ Using any sperm, eggs, embryos, or tissue for research. "Tissue" can mean fluid from follicles, endometrial tissue, or anything else removed at the time of retrieval or transfer.

✔ Freezing of any embryos not transferred on a fresh transfer. Some people have religious objections to embryo freezing, and they want to inseminate only a few eggs, so that they can use up all their embryos and not have any left to freeze. Discuss this step ahead of time with embryology to make sure that everyone understands exactly what will be done.

If you have objections to anything in the consent forms, address them before the morning of your egg retrieval. If your clinic has a problem with your requests, it could delay or cancel your retrieval.

Meeting the retrieval team

A whole new group of unfamiliar people will be with you for the egg retrieval — how wonderful. During the egg retrieval, a nurse or a medical assistant may be in the room helping the doctor. An ultrasonographer may be present, and the embryologist will be very nearby. Hopefully, you'll know the ultrasonographers and the nurse. With any luck, you'll know the doctor, too, although, the doctor you had an initial consultation with may not do your egg retrieval. The person you may be most interested in as you arrive in the IVF area (which you probably have never seen before) is the person who will give you the medication for your retrieval.

Previewing what happens in an egg retrieval

Different centers do things different ways, but in most centers, you're taken to the IVF suite, a part of the building you've never seen before and had no idea existed. You'll change into a gown, hat, and shoe covers because the IVF suite is a sterile area where an attempt is made to keep outside germs from entering.

An intravenous (IV) infusion is started. The purpose of the IV is mainly to have access for giving you medication, but it's also there in case any complications require you to be given large amounts of fluid quickly. If you know that certain of your veins are better than others for the IV, don't be shy about informing the person starting your IV!

The embryologist usually comes in to see you before the procedure starts to ask you to verify your name, Social Security number, and information about your partner. The purpose of checking this information is to prevent any type of mix-up with eggs, sperm, or embryos.

The doctor generally comes in the room at the last minute, hopefully introduces herself if you don't already know her, and instructs the person giving you medications to start giving them. The doctor inserts a speculum and washes the vagina and cervix thoroughly, trying to keep the area as clean as possible.

You won't remember the rest, so we explain what happens next. The doctor inserts the vaginal ultrasound probe into your vagina. On the top of the probe is a needle guide along which a long metal needle slides. The doctor locates your follicles on ultrasound with the probe and then punctures the back of the vagina with the needle, entering each follicle and sucking out the fluid. The follicular fluid is given to the embryologist, who examines it under a microscope and says, hopefully, "Egg one, egg two" and so on. When the follicles are all emptied, you'll wake up and be taken to a nearby bed for a short time to recover. An egg retrieval usually takes about 30 to 40 minutes from start to finish, and you'll be asleep the whole time.

Knocking you out: Anesthesia choices for the retrieval

IVF centers vary considerably in their methods of anesthesia for egg retrievals. Some centers do all their retrievals in a hospital operating suite, so a nurse anesthetist or an anesthesiologist (a doctor who specializes in giving anesthesia) gives your medications. Smaller centers may have only an assistant or the nurse giving medication under the guidance of your doctor. Still others offer you a choice between conscious sedation and MAC, or monitored anesthesia care.

With conscious sedation, you receive some version of medication in the valium family, possibly Valium or Versed, and also some type of narcotic, such as Demerol, fentanyl, or morphine. The degree to which you're awake during your procedure varies quite a bit between individuals. If you've taken narcotics frequently in the past, you may develop a tolerance to them, and they may not make you comfortable. Some women are much more sensitive to all drugs and need very little medication to put them to sleep. Your vital signs, including your heart rate, blood pressure, and respirations, are carefully monitored during your procedure.

If you have MAC, an anesthesiologist or a nurse anesthetist must give it to you. Either of those professionals is qualified to give the medication propofol (Diprivan is the brand name), which will put you in a deep sleep for your retrieval.

Certain medications, such as Versed, have amnesiac properties, which is a fancy way of saying that you won't remember what went on during the retrieval. This effect lasts for a short time after the procedure as well. Nearly every IVF patient wakes up after the procedure and asks, "How many eggs did I get?" at least three times before she's actually awake enough to remember the answer! You may not remember walking from the table to a bed, either, but you did!

Looking for the perfect egg

Eggs can come in many different shapes and sizes, but what your embryologist hopes to see at the time of retrieval is an egg that is round, surrounded by corona cells and cumulus, with a polar body attached to it. See Figure 12-1 for a normal, mature egg.

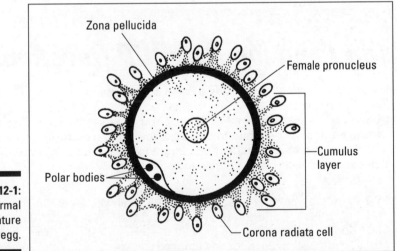

Figure 12-1:
A normal mature human egg.

Some eggs at retrieval time are still small and may be classified as immature. Often, immature eggs mature by the next day and can be inseminated with sperm then. Immature eggs won't fertilize properly.

Eggs that are dark and grainy, or elongated in shape, probably won't fertilize. See Chapter 13 for some examples of abnormal eggs.

Doing His Duty: Your Partner Is Busy, Too

While you're snoozing away in the IVF suite, your partner will be watching the movies most centers helpfully provide to make it easier for him to masturbate to produce a semen specimen. This can be a tricky issue for some men and downright impossible for others. If you think that your partner is going to suffer from performance anxiety on retrieval day, consider the following ways to take the pressure off:

✔ You can have him freeze a specimen ahead of time. Most centers prefer to use fresh sperm, but if your partner knows a frozen backup is available, he may have an easier time in the producing room.

✔ He can go to a nearby hotel, or home, if you live close enough — within 15 to 20 minutes away — use a sterile cup the andrologist will give him, and produce there.

✔ You can help him produce. You may feel uncomfortable going in with him, but believe me, it's no big deal — people do it all the time. But andrologists enforce two rules: no saliva and no lubricants. Either one can mess up the semen specimen.

Answering Common Post-IVF Questions

After a retrieval, almost everybody asks these questions:

✔ **Can I see my eggs before I go home?** You can't see your eggs because they can be seen only under a microscope, and no embryologist in the world is going to let a patient still lurching around in an anesthesia daze mess around with his extremely expensive microscope or those precious eggs!

✔ **Why can't my partner come back to the retrieval room?** In some centers, partners are allowed to be present at the egg retrieval. Other centers don't allow anyone else to be in the room for the retrieval, although they're often allowed in for the embryo transfer. Usually the rooms are too small to allow extra people, and no one wants partners feeling woozy in the retrieval room and knocking over the ultrasound equipment if they fall.

✔ **Do I have to have an IV?** Yes.

✔ **Are you *sure* you won't mix up my eggs (or sperm or embryos) with someone else's?** Yes.

With several mix-up cases in the news recently, most centers are anxious to reassure patients on this topic. Mix-ups with sperm, embryos, or eggs happen only when someone is extremely careless, and all centers are very aware of the recent cases in the news and are being extremely careful to avoid such an incidence.

Most centers label all dishes, collection cups, and so on with the patient's name, Social Security number, patient number, and sometimes a color code. Egg retrievals and embryo transfers are done one at a time — never two at the same time. Catheters used for embryo transfer are never reused, so someone else's embryo won't be stuck in your catheter!

After an embryo transfer, the catheter used is examined again to make sure that none of your embryos decided to stay behind. All those little guys should be in the uterus, where they belong!

✔ **Where do you keep the eggs?** Eggs are incubated overnight with sperm in a petri dish and then checked in the morning for fertilization.

✔ **Where do you keep frozen embryos?** Frozen embryos are kept in a liquid nitrogen tank.

✔ **What happens if your power goes out? How do the embryos survive?** Nitrogen tanks don't use electricity. For everything else, centers have backup generator power.

✔ **How many eggs did you say I got?** Sigh.

Chapter 13

Creating an Embryo: Amazing Teamwork in the Lab

The medical advances that enable IVF (in vitro fertilization) clinics to fertilize eggs and grow embryos in a lab is a science, but it's also an art. The embryology team is skilled in working with the most precious of all biologic material: the eggs, sperm, and embryos that have the potential to become your child.

After you've completed an IVF cycle and gone through an egg retrieval, everything is in the hands of the members of the embryology team. They're the ones who check your eggs, ready the sperm for fertilization, and keep those embryos growing until the day of transfer. They're the bearers of all good news and bad news, and you want to know everything they're doing.

In this chapter, we tell you what goes on in the lab, what the embryologists want to see, and what they *don't* want to see in eggs, sperm, and embryos. We also review your instructions for transfer, explain why you're taking certain medications, and give some insight into how many embryos you may want to transfer.

Recognizing a Good Egg When You See One

Before you go home after retrieval (see Chapter 12), embryology can take a look at your eggs and let you know whether they're mature, postmature, or immature. Mature eggs are needed for fertilization to occur, but immature eggs will often mature within 24 hours after retrieval. An egg retrieval may yield eggs that are both mature and immature, especially if you made a lot of follicles. If your eggs are postmature, they may not fertilize.

A mature egg is one that has a fluffy cumulus layer, a dense outer layer called the corona, which a single sperm will need to break through for fertilization to occur, a polar body, and no germinal vesicles (immature cells). Polar bodies (there are two) are the "leftovers" after an oocyte has completed its final cell division, which leaves it with just 23 chromosomes. The first polar body is eliminated at the time of ovulation, and the second at the time of fertilization. A mature egg is ready to be fertilized because it has already completed one of the last stages of cell division, called *meiosis;* it now contains 23 chromosomes. (Refer to Chapter 12 for a picture of a mature egg.)

An immature egg usually doesn't have a polar body, and it will have germinal vesicles, meaning that it hasn't yet completed the division to 23 cells.

Postmature eggs may be dark and grainy-looking.

If you're doing normal insemination, some of your eggs (usually six to eight) and sperm will be placed in a *petri dish,* a flat-bottomed round glass or plastic dish, which will be labeled with your name, lab number, the date, and the number of eggs in the dish. This is done after the sperm are washed and the egg is stripped of the cumulus and coronal layers. The dish is placed in an incubator so the eggs and sperm can be kept at body temperature.

Most of the time, conventionally inseminated eggs are left alone for 16 to 20 hours. The day after the retrieval, embryology takes the dish out of the incubator and checks the eggs; what they hope to find is two pronuclear (2PN) embryos, or embryos that have two visible circles lined up next to each other (see Figure 13-1). These embryos contain the genetic material from each parent.

If you're planning to freeze some or all of your embryos for use at another time, your clinic may freeze them at the 2PN stage. Some centers grow all your embryos out to blastocyst stage and freeze only those that make it to blastocyst.

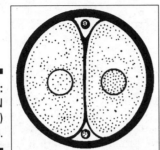

Figure 13-1:
A 2PN
(pronuclear)
embryo.

Congratulations! You've got embryos!

Looking at what can go wrong when egg meets sperm

Good fertilization depends on the quality of the sperm and egg. At most centers, the fertilization rate is about 70 percent. When embryologists look at the other 30 percent of the eggs, they may see things they'd rather not. For example, they may see the following:

✔ Your embryos may be *polyploid,* meaning that they contain more than two pronuclei. This can occur when more than one sperm has entered the egg, or when the egg doesn't throw off the second polar body (which should occur at the time of fertilization). These embryos are never normal, because the egg or the sperm that created them isn't normal.

✔ The egg may show no signs of fertilization. In this case, the egg might be reinseminated the next day by using intracytoplasmic sperm injection (ICSI).

Injecting for male factor, if necessary

If you need to do ICSI for male factor (explained in Chapter 7), the embryologist removes the cumulus and the coronal layers from the egg, washes the sperm in a special solution, and then sits down at the microscope for a long and tedious task. ICSI is done under a high-powered microscope, under the most sterile conditions possible; your embryologist wears a cover suit, a mask, hat, and booties while peering through the microscope trying to pick out the best sperm possible.

This task can be time consuming, and if moving, active sperm aren't available, the embryologist tries to pick out sperm for fertilization that are at least "twitching."

ICSI is done with a very fine-gauge needle. The sperm is sucked into the needle, your egg is stabilized, and the needle point is slowly inserted into the egg. ICSI requires very steady hands and a good eye for picking the best-looking sperm.

The process afterward is the same as conventional insemination. The ICSI eggs are left overnight and checked in the morning for fertilization. If the eggs haven't fertilized, ICSI can't be redone.

Some studies have shown that ICSI embryos have a higher than normal rate of *aneuploidy,* or abnormal chromosomes. This higher rate may occur because men with severe male factor have more chromosomal abnormalities, such as Klinefelter's syndrome.

RICSI, or rescue ICSI, is done the morning after conventional insemination if the eggs haven't fertilized. Success rates from RICSI are very low, not only for fertilization but also for pregnancy. The pregnancy rate with RICSI is about 5 percent.

Answering the Call from Embryology

An embryologist usually calls the morning after your egg retrieval to let you know how many embryos you have and to discuss how many to transfer. If you're going to freeze some, the embryologist also gives you some help deciding how many to leave out to grow a few days before picking the best few to transfer. Some centers suggest letting six to ten embryos, if you have that many, grow for a few days. They then pick the best two or three to transfer and freeze the rest, sometimes growing the remaining embryos to blastocyst stage before freezing all that survive.

The embryos that are frozen after a few days usually have two to eight cells, and their thaw rate may not be as good as 2PN embryos (embryos frozen the day after egg retrieval).

Two days after retrieval, embryology may call again, this time to tell you how your embryos are growing. Hopefully, they've now reached the two- to four-cell stage. Figure 13-2 shows a four-cell embryo.

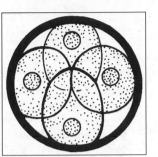

Figure 13-2:
A four-cell
embryo.

You may get a third call from embryology the third day after retrieval, if you're doing a three-day transfer. Some centers still do transfers two days after retrieval, and some do most transfers five days after retrieval — at five days, the embryo should have reached the blastocyst stage. (We discuss blastocyst transfer in the section "Blasting Off! Considering a Blastocyst Transfer," later in this chapter.) If your embryos are now four to eight cells, they're ready for transfer. In addition to being graded by the number of cells, embryos are also graded by the equality and roundness of the cells and by the amount of fragmentation, or broken pieces, that are in the embryo. Figure 13-3 shows an embryo with a high degree of fragmentation.

Although a funny-looking embryo doesn't create a funny-looking kid, most embryologists do feel that an embryo with less fragmentation and more even-looking cells has a better chance of implanting. If you do get pregnant from fragmented embryos, the fragmentation does *not* mean that your baby will be abnormal in any way. Some centers remove the fragmented pieces before the embryo is transferred.

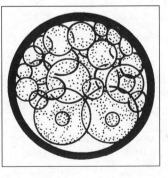

Figure 13-3:
An embryo
with a lot of
fragmen-
tation.

Grading an embryo

At some centers the best-looking embryos are graded as a 1A, with 1 through 3 being the size of the cells and A through D being the degree of fragmentation. Different centers grade embryos differently, so make sure you understand you particular clinic's grading system.

Does a great-looking embryo improve your chance of getting pregnant? Most embryologists would say a cautious yes, depending on your age, uterine cavity, general health, and many other factors.

Occasionally, if you're doing a three-day transfer, your embryos may already be *morulas,* or embryos that have 10 to 30 cells. Morulas usually have a very high rate of implantation, similar to blastocysts; in fact, they're the embryo stage right before blastocyst (see the section "Blasting Off! Considering a Blastocyst Transfer," later in this chapter).

Should you transfer that embryo?

Not all embryos are eight-cell, 1A embryos. In fact, most aren't. But most embryos that are at least four cells and graded 2B or C have a decent chance of implanting, and every embryologist has seen terrible-looking embryos that went on to become beautiful children. Embryologists suggest discarding the following types of embryos, however, because they're generally chromosomally abnormal:

- Multinucleated embryos, which contain three or more "bundles" of genetic material: At least 75 percent are abnormal.
- Embryos with uneven pronuclei: About 85 percent are abnormal.
- Embryos that develop too rapidly: Many of these have an abnormal number of chromosomes.

That's your baby . . . err, babies!

Many centers will give you pictures of your embryos to take home with you. How crazy is it to frame your embryo picture? We discuss that at the end of this chapter!

Looking at Your Uterine Lining

Embryos will implant only if the uterus is ready for implantation. Many centers look via ultrasound at the uterine thickness and also the appearance of the lining, called the pattern, to decide whether your embryos have a good chance of growing. Your lining may be described as triple lined, also called tri-laminar. This pattern description is shortened to TL in most centers and describes the lining most clinics like to see before embryo transfer. Fertility centers differ on what's considered a good thickness, but most prefer to see a thickness of at least 7 millimeters.

The next best lining is an isoechogenic (IE) pattern, and the lining that has the lowest implantation rate is a homogenous hyperechoic (HH) pattern. Different clinics place varying amounts of importance on lining patterns, and your clinic may not even check the pattern.

Most centers, however, do check the lining thickness before transfer; anything over 7 millimeters thick is considered adequate, although pregnancies do occur with thinner linings. Your center's emphasis on the importance of the lining thickness or pattern will vary.

Hatching Embryos — Come on Out, You Guys

Around 1994, embryologists came out with a new technique called *assisted hatching* to help human embryos implant in the uterus. The majority of IVF centers do hatching on at least some of their embryos.

Assisted hatching (AH) is done the morning of your embryo transfer. The embryologist takes a tiny needle with acid on the end of it and barely touches the shell of the embryo, creating a small hole. This helps the embryo "break through" the *zona,* or hard shell, and attach to the uterus, an action that must happen a day or so after the embryo reaches the uterus in nature. Embryos created in the lab often have harder shells than are seen in natural conception, so the little hole hopefully gives them a head start on breaking out and hunkering down where they belong.

Hatching was originally done only on embryos whose zona, or outer shell, was thicker than normal, or on embryos from women over age 37, whose embryos might have a harder time breaking out of the shell. Now, some centers do assisted hatching on almost all their embryos; others still do AH only on certain patients.

Making embryos stick: Why superglue doesn't work

Several IVF centers have come forward with new ideas for "sticking" embryos to the uterine lining. They either coat them with a sticking substance or dig a little hole in the endometrium to put them into. The IVF community hasn't gone crazy over these ideas because failure to implant usually isn't due to the embryos not sticking to the lining. It's a problem with the embryo or the lining itself. If the embryos, for whatever reason, aren't capable of growing into normal human beings, or the lining itself isn't capable of supporting their growth, forcing the embryos to attach to the lining won't make them grow.

Deciding How Many Embryos to Transfer

Deciding how many embryos to transfer can be difficult. Some centers and some parts of the world don't give you any say in the matter. For example, in England, you transfer two embryos if you're under age 40 — no exceptions. Some centers allow transfer of two embryos for women up to age 30, three embryos between ages 30 and 35, four embryos over age 35, and six or more embryos if you're over 40.

The ideal situation is discussing at your first doctor's appointment how many embryos to transfer, but the trouble is, you won't know at that point how well you'll stimulate, or how your embryos will look. Spending an hour debating about transferring four embryos is silly when you may get only three. If you end up with five embryos with a lot of fragmentation, most doctors suggest transferring more embryos than if they all look "good." Some centers don't freeze extra embryos, usually because their labs don't do freezing well. You may have to use 'em or lose 'em, and you may not be willing to discard embryos. At the very least, you can find out your clinic's policies about transfer at your first visit, and keep thinking ahead as you go through IVF about what you'll do at transfer time.

Blasting Off! Considering a Blastocyst Transfer

A few years ago, IVF centers became alarmed at the large number of higher-order multiples (triplets or more) their patients were delivering, and they started looking for ways to transfer fewer embryos and still maintain the all-important high pregnancy rates.

In most centers, the percentage of live-birth twins is about 25 percent of total births, and triplets a little less than 10 percent. Quadruplets and higher are considered a problem at almost all clinics, because the complication for both mother and babies is very high, and many babies die of prematurity or are miscarried.

Out of that concern came the *blastocyst transfer,* the transfer of a five-day-old embryo. Because only 30 to 50 percent of embryos grow to blastocyst stage (see Figure 13-4), centers felt that only the best embryos were going to be transferred. As it turned out, blastocyst transfer of two embryos results in pregnancy about 70 percent of the time in those under age 35, compared to 50 percent in a three-day transfer of three embryos.

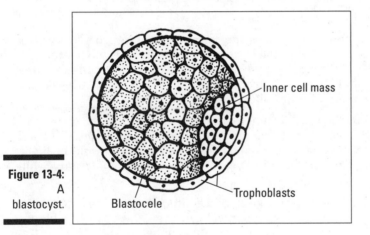

Figure 13-4:
A
blastocyst.

Inner cell mass

Trophoblasts

Blastocele

Blastocyst transfer isn't for everyone. Because blastocysts are more complicated to grow than three-day embryos, requiring multiple media changes to keep up with their increased nutritional needs, many centers find it too difficult to grow enough blastocysts to get to transfer. So if your center transfers only blastocysts, you may end up with nothing to transfer.

The second problem comes from the blastocysts themselves. Because they're already "hatching" out of their shells at the time of transfer, blastocysts seem unusually likely to split into identical twins. Although on the surface, having identical twins doesn't seem much different than having fraternal twins, the fact is that identical twin pregnancies are much more problematic than fraternals. Because identical twins share the same placenta and sac, *twin-twin transfusion syndrome,* in which one twin gets too many nutrients and the other not enough, is more common, as are cord accidents, in which one baby gets tangled in the other's umbilical cord. The incidence of identical twins is about four to five times higher in blastocyst transfer than in normal conception. Of course, if you transfer two blastocysts and one splits, you're right back to the problem of higher-order multiples again. For these reasons, some centers have stopped doing blastocyst transfer on all patients and instead use it selectively, for patients who have had several IVF failures.

Taking Postretrieval Pills and Potions

You may think that you're all done with medication after your egg retrieval, but you'll receive a sheet full of instructions about everything you need to take starting the day of your retrieval. Yes, the pills and potions go on after retrieval, but most are designed to help your embryo grow. Here's what you'll probably be given:

✔ **Antibiotics:** An egg retrieval is surgery that goes through a "dirty" area: your vagina. Yes, your vagina is considered a dirty area no matter how personally dainty and clean you are. So your doctor will probably give you antibiotics for several days, starting the day of your retrieval. Make sure that you mention any allergies or sensitivities.

If you're prone to yeast infections, you can take an over-the-counter pill called acidophilus, which maintains the balance of good and bad bacteria in your vagina. When the good bacteria are killed off with the bad ones, you get an overgrowth of yeast, which causes itching and a white cheesy discharge.

✔ **Steroids:** These may seem like an odd addition to your pill arsenal, but steroids are given to protect your embryo from attack by white blood cells after transfer. Steroids decrease the number of white blood cells in your blood. The dose given is very low and usually for just a few days.

✔ **Progesterone:** When it comes to progesterone supplements, you may be given pills, gels, suppositories, or — can you stand it? — injections. Some centers give progesterone injections to everyone, because injections are the best absorbed. But progesterone injections do have a downside:

• **They hurt.** The needle used for progesterone needs to be at least a 22-gauge (relatively thick) variety because the progesterone is very thick, or viscous, and won't flow through a smaller needle. The progesterone is mixed in sesame or peanut oil, and a fair number of women have allergic reactions to the oils.

• **They're hard to find.** Commercially made progesterone in oil is very hard to find. Some small compounding pharmacies make their own, as do some of the large mail-order pharmacies that specialize in fertility medications.

- **Insurance doesn't always cover the cost.** Some insurance companies don't feel that progesterone injections are medically necessary. Costs are reasonable — about $45 a bottle — but can add up if you're using a bottle every five days for several months.

On the other hand, some centers use vaginal suppositories. The downside of these are

- **They're messy.** The suppositories leak, making it necessary to wear a pad.

- **They can cause yeast infections.** Because they keep you continually wet, you're more likely to develop a yeast infection or rash, which can be more than a little annoying.

- **They're hard to find.** Specialty pharmacies usually make them themselves, which means that the amount of medication delivered can vary.

Other progesterone options are the following:

- **Crinone:** This is manufactured by Serono, a drug company that makes many fertility medications. Crinone is a gel and causes less leakage and irritation than suppositories. It comes in an applicator that is inserted vaginally. Crinone is more expensive than vaginal suppositories.

- **Prometrium capsules, or compounded capsules:** These are pills, which means that they pass through your liver after being digested in the stomach. The main disadvantage is that the way they're metabolized causes drowsiness, which can be severe. Some women also complain about dizziness or nausea.

Transferring Your Embryo

When you arrive for your embryo transfer, you'll be taken back to the IVF suite. Many centers allow your partner to come with you, and you'll both change into sterile gowns and coveralls. Some centers give you Valium before your transfer, primarily to reduce cramping after the procedure, although relaxing you is a side benefit.

Studies have shown that reducing cramping that you can't even feel can boost the pregnancy rate by 50 percent.

You'll be instructed to lie on an exam table that can be tilted. The worst part of the transfer in most clinics is that you're lying there with a full bladder. A full bladder, uncomfortable as it is, makes it easier to see your uterus under ultrasound guidance, and many centers now do embryo transfers under ultrasound guidance rather than blindly placing them through the cervix.

Your bladder, lying right under the uterus, pushes your uterus up when it's full; it also straightens the path into the uterus, making the transfer easier. A full bladder is especially helpful if you have a retroverted, or tilted, uterus.

An embryologist or your doctor may come in to speak with you before the transfer. That person will tell you how your embryos look today, may show or give you pictures, will verify your identity, and will confirm the number of embryos you want to transfer. You'll most likely receive something to sign that says that you agree to transfer X number of embryos, that you understand the risks of multiple birth, that you realize there's no guarantee of success, and that you are who you say you are.

An ultrasonographer (if your clinic uses ultrasound guidance) will place the probe on your abdomen so that the uterus can be visualized. The doctor or associate (nurses do embryo transfers in some centers) will wash your cervix and remove any mucus from the opening. Leaving a speculum in place, the doctor will let the embryologist know she's ready. Here come your embryos!

Your doctor will slide the catheter through your cervix, which may cause a little cramping. If your clinic uses ultrasound guidance for the transfer, the ultrasonographers will let the doctor know how far away from the top of the uterus the catheter is before the embryos are slowly injected into the uterus. The catheter is slowly removed and handed back to the embryologist, who examines it under a microscope to make sure that no embryos are still in the catheter.

A transfer that's traumatic in any way, causing bleeding or severe cramping, may decrease your chance of pregnancy. If you've done a mock transfer (in a mock transfer, a soft catheter is inserted into the uterus, and the depth of the uterus and the angle required to get into it are recorded) before starting IVF, the doctor has a "map" of your cervical canal and uterine opening so trauma is less likely. Ultrasound guidance also makes it easier to see the curves in your anatomy, so your center may not do a mock transfer if it's using ultrasound guidance for your embryo transfer.

After your embryos are in the uterus, you may need to stay on the table with your feet tilted up for a half hour or so. Clinics vary widely in their bed rest requirements, and they may keep you anywhere from no time at all to up to four hours. After you go home, you'll be instructed to maintain bed rest for a specified time. Most clinics suggest two days. Others recommend up to a week, and some clinics don't feel that any bed rest is justified.

Embryos are placed directly into your uterus; emptying your bladder or bowels isn't going to dislodge them! In fact, not going when you need to can increase uterine cramping, which *can* have a negative effect on your getting pregnant.

Keeping Your Feet and Your Spirits Up After the Transfer

After you're safely home, you may be on restricted activity for a period of time, depending on your clinic's policies. Try not to compare what you're doing to what anyone else is doing, because different centers have different policies. If you don't follow your center's policies, you're bound to feel guilty if you don't get pregnant, so follow your instruction sheet.

Restricting your activity

If your center restricts activity after the transfer, you'll be lying around on the bed or couch, getting up only to use the bathroom and eat meals. After your strict rest period is over, many centers still ask you not to lift anything heavy (over 15 pounds is typical), not to do any strenuous exercise, and not to have sex.

Sex is restricted because it can cause uterine contractions, especially if you have an orgasm, so the no-sex rule applies to *any* activity that could cause an orgasm, not just intercourse. Yes, this restriction does include vibrators!

Heavy lifting is another prohibition that can cause concern, especially if your job requires it or if you have a small child. Most centers will gladly write you a note restricting your work activity, but your 1-year-old probably won't understand a note saying you can't lift him into his high chair. If you have to lift a child, bend with your knees, trying to keep your back straight when you lift rather than bending at the waist and straining your abdominal muscles. This form is good body mechanics, and you should pick up heavy objects, such as children, this way all the time if you want to keep your back in working order.

Mild exercise, such as a leisurely walk, is fine, but forget about aerobics for a while. Use common sense about yoga, tai chi, or whatever else you do to decrease stress and increase endorphins. If you feel guilty doing it, you probably shouldn't be doing it!

Dealing with your partner

After all of the running around for blood work, ultrasounds, retrieval, and transfer, two days of bed rest may sound like an ideal antidote. And it very well may be. However, take heed before inviting anyone to keep you company.

Most women recuperate from their transfer at home, while some who are traveling for the procedure may find themselves in a strange hotel room. Either way, the same rules apply. Generally speaking, this is *not* the time to entertain your relatives, host a slumber party for your friends, or plan on long, soulful discussions with your partner. The truth is, you'll probably spend much of the transfer day itself relaxing if not sleeping, as a result of the pre-transfer medication often used to calm you and your uterus. After you wake up, you should feel fine, but you may be excited, nervous, restless, or all of the above.

You've gone through a lot to get to this point, and you need time to unwind. Make your two days of bed rest about you, not your partner, mother, or best friend. Surround yourself with a person, persons, or professional who can prepare your meals, dispense or administer your post-transfer medication and shots, and run interference between you and the pesky world outside. Your partner may be this person, or he may not be. Some folks do better than others at tending to the bedridden (generally they're called nurses). Others, such as my husband (coauthor Jackie here), become antsy at the mere thought of sitting at home for two days with nothing to do.

For those whose partners fall in the latter group, this isn't the time to try and train your partner to enjoy quiet time; engage in long, meaningful conversation; or contemplate whether your navel is growing. Your partner has also experienced a range of emotions as a result of all the activity leading up to this point. He may need a bit of his own time and space to relax as well, in a way best suited for him.

Allow your partner time off for good behavior. He may welcome the opportunity to get out and do the grocery shopping or pick up the dry cleaning, a good book (for you!), or a pizza. If need be, arrange for a friend to fill in during these absences.

If you haven't prepared for ways to keep yourself entertained (and horizontal) during this period, consider dispatching your partner, friend, or relative to pick up a good magazine (or six), a book, or the rental movie you've been meaning to watch. You can pay as much or little attention as you can muster with these forms of entertainment. This is generally not the case, however, when you're trying to fill time with the company of others.

This two-day period is also not the best time to try to catch up on a backlog of work, phone calls, or bills. Consider this instead as a short respite for relaxation and recovery. Besides, you'll have plenty of time during the remainder of the two-week wait (the time between your embryo transfer and your pregnancy test).

Pinning your hopes on your embryo picture

Is it crazy to frame your embryo picture? Well, that depends on your definition of crazy. Keep in mind that embryos don't have a lot of distinguishing characteristics. Nothing shows whether your embryo is a boy or girl, blond-haired or dark-haired, brown-eyed or blue-eyed, or short or tall. In fact, an embryo picture doesn't have much that would even identify it as human.

And yet, you may find yourself staring at your embryos as if they held the secret of life itself. You'll scrutinize every angle, bump, lump, or dent as if this embryo will somehow reveal itself to you if you study it long enough. "Who are you?" you may find yourself asking. "Please live," you may whisper, over and over. "Please come home. We're waiting for you."

Some people even name their embryos, not formally of course, but with cute little nicknames, almost as if they're embarrassed to be caught humanizing their embryos.

You may at times think of yourself as crazy for doing this, but rest assured that you're not. This picture is the only visual affirmation you have of all your hopes and dreams. Even though it resembles a mouse as much as — or more than —it does a blue-eyed baby, it is something tangible. By all means, frame the picture. Keep it in your bedroom if you're afraid what people will think. Allow yourself your dream.

Chapter 14

Waiting, Waiting: Surviving the Two-Week Wait after an IVF Cycle

Finishing up an in vitro fertilization (IVF) cycle brings a whole host of emotions. You're happy that the procedure itself was successful and that the shots are finished or at least greatly diminished. You're ecstatic about having your life back, without the frequent blood draws, ultrasounds, and phone calls. On the other hand, you may feel adrift when the intensity is over and you've gone from constant monitoring to being almost ignored by your clinic.

Now it's time to wait for your pregnancy test. Because the test results won't be accurate for almost two weeks after your embryo transfer, this time period is often referred to by patients as "the two-week wait."

In this chapter, we review some of the do's and don'ts of the two-week wait, and peek a little into the future when you'll have an answer to the big question — am I pregnant or not? — and what you'll be doing in either case.

Technically, You're Pregnant — Waiting for the Proof

From a purely technical viewpoint, after the embryos are placed into your uterus, you're pregnant — in the loosest sense of the word, at least. You have embryos floating around where they belong, and all they have to do is attach and grow.

This is probably the first time in your infertility history where you can say without a doubt that you've formed an embryo and that it is where it needs to be to grow. You may have known that you made a follicle, and been fairly sure that you got sperm where it needed to go at the right time, but you never knew for sure that the egg and sperm got together. Now you do.

Now comes the waiting period. The two-week wait is a time of "what ifs" and "if onlys" like no other time you've probably experienced.

As a fertility patient who has spent no less than two years in the two-week wait, I (coauthor Jackie) can attest to the fact that this is truly the time when the mind runs wild. A friend and fertility cohort finds the two weeks of waiting to be restful. This attitude is certainly one worth noting. By the time you get to this waiting game, you have done everything you can do to get pregnant. Even if your doctor is the kind who checks your blood work midluteal phase (translated: after week one of the two-week wait), keep in mind that although higher estrogen and progesterone levels may be more suggestive of a pregnancy, these are not a reliable indicator. Or in the words of an oft quoted fertility doc, "If midluteal numbers were so accurate, we'd call it a pregnancy test." So, whether your doctor orders midluteal tests or not, you're pretty much left with your thoughts and your progesterone to keep you company.

Dwelling and worrying do you no good and have no impact whatsoever on the final outcome. Enjoying yourself and keeping busy with your day-to-day responsibilities will help to keep your life manageable and put you in a better place for whatever news you receive. Remember, at the end of the day, or at the end of the two-week wait as the case may be, you will have passed through two very valuable weeks of your life. Why waste them on worry?

Although you may be tempted to just relax and wait, unencumbered by other responsibilities, the truth is that sitting around waiting is hard work, a lot harder than keeping yourself busy with everyday tasks. Waiting for water to boil and staring at it as well is a quick recipe for instant irritation, and so is staying idle during these two weeks.

Try to plan as many activities as you can manage (after your post-transfer rest period). If you work, consider it a blessing and immerse yourself in your responsibilities. Many women suggest reading a good book to get you through this time. Try to keep the book as far away from the topic of fertility as possible. Exercise is also a good way to keep busy, but before you plan on running marathons, check with your doctor. Most doctors recommend keeping your heart rate less than 140 while trying to conceive. Many couples find that the two-week wait is a great time to take a vacation. What better way to distract yourself than with a little R&R?

Some women say that the optimism of the two-week wait can make this a great time to check in with pregnant friends or friends with children who may have been difficult to talk to during the trials of fertility treatment. During the two-week wait, even those of us who are fertility patients are going through essentially the same thing that any other woman trying to conceive goes through. Our stakes may be a bit higher, but our impatience is similar.

Don't think that waiting as a couple is any easier. Staring at each other while waiting for the phone to ring is hardly the definition of quality time. Rather, it provides fertile (pun intended) breeding ground for arguments large and small. At times, I (Jackie) found myself annoyed at my husband for giving off the appearance of calm. The truth was that he actually *was* calm, or calmer than I was! He took this time to remind me that two of us "co-stressing" didn't help matters. He used the two-week wait to immerse himself in work and generally keep his mind off all matters regarding baby. As a result, at the end of the two weeks, he often emerged far saner than I. Granted, to conceive or not to conceive was going on in my body. However, his attitude was far more beneficial for both of us. As best you can, go about your business, as individuals or as a couple.

I (Jackie) passed many a two-week wait talking with fertility friends whom I had met either online or through support groups. We would wile away our lunch hours comparing symptoms and poking at our breasts periodically to see whether we felt any of the classic tenderness associated with pregnancy. I recommend limiting this poking activity to private times, as other motorists have a tendency to stare at this odd rite of passage.

If all else fails, visit one of the many sites that list all the standard pregnancy symptoms . . . and then some. Sites such as `www.onna.org/information/pg-signs.html` give you at least a symptom a day to obsess over.

If the tension does begins to run high, assemble your backup plan. What will you do next, pregnant or not? This type of planning often alleviates the fear and uncertainty that accompany the two-week wait.

Seeking support during an uncertain time

Going through the two-week wait is something best done with lots of support. Your doctor will take care of the medical end of this equation, but you'll undoubtedly need a little help from your friends to keep your mind on track. If you've shared your story with friends and family, you can hopefully lean on them during this period of waiting. If you've kept those around you in the dark, consider sharing your anxiety with a professional, such as a therapist, a religious figure (your minister, priest, or rabbi, for example), or a support group.

If anonymity is your bag, consider the online resources discussed in Chapter 5. Many online bulletin boards have specific sections devoted to the two-week wait, which reassure you that you're not alone. You can find one such example of this at www.inciid.org (the InterNational Council on Infertility Information Dissemination). At sites such as this, you can share your hopes, fears, and daily symptoms with legions of women going through the same thing. This type of camaraderie can actually make waiting fun.

Making your to-do or not-to-do list

Taking care of yourself during the roller coaster ride of trying to create a baby is crucial. For some women, this may mean a trip to the hairdresser, manicurist, gym, or all of the above. But you should consider a few limitations as you wait out these last few weeks before your pregnancy test.

Coloring your hair

For those whose follicle challenges begin at the top of their heads, hair coloring is more than just a luxury; it's a way of life. To color or not to color has been a long-time topic of discussion among the newly pregnant. According to the American College of Obstetricians and Gynecologists, hair coloring *is* safe during pregnancy. Based on this opinion, coloring your hair during the two-week wait is also presumed to be safe (unless of course your colorist turns your hair orange!). However, keep in mind that the two-week wait is only two weeks. If you're at all concerned, staying off the bottle (of color, that is) for the time being may be the best advice for you.

Having manicures and pedicures

The greatest danger that we know of in manicures and pedicures is for those who give them. You may have noticed that many manicurists now wear masks to protect themselves from the fumes and toxins generated by the products. A simple polish-and-go won't hurt you during the two-week wait. Those with acrylic nails are advised to refrain from having this service during the two-week wait, and those who don't have acrylic nails but want them are best waiting until after the two-week wait, and after the first trimester of pregnancy for that matter. If you already have acrylic nails, don't panic, but you may consider having them removed before your cycle.

Getting your exercise

Exercise can be a great way to take your mind off your waiting and your worries during the two-week wait. Here are two basic rules to remember with exercise during this time:

 ✔ Don't start up a brand-new routine during the two-week wait. In other words, if you're not a runner, don't become one now. Keep your exercise routine consistent with that which you engaged in before.

> ✔ Keep your heart rate equal to or lower than 140 beats per minute. This rate is also recommended during pregnancy, so this is a good time to get used to keeping track of it. Most fitness stores sell inexpensive heart rate monitors, and certain exercise machines (such as particular brands of treadmills) have a built-in monitor that can read your heart rate when you grasp the metal sensors on the handle bar.

Keep in mind that moderation must become your middle name, in judgment and in exercise. Should you choose the two-week wait as the ideal time to scale Mount Everest? We think not. Nor do we recommend skydiving for novices (or even experts) during this time. Both activities, aside from being highly dangerous, also pose the added risk of high altitude, which may be hazardous for those unaccustomed to it. However, if you live in Denver, the mile-high city, you don't have to move. The two-week wait calls for maintaining the status quo. Leave the new stuff for later.

Having sex during the two week wait

For those going through the two-week wait after in vitro fertilization, sex is considered a no-no (at least by most doctors). You've had surgery (albeit minor), and the risk of infection is greater, so hands (and other body parts) off during this time. Another concern is that female orgasm may cause a series of uterine contractions, which are not ideal in creating a hospitable environment for baby embryo. Read a good book instead.

Sensing Every Little Twinge: The Truth about Pregnancy Symptoms

Of course you're anxious. Of course you're anxiously examining every twinge and cramp you have for some indication of whether you're pregnant. If you're taking progesterone, as you most likely are after an IVF cycle, the symptoms of pregnancy can easily be confused with symptoms of progesterone supplementation, because an increase in progesterone is associated with many common pregnancy symptoms. What might you experience, and which signs are good, bad, and meaningless? Here are some symptoms you may experience and what they mean:

> ✔ **Sore breasts:** Tender breasts are almost a universal sign of pregnancy, with or without feelings of heaviness or tingling in the nipples. Unfortunately, sore breasts are caused by increased progesterone and estrogen, so sore breasts may be caused by your suppositories rather than by a growing embryo.

✔ **Spotting:** This symptom is very common in very early pregnancy, whether or not you've undergone fertility treatment. Spotting may be caused by an embryo burrowing into the uterus and causing leakage of blood from small blood vessels. If you're taking progesterone suppositories, irritation from the suppositories can also cause some spotting.

✔ **Cramping:** This discomfort is typical in the two-week wait and may be caused by the enlarged ovaries if you've done a medicated cycle (taken ovarian stimulating medications, as discussed in Chapter 9). Some centers believe that cramping is a sign of low progesterone, and they increase your supplements if you have continued cramping.

✔ **Fatigue:** This symptom is often related to higher than normal levels of hCG (human chorionic gonadotropin, the injection given 36 or so hours before an egg retrieval) and progesterone, both of which can be from the growing embryo or from your hCG trigger shot. Progesterone pills are particularly noted for causing extreme fatigue. Progesterone also raises your temperature, which may make you more sluggish than usual.

✔ **Nausea:** This symptom is fairly common with progesterone, especially in pill form, and also with high levels of hCG. Higher than normal levels of estrogen can also cause nausea.

So how can you tell whether you're pregnant in the two-week wait? Unfortunately, you really can't. I (coauthor Sharon) can name at least a dozen patients who swore they weren't pregnant and were, along with many patients who were sure they were but weren't. Continue taking your meds even if you're *sure* you're not pregnant, because there's a good chance you're wrong!

Don't be so sure you're not pregnant!

Patients who quit taking their medications such as progesterone on their own when they assume that they're not pregnant make me (coauthor Sharon) want to pull my hair out. I usually find this out when I call a patient (I'll call her Mary) who inexplicably never came in for her pregnancy test a week or so ago. When I ask her why she never came in, she says, "Oh, I got my period, so I stopped my meds." At this point my hair starts to stand on end, and I ask if she got a full flow period. She may say yes, but more often she says no — it was lighter than normal. Some women have a very light period even though they're pregnant, so this raises my voice a few octaves, and I tell her to have blood work done. Today. Right now, in fact. Mary voices extreme surprise and a little irritation at this, and says she knows she's not pregnant. And besides, she has something else to do today. You would think that people who just spent thousands of dollars trying to get pregnant wouldn't do something like this, but you'd be wrong. And so is Mary, quite frequently. Don't stop taking your medications until you have your pregnancy test done!

Send me a sign! Looking for a miracle during your wait

In many aspects of life, people are looking for a sign. In the two weeks between embryo transfer and pregnancy test, every rainbow, shooting star, or burning bush may be interpreted as a sign, by even the most pragmatic of folks, that pregnancy has occurred — or not occurred.

For the record, we've seen and heard of women in the two-week wait experiencing everything short of the earth moving (and I'm sure quite a few women who live on fault lines can claim that one too), while others writhe in fear whenever a black cat crosses their path. Keep such signs in perspective. Looking for symbolism in the two-week wait can be fun, but remember that the only sign that matters is the one that appears after your pregnancy test.

I (coauthor Jackie) experienced almost every bad luck talisman imaginable during the two-week wait that followed my successful cycle. Before that, I had been convinced numerous times that the good luck that came my way during previous two-week waits was an omen. Perhaps it was. In my case, however, it would have been a sign to appreciate my good luck in other areas of my life as I recorded one negative pregnancy result after another. So if good luck comes your way during the two-week wait, enjoy it for what it is and let the rest of the cards fall as they may.

But What If? Having a Plan B

So you're as positive as the day is long. You've kept yourself active and busy. You have benefited from the support of everyone, both in real life and in cyberspace. Still, the question keeps coming back: But what if you're not pregnant after the two-week wait? As you turn over this question for the 40,000,000th time, we suggest that you develop an answer. Of course, you don't want to dwell in the negative, but often having a Plan B can provide you with a sense of direction and confidence. As one saying goes, "The success of your life is measured by how well you adapt to Plan B." The two-week wait might also provide you with some time to consider your options.

Will you try again? Will you continue down the high-tech highway or go back to more intermediate measures. (Many women have failed at IVF only to find themselves pregnant naturally or by lesser means in the months to follow.) Will you consider other alternatives, such as donor egg, donor sperm, or adoption? Do you want to just get away from it all for a while? Any and all of these are acceptable courses of action. You may decide on one path and find yourself veering off in another direction. That's okay. Sometimes, the mere process of just choosing something — anything — can be a relief as well as an acceptable backup plan.

For the more immediate future, we have found that a Plan B is a good idea in planning for the day when you receive your news. If the news is positive, you'll no doubt celebrate. But what if it's not? Consider planning a comforting alternative for the day. A great movie, a soothing meal, or a night on the town may help you and your partner deal with the news. Just having a direction can help you cope with the uncertainty of a situation that doesn't go as planned. This day is neither the beginning nor the end of your life. It's simply a day to use as you choose. Choose wisely.

Saying No to Home Pregnancy Tests

Most women find the temptation of a home pregnancy test (HPT) impossible to resist. Those little packaged sticks promise immediate results and an answer to the question "Am I pregnant or not?" Before you go out and buy up your druggist's supply of home pregnancy tests, consider the following:

- Many home pregnancy tests require a minimum amount of hCG in your system in order to register a positive. Early pregnancy may not result in this high of a number, leaving you with a negative result, even in a positive situation.

- You were most likely given an hCG shot to trigger ovulation before your IVF retrieval. That shot of 10,000 units of hCG doesn't leave your system overnight. Furthermore, it's the same hormone (the pregnancy hormone) measured in home pregnancy tests. For some women, the traces of the hCG shot can take 10 to 15 days to disappear. Your HPT doesn't know that though! This can result in a false positive and a big letdown when the moment of truth arrives.

- Home pregnancy tests generally require the first morning's urine, which contains the highest concentration of hCG, for greatest accuracy. Many women, pregnant or not, awake in the middle of the night to urinate, making the first morning's urine not the first after all. Unless you want to subject yourself to 3 a.m. wake up calls for home pregnancy tests, this is yet another reason to "skip the stick."

- Home pregnancy tests are, first and foremost, over-the-counter devices. They do not replace a *beta sub unit (BSU)* — a blood test that measures the level of hCG, also known as the "real pregnancy test for serious reproducers." Do not expect the same accuracy or reliability from drugstore pregnancy tests.

Many women get on the HPT roller coaster, allowing their emotions to rise and fall with each subsequent pee stick. It isn't worth it. Wait for the real thing, as hard as the waiting may be. You have no reason to subject yourself to a test that could very well yield incorrect results.

Waiting for the Phone to Ring

It's beta day — the day your blood tests reveal whether you're pregnant or not.

Waiting for the phone to ring is almost always an unpleasant experience whether waiting for a date to call or a nurse to deliver news of whether your baby is on its way. But modern technology has given us answering machines and voice mails so that you don't have to sit by the phone! Take advantage of this technology. Sitting by the phone is a thankless job. Let someone (or something) else do it.

Deciding where you want the call

If you choose not to be home when the phone rings, alert the nurse or doctor who will be calling you with your results. Do you want that information left on your answering machine? Is there a chance that your little sister, mother, or cleaning person might hear the results instead, and perhaps forget to tell you? Work out these details ahead of time and communicate them to those who'll be delivering your results. Planning to receive this call at work may not be the best idea, unless you have a private area and/or supportive people around you. If you don't want to be called at work, make this fact very clear to the nurses and/or doctor as well. Some choose to have their partners receive the news. If you feel that hearing the news from someone close to you would be easier, consider this option and put it into action. You can't control the news you'll hear, but you can control the way you hear it.

Understanding chemical pregnancy and false positives

False positives are rare in pregnancy tests. You're most likely to get a false positive result on either a home pregnancy test or a beta subunit if it's been less than two weeks since you took hCG. Some doctors give hCG "boosters" during the two-week wait because it helps the corpus luteum, the remnant of your follicle that produced an egg, put out more progesterone.

Sometimes the BSU comes back positive, but it's a very low positive, less than 50 IU. Some doctors don't consider a BSU positive if it isn't at least 20 or so, while others consider anything over 5 to be positive and will keep you on progesterone supplements in hopes of keeping a tentative pregnancy going.

Although anything over 5 IU is a positive test, the chances of a pregnancy with such a low starting level succeeding are less than if the BSU was higher. However, sometimes a pregnancy may implant a few days later than normal, giving an initial low positive. These pregnancies may pick up steam quickly, and the beta will start rising appropriately.

A BSU that is positive for only a few days may be called a chemical pregnancy by your doctor; a *chemical pregnancy* is one in which the embryo starts to implant but fails to grow normally, so that a low level of hCG may be picked up for a short time. The beta in these cases may be negative a few days later if you repeat the test.

Most clinics urge cautious optimism if the first beta level is lower than they would like to see it. Don't broadcast the news to anyone except those closest to you if your initial beta isn't very high.

Responding to Positive News

After you get the call from your center that your test was positive, your initial elation may quickly change to worry: Will everything go well? Are your numbers too high or too low? Should you tell anyone yet? After almost constant contact with your clinic for weeks or months, it can be scary to think that you'll soon be leaving the people you've come to know and trust.

Don't panic. Most clinics continue to see you for a few weeks after your first positive test to make sure that your pregnancy is going well. Some centers even have nurses on staff who deal only with the center's pregnant patients.

Continuing the tests

Some centers continue to check your beta and your progesterone levels for several weeks to make sure that your pregnancy is a good one. Because you may not be able to see an obstetrician for a few weeks, this monitoring ensures that if you have an ectopic pregnancy, you'll be diagnosed promptly, to avoid life-threatening complications.

Your clinic usually wants to see your beta double every two to three days for the first few weeks. The following numbers are typical milestones based on a day-three embryo transfer (three days after the egg retrieval). If you transferred blastocysts on day five, subtract two days. Obviously there are many exceptions to the "rules" here. This list gives only the averages.

✔ **9 days post-transfer:** Average BSU 48; range 17–119

✔ **10 days post-transfer:** Average BSU 59; range 17–147

✔ **11 days post-transfer:** Average BSU 95; range 17–223

✔ **12 days post-transfer:** Average BSU 132; range 17–429

✔ **13 days post-transfer:** Average BSU 292; range 70–758

✔ **16 days post-transfer:** Average BSU 1061; range 324–4130; yolk sac may be visible

✔ **By the sixth week of pregnancy:** Average BSU 17,000; heartbeat seen by end of sixth week

✔ **End of sixth week:** Average BSU 30,000; embryo seen

If your beta isn't rising appropriately, no one can do much but wait to see what happens. Some clinics monitor your progesterone levels and add more progesterone if your numbers are a little low, but adding progesterone won't save a bad pregnancy if the issue isn't a lack of progesterone.

When will you get to see your baby on ultrasound? Some clinics schedule an ultrasound around six weeks, or two weeks after you've missed a period. Don't expect to see much at this point. The enthusiastic ultrasonagrapher may be able to point out the fetal pole and the yolk sac to you, but these features resemble a blob much more than a baby.

At this point, you should know whether you have more than one baby, but keep in mind that many times one twin or triplet will disappear by the next ultrasound. Very early losses of one or more embryos are very common, so wait until 12 weeks or so before you tell all the neighbors you're having twins or triplets.

By six to seven weeks you should be able to see a heartbeat, which you may actually recognize on ultrasound as a little flicker, and the embryo will be visible. At this point, your baby will resemble a fish more than a human being. No one will be willing to guess if you're having a boy or girl for another seven or eight weeks. Remember that ultrasound guesses aren't always accurate, so don't decorate the nursery in pink or blue just yet!

A BSU that is rising much faster than normal may indicate a *molar pregnancy,* one in which there is no embryo, only a very fast-growing, possibly cancerous placenta. (See Chapter 6 for more on molar pregnancies.)

A beta that rises very quickly may also mean a twin or triplet pregnancy. In one very unusual case in the clinic where I (coauthor Sharon) work, a very high first and rapidly rising beta was caused by a pregnancy growing in an ovary. This is an extremely rare type of ectopic pregnancy.

Fetal heartbeat and health

The first fetal heartbeat is usually detected around five weeks, and averages 97 beats per minute. By six weeks, the heart rate is about 120, and by eight weeks, the baby's heart beats about 160 times per minute. The heart rate should increase 3.3 beats per minute on average during the first week a heartbeat can be detected. Several recent studies have indicated that a heart rate of less than 90 beats per minute in the first 12 weeks is associated with a high (80 percent) miscarriage rate. By the end of your pregnancy, the baby's heart rate will range between 120 and 160 beats per minute.

One of the most accurate ways of making sure that your baby is growing the way it should is to measure the crown-to-rump length. The embryo can first be measured around five and a half weeks, when it's 2 millimeters long. Fetal growth in the first 12 weeks is very exact, and your baby's exact age can be determined from the crown-to-rump length. Here are what the measurements should be at different stages. These time frames are based on your last menstrual period and are accurate only if you had your embryo transfer around day 17 of your menstrual cycle.

- **Six weeks:** 4 millimeters
- **Seven weeks:** 10 millimeters
- **Eight weeks:** 16 millimeters
- **Nine weeks:** 23 millimeters
- **Ten weeks:** 31 millimeters
- **Eleven weeks:** 41 millimeters
- **Twelve weeks:** 54 millimeters

Celebrating your success, within limits: Restricting sex, drugs, and alcohol

Congratulations, honey, we're pregnant! How will you celebrate? If you can't have sex or alcohol, is there anything left to celebrate with? How about a nice dinner out? Of course, now that you're pregnant, you should be eating a healthy diet and watching those empty calories!

The first few weeks of pregnancy can be dangerous for your embryo's health, because the rapid cell divisions mean that normal development can be disrupted by a number of outside influences. During this time, you need to be vigilant about what you ingest, breathe, or otherwise come in contact with.

Prescription medications are usually classified as Category A, B, C, D, and X in regard to pregnancy. Categories A and B are safe to take, Category C may cause adverse affects in animals, Category D is associated with birth defects in humans, and Category X should not be taken. Some drugs known to cause birth defects are Accutane, an acne medication, and Thalidomide, used in the 1960s to treat morning sickness.

Generally speaking, a drug should be safe to take as long as your doctor is aware that you're pregnant when taking it. All prescription medications are listed in the *PDR (Physicians' Desk Reference),* and can be checked for safety before being prescribed for you.

Taking medications that haven't been prescribed specifically for you is dangerous, but a whopping 3.7 million women took prescription drugs for non-medical reasons last year — medications that either weren't prescribed for them or weren't necessary. Don't take anything that wasn't prescribed for you by a doctor who knows you're pregnant.

When it comes to illegal drugs and pregnancy, the advice is, don't use them. Nine million women used illegal drugs last year, and undoubtedly some were pregnant at the time. But there are *no* safe illegal drugs! Some drugs are linked with prematurity or an increased chance of miscarriage; others may cause your baby to be born addicted and to go through painful withdrawal. Cocaine can cause the placenta to separate from the uterus, so that the baby loses its blood supply and must be delivered immediately.

Alcohol is legal, but you should eliminate its use in pregnancy altogether. A very occasional glass of wine in the last trimester is unlikely to cause harm, but daily heavy drinking, especially in the first few months of pregnancy, can cause fetal alcohol syndrome, which causes lifelong physical and behavioral problems.

Why the restriction on sex in early pregnancy? Not all clinics impose this restriction, but many clinics worry that orgasm may cause uterine contractions, which might "push" a tentative pregnancy over the edge.

Smoking cigarettes is also linked with increased miscarriage rates, so if you're looking for that extra incentive to quit, being pregnant may help your resolve. And if possible, plan to quit permanently, not just while you're pregnant; babies whose parents smoke have more respiratory problems and are more likely to suffer from asthma.

Saying goodbye to your fertility doctor

Some fertility clinics monitor you through the first few weeks after you become pregnant; others wave goodbye with your first positive beta test. Most clinics don't want to keep you too long as a pregnant patient because malpractice insurance for doctors who treat pregnant patients is much higher than for reproductive endocrinologists. But you may have a hard time getting an appointment with an obstetrician until you're ten weeks pregnant or so, leaving you in sort of a no man's land of medical care.

Establish yourself as a patient of an obstetrician even before you get pregnant. That way, if you have any problems in the first few weeks, such as spotting, cramping, or severe pain (as in a possible ectopic pregnancy), your obstetrician can take care of you, if your clinic doesn't deal with these issues.

Defining high-risk pregnancy

Don't think of yourself as a high-risk pregnancy just because you did IVF to get pregnant. Most of the time, IVF doesn't increase the risk of complications in pregnancy. The complications come from whatever caused your infertility, such as your age, uterine shape, or other health issues.

Most doctors consider you high risk for the following reasons:

- You're over age 35.
- You have a uterine malformation that may make it hard for you to carry the pregnancy.
- You have multiples (twins or higher).
- You have a health history of cancer or a disease such as diabetes, lupus, or heart disease.
- You have a history of incompetent cervix (see Chapter 6).
- You have had several previous cesarean sections.
- You're significantly overweight.

If you're a high-risk patient, you'll probably be seeing your obstetrician more often than once a month in the first trimester. You may be doing additional testing, such as chorionic villus sampling (CVS), to check for chromosomal abnormalities in the first three months.

CVS or amniocentesis?

For many years, the only way to evaluate chromosomes in an unborn child was to wait until the uterus grew large enough that the fluid surrounding the baby could be withdrawn through a needle under ultrasound guidance. This procedure, called *amniocentesis,* generally wasn't possible until after 16 weeks of pregnancy; if a problem was found, the fetus was too large to abort with a dilatation and curettage, and a mini-labor was needed for the baby to be delivered. A newer technique, done between 10 and 12 weeks of pregnancy, is called chorionic villus sampling (CVS). Your doctor aspirates a small amount of the tissue that attaches the sac to the uterine wall. This can be done through the abdomen or through the vagina. If you have a tipped or retroverted uterus, the procedure may be safer to do abdominally. The risk of miscarriage is small, less than 1 percent. CVS was done earlier, before ten weeks, when the technique first came into use, but a small percentage of babies born had limb defects. Now CVS is done after ten weeks, and the risk to the fetus has been negligible. The risk of miscarriage after amniocentesis is less than .05 percent, or about 1 in 300.

Finding more resources online to see you through

After spending days, weeks, and months exchanging posts and pleasantries with my newfound friends on the infertility bulletin boards online, I (coauthor Jackie) had a pregnancy to celebrate, and my darling husband had a question to ask: What was I going to do now without my (online) High FSH support board? With a smile on my lips, I walked my husband over to the computer, typed in a few lines, and voilà! There appeared the Pregnant Despite High FSH bulletin board! After shaking his head a few times, my husband abandoned the idea of *ever* separating me from my computer. (Yes, folks, there is a High FSH Playgroup for after baby is born as well!)

But seriously, after so many trials and tribulations, a pregnancy doesn't suddenly makes you footloose and fancy free. No, it only provides a new category of things to worry about. Luckily, resources are available where you can share your worries at this stage as well. For example, if high FSH is your problem, you can find support at Pregnant Despite High FSH (www.network54. com/Hide/Forum/47599). You can turn to the INCIID bulletin boards (the InterNational Council on Infertility Information Dissemination at www.inciid. org). There you will find chat rooms to hang in while you wait for your beta to rise, support for those carrying multiples, help for high-risk pregnancies, and sites specifically dedicated to women due to deliver in any given month.

If online isn't your thing, you can find support from friends and family, who now may feel safer discussing your pregnancy. Pregnancy, particularly early on, is often a time fraught with worry, whether you have undergone fertility treatments or not. You may be surprised by how many other women have shared or are sharing your feelings during this critical time. This support alone can help ease your mind and allow you to enjoy your pregnancy from the get-go.

Considering the Next Step If IVF Doesn't Work

Every day, a patient asks me (coauthor Sharon) how she could *not* be pregnant. "But my embryos looked perfect. My lining looked great, and I did everything I was supposed to. How could it not work?" women say.

Unfortunately, most of the time the answer is, "We don't know." Statistically speaking, if you have a 50 percent chance of getting pregnant, you have an equal 50 percent chance of not getting pregnant, but this isn't the answer a disappointed patient wants to hear. You want an answer, something you can fix in the future. But the truth is that medicine doesn't have all the answers.

Figuring out what happened

What happened? One of several things happened if your pregnancy test was negative. The embryos may not have implanted at all. Sometimes this happens because the lining of the uterus and the embryo were *asynchronous,* meaning that the lining and the embryo weren't developed in synch with each other. Like a flower planted in January, an embryo planted at the wrong time won't grow. Because IVF is an artificial process, you can't be sure that your lining is at the exact right stage for implantation when the embryos are transferred. The doctors can look at the lining through an ultrasound, but the only way to truly tell what stage the lining is at is to do an endometrial biopsy, a procedure in which a little piece of lining is scraped off and sent to pathology to see if it was growing properly. Obviously, a biopsy can't be done if you're trying to get pregnant at the time, because the bleeding caused by the biopsy disturbs the lining.

Another possibility is that the embryos started to implant and then stopped. Usually this happens because the embryos are abnormal chromosomally. The only way to tell whether embryos have the right chromosomes is to do preimplantation genetic diagnosis (PGD), a procedure in which one cell is removed from the embryo before implantation and its DNA is analyzed for abnormalities. This procedure is expensive, and not all centers do PGD.

Sometimes embryos stop growing because of the level of progesterone, a hormone that helps the uterus nourish the embryo. Progesterone supplements are usually given after an IVF cycle, and the leftover corpus luteum also produces progesterone, but some people need much higher doses than others to keep the lining optimal. An endometrial biopsy is the only way to assess this.

Because IVF is a mechanical procedure, the embryos could be damaged during the process of growth in the lab and in the actual transfer itself. Manmade processes are never going to be as effective as nature intended, and occasionally, a bad batch of medium, which is used to nurture the embryos before transfer, causes the embryo not to grow the way it should.

Questions for God and your doctor (who are not one and the same)

An unsuccessful attempt at IVF can be devastating financially, physically, and emotionally. It opens up the floodgate for a host of worries and fears that can be overwhelming. For this reason, your best thinking probably doesn't come on the day of or the day after an unsuccessful attempt. You need to put some time and space between the cycle and your next steps. Remember that your hormone levels are probably off kilter as well. They'll eventually return to normal and probably your mood will, too, as the days pass.

Your doctor will probably also refrain from any immediate action. Don't panic if your doctor doesn't schedule your follow-up visit for a few weeks after receiving your results. Your doctor has experienced this scenario time and again and is probably giving you time to heal as well as a chance to collect your thoughts and your questions. Give yourself and your partner a break, and take advantage of this time, before rushing to ask, "What went wrong?" You may find that the more immediate questions you have become less important in a week's time, while other, more pertinent questions come to the surface.

Your doctor is preparing as well during this time. The lab reports have to be complete and compiled before your doctor can review them. Give your doctor the necessary time to do a thorough examination of your cycle so that you can have the best possible explanation.

As you prepare your list of questions for your doctor, try to be as specific as possible. "What went wrong?" may be a good question to start with, but you're better off breaking this broad question down into more specific questions, such as the following:

- Did I respond as expected?
- How was my egg quality?
- What particular stage in the process did you feel posed the most problems?
- What did you learn about me and my situation through this process?
- What would you recommend as a next step? Why?

As you prepare your questions, think of your cycle in stages as well. Ask your doctor about your particular preparation for your IVF cycle (Lupron and birth control pills), your follicular phase (as the eggs mature), ovulatory phase, and luteal phase (the stage in which your body either accepts or rejects the embryo). What area would your doctor focus on or change for your next cycle? Why? Would your drug protocol be different? How and why?

You may find that your doctor has garnered a great deal of information about your body and its reproductive abilities through this IVF cycle. Those findings may suggest a different course of action, either less technological (if your doctor feels that IVF isn't warranted in your case) or more technological (through the use of third-party reproduction, a topic we discuss in Chapter 16). Your follow-up meeting is a good time to inquire about this and find out what your doctor believes is the best plan for you.

Remember that your doctor is not God and doesn't have all the answers that you may want. Fertility is a numbers game, under the best of circumstances. If doctors knew exactly why or why not it all worked, they would save you and themselves a lot of time and make a lot more money. Unfortunately, medicine doesn't have all the answers, for anything, including fertility.

Your doctor may also be a great source of comfort, but consider taking the "Why me?" question to a therapist, a religious person, or God. Your doctor is undoubtedly well aware of your pain and would do anything in her power to relieve it. Like all of us, however, your doctor has limitations. Use your doctor for the knowledge that she does have and seek other avenues for the answers that your doctor doesn't have.

Going through the grief process

Perhaps the best way to deal with the morass of emotions brought on by an unsuccessful cycle is by looking at the grief process. Elisabeth Kubler-Ross, the author of *On Death and Dying,* identified the five stages of grief following the death of a loved one: denial, anger, bargaining, depression, and acceptance. The death of a dream, even if it's only a temporary condition, is much the same. You can treat this disappointment as a loss, and some women even liken it to miscarriage. Consider the following stages and how they may apply:

- ✔ **Denial:** "Maybe the test results are wrong, and I really am pregnant," you may say. Denial is perhaps one of the most time-honored human traditions in dealing with painful situations. Although denial provides you with a brief respite from your pain, it isn't something that can successfully carry you out of your grief. Realizing that you're not pregnant (after your doctor has confirmed it), no matter how much you want to be, is the first step.

- ✔ **Anger:** "My doctor doesn't care" or "Somebody messed up" may be a typical response. Anger is also a perfectly natural and understandable response to grief. Perhaps your anger is justified, and you do need to take some action. Now is probably not the best time to do so. Instead, work on taking the sting out of the anger. If you do need to take some action, you can wait for a few weeks. You may find that, as your emotions (and hormones) subside with time, your anger may not seem as urgent. Remember that physical force or verbal intimidation are never appropriate, no matter how angry you are. If you feel this way, you need some time to cool off and perhaps some professional help to do so.

- ✔ **Bargaining:** "If only I could be pregnant, I would never again (pick one) yell at my mother, slack off at work, speed, or engage in any other bad habits." Bargaining is similar to foxhole prayers, those pleas for help that come at desperate times. It's also a normal reaction to grief, albeit not a very useful one. Allow yourself time to move through this stage (as with all of the stages that you experience). This too shall pass.

- ✔ **Depression:** "I'm not pregnant. I'll never have a baby. My life is worthless." Also known as "stinking thinking," depression can cast a cloud over your thoughts and feelings. This is another (normal) stage of grief that often doesn't let you take into account the positive realities in your life. Try to remember that, when depressed, you're likely to paint your circumstances in a particularly dim shade of gray. If your depression lasts longer than two weeks, consider seeking professional help, whether from your doctor or a therapist. They may prescribe antidepressants to get you through this difficult time. Your feelings are real, but they're also temporary.

- ✔ **Acceptance:** Remember that acceptance doesn't equate to agreement. You may accept your circumstances as they are today and yet continue to feel that the situation is unfair — and it is. Remember that you can change your circumstances now that you've passed through your period of mourning.

You may go through these stages of grief more than once. You may skip a stage or repeat it twice before you come to accept what has happened. Regardless, don't rush yourself. You'll get there when you get there, and not a moment sooner.

Taking time out for you and your partner

While you're grieving, your partner may be grieving as well. Or he may be stuck in a particular stage of the process, such as denial or anger. Keep an eye on him. Look for signs that he may need some additional help to work through his feelings.

After you're both past the initial shock and grief, consider taking some time out to relax and regroup, in that order. Although you may be tempted to resume your normal routine, your body, mind, and spirit will benefit from a little R&R. Your relationship will, too. Grief can be a very personal thing and one that isolates you from the most important people in your life, including your partner. Take the time to reconnect with one another and appreciate those things that you love in each other. This is a great time for a fertility-free holiday, whether that is an exotic destination or your own backyard. Either way, give yourselves the time off to relax. A one-month hiatus will not make a difference in the big picture. However, not taking the time to recoup and renew yourself and your partnership could have lasting effects.

Use your follow-up doctor's visit as a springboard to discuss your future plans with your partner. Remember that you're both playing on the same team. If your goals appear to be different at this point, give one another the space and time to consider both sides. If you need help arriving at a mutually agreeable decision, you may want to consider visiting a therapist or a religious adviser. If your partner appears to be reluctant to try again, listen to his point of view and give him some time. More than likely, time will help to bridge differences in opinion and heal hurt feelings.

Chapter 15

Trying IVF More than Once

. . . .

. . . .

Maybe your first attempt at in vitro fertilization (IVF) failed, and you're wondering whether it's worth trying a second time. Or maybe you got pregnant right away, have a brand-new baby, and wonder whether you should get started right away on number two, just in case getting pregnant takes a while.

In this chapter, we look at the decision to try IVF two, three, four, or more times. We also look at some really high-tech additions to the IVF mix that may increase your chances — or just deplete your pocketbook. The jury's still out on some of the controversial options.

Looking at the Odds: Success Rates per IVF Cycle

If your IVF cycle ended in a negative pregnancy test, your first question, after "Why didn't it work?" may be "What are my chances next time?" Most doctors feel that your chances of success don't drop in your first three cycles; in other words, if you're in an age group in which 40 percent get pregnant doing an IVF cycle, your chance of getting pregnant is 40 percent in each of your first three tries. After three failed attempts, something may be going on to prevent you from getting pregnant, and your doctor may want to change your protocol or do more testing.

Statistics are averages. Many people have gotten pregnant on their fourth or fifth attempt without changing anything. Others get pregnant the first time they change everything, including doctors. That doesn't mean the change was what did the trick; they may have gotten pregnant that cycle no matter what drugs were used or what doctor did the embryo transfer.

If you're over 40, the three-tries rule may not apply, because your chance of getting pregnant in each cycle is less. If you're over 40, the secret to success may be getting a chromosomally normal embryo, and that's more difficult to achieve because so many eggs are chromosomally abnormal at that age. For this reason, your doctor may suggest that you transfer more than three embryos at a time, hoping to get at least one good one in the bunch.

Going Back for Seconds? Considering Your Options

If you've had one failed cycle, you may be anxious to jump back in and try again right away. This step is pretty simple if you have frozen embryos; you'll usually take medication to thicken your lining for a few weeks and then transfer the embryos back. The monitoring is much less frequent than a stimulated retrieval cycle (see Chapter 12), the drugs cost almost nothing, and the cost of the transfer is usually much less than the cost of an egg retrieval cycle.

If you don't have embryos frozen, you need to go through the entire IVF process again, with frequent monitoring, daily injections, and an egg retrieval. How soon you want to try again depends on your finances, your emotional state, and your clinic. Some clinics cycle only at certain times of the year or every few months.

If you need another egg retrieval, most clinics ask you to make another appointment with your doctor to talk over what might have gone wrong and what can be changed. If you have frozen embryos, many clinics let you start a frozen embryo transfer cycle right after your first failed cycle because the protocols for frozen transfer are fairly standard.

If you get pregnant and deliver, you may want to go back for seconds in another sense: baby number two. Most clinics want you to do a full-consult appointment with your doctor; usually the clinic will redo the mock transfer (see Chapter 13) because your uterine measurements will have changed after pregnancy, and your infectious blood work may also need updating.

If you still have frozen embryos, you'll probably use them up instead of doing another retrieval cycle. A frozen embryos cycle involves far fewer medications and less monitoring.

Deciding when to start another cycle

Some doctors believe that taking stimulating gonadotropins back to back, that is, two or more months in a row, doesn't allow your body to return to a resting state and may decrease your response to the medications. Others worry that taking gonadotropins for too many cycles in a row may increase the risk of developing cancer down the road.

Whether your clinic encourages another cycle after a negative pregnancy test depends on your clinic's thinking. If you're going back for your second child and have no frozen embryos left, most doctors don't want you to do an IVF cycle until your first child is no longer breastfeeding. Some doctors want you to have resumed regular periods, but other doctors don't consider it important as long as you have one period, which can be brought on artificially, before starting again.

Many couples embark on pregnancy number two with the attitude that it may take a long time to get pregnant again, and then they're shocked when the first attempt ends with a positive pregnancy test. Be sure that you're ready for baby number two before you get started again!

Switching doctors and protocols — or not

When something doesn't work, many people go to one extreme or the other: They either do nothing or do something entirely different. Often, the answer or solution lies in the vast area between the two extremes. Because the difference between success and failure when a fertility treatment doesn't work can be as microscopic as a single cell, remember this before chucking your old doctor in favor of someone new.

The odds of success, even in the best circumstances, are not in your favor when it comes to reproduction, regardless of whether your method is no-tech or high-tech. Based on this fact, an unsuccessful cycle merely reflects the odds that you're dealing with, not necessarily the ability of your doctor. Some women doctor-hop with the thought that this continual infusion of new information and new approaches helps speed up the process. This approach, however, can work against you. Each time you switch doctors and practices, your new team must relearn everything there is to know about you and your system. Sure, they can review your records, but doing so doesn't take the place of hands-on experience and the knowledge that your former doctor had been accumulating. Other women assume that the search for the best doctor will ultimately lead them to baby as well. Remember, the "best" doctors generally take their information and knowledge from the same pool available to all doctors. They also may be a great deal busier than the doctor next door, resulting in less personal time and attention to your individual case.

Frozen embryos and their expiration dates

No one knows for sure whether embryos have an expiration date, because embryos frozen up to ten years have produced normal children. Many clinics, however, impose time limits on embryo use based purely on storage space available. Some clinics have decided to keep frozen embryos only five years before discarding, unless the prospective parents make other arrangements.

If you have embryos frozen, you'll probably pay a storage fee each year. Most centers send out a bill reminding you that your embryos are still there. If several years have passed since your last transfer, in addition to seeing your doctor to make sure everything's okay to proceed with an embryo transfer, you should also contact the embryology department just to make sure how many embryos you still have frozen.

If you have twins or triplets and don't think you'll ever want more children, don't be too quick to decide to donate your remaining embryos to your clinic. The clinic where I (coauthor Sharon) work has had several cases where parents who delivered triplets decided five or more years later that they wanted to try again — for *one* baby! In one case, the patient transferred only one embryo, not wanting to risk multiples again, and did have one baby. In another case, several one-embryo transfers failed, so the couple decided to transfer two. No pregnancy. They increased the number to three, and — you got it — triplets again!

Other women believe that the latest protocol is the best or that the protocol that got their neighbor pregnant can do the same for them. Again, this isn't always true. Cutting-edge protocols may turn out to be the greatest thing since sliced bread. They also have an equal probability of being totally useless, or even detrimental. New is not always better. Other people's protocols may not be the answer for you, either. Every woman's body is different, as is her response to medicines and techniques. Some women do wonderfully with a protocol involving the drug Lupron. Others find that their systems shut down entirely from this drug.

 If you're curious about a new method or protocol, bring it up with your doctor at your follow-up meeting. If you have found material online or in a magazine or journal describing this new technique, bring it with you. Many doctors are willing to look at something new and even try it, *if* they believe it will be beneficial to you. Recognize that your doctor may determine that this new protocol is a valid one, but not likely to be effective with you. Whether you like or agree with your doctor, he or she has significantly more experience in the field than you do, if based only on the number of patients seen!

You may, however, feel that you have given your current doctor enough time and opportunity. You may have found that your doctor is unwilling to think outside the box and try anything different. Perhaps it's time for a change of venue. Arrange a consultation with a new physician before kicking your old doctor to the curb. You may find that your doctor's practices are the norm.

Be a savvy shopper. Don't just fall for any doctor who tells you that he or she can bring you a baby. On the contrary, these claims should strike you as suspicious. Instead, ask your doctor for materials, published articles, studies, and sample protocols that support what he or she is proposing. Some things (or people) that appear to have fallen from heaven are, in reality, not the miracle that you think they are.

Reaching out for more help

Whether you're trying to decide whether to stay with your current doctor or punt, or contemplating how, when, and why you're going to try again, remember that you don't have to go it alone.

This is an ideal time to reach out to relatives, friends, online resources, your medical network (including your family physician), or a professional association to help you determine the next right thing to do. Some sites (`www.highfsh.org`, for example) publish fertility doctor reviews where you can check out your current and potentially future caregiver. Online resources such as PubMed (`www.pubmed.com`) offer a search engine where you can check out medical publications about a variety of protocols, conditions, or doctor studies.

Some people say that "it takes a village" to raise a child. I (coauthor Jackie) believe that it also takes a village to *make* a baby. When my husband and I were trying to conceive, one of the most helpful people to us was not a formal part of our medical team. Rather, it was our local pharmacist, who helped us decipher much of the medical lingo, provided us with our medications at the proper time, came through with last-minute requests, and encouraged us along the way. Consider infertility as an opportunity to widen your network and recognize just how important the people in your life are, whether they play a big role or not.

You can also find emotional support through support groups filled with others experiencing the same thing. There is no substitute for the understanding and compassion that those who truly walk in your shoes can provide. You can use all the support you can get. Now is the time to get it from as many sources as possible.

Resisting the Urge to Write Your Own Protocol

Often, the more you learn about something, the less you realize that you actually know. Consider this fact before trying to dictate your own treatment or protocol. You may be tempted to believe that the information that you garner throughout the infertility process makes you an expert in the field, or at least an expert in yourself. Nothing is farther from the truth. Although the portion of the process that you actually see or experience may seem as simple as writing a prescription and injecting a drug, it is far more complex. Doctors have an education in and an understanding of your reproductive system and how medications and treatments interact with your reproductive and other anatomical systems. They acquire this information through long years of study and daily practice of their skills.

Fertility patients, often more so than others, may believe that they're truly on top of their needs, responses, and reactions. This attitude may be due, in large part, to the fact that fertility patients are generally more involved in the hands-on details of their care. This care includes giving their own injections, charting their basal body temperature, and monitoring their LH (luteinizing hormone) surge. Many fertility patients are very educated in the process and often have a good working knowledge of what is going on. It's the "why?" that separates the devoted amateur from the professional. Think you can dictate your own protocol? Consider how little you may know about how your liver or kidneys metabolize any given medication.

Want to start prescribing your own herbs? Realize that you're probably largely unaware of how herbs interact with other medications that you may be taking or what their biochemical makeup is and how this may affect your individual system. In other words, medicine is *not* a do-it-yourself science. Use the knowledge that you gain to become a more informed patient, and perhaps a more proactive one. If you want to lead the process, consider making it a profession, not a hobby.

I'm Okay, You're Okay — Checking on the State of Your Union

Where's your partner in all of this treatment process? The state of your union must remain an important component throughout the process of baby makes two, three, or more. The idea is to *add* to your life, not have a baby at all costs, including your sanity, your health, or your relationship. A baby doesn't transform a miserable existence or relationship into a blissful one. It merely provides a temporary diversion from whatever relationship issues you face today, and adds a significant amount of responsibility into your life and/or partnership.

Before rushing out to interview the next world-renowned specialist in fertility or researching the latest, greatest advances in the field, consider a quick (or not so quick) check on your own feelings and state of mind, as well as that of your partner's. Ask yourself these questions:

✔ How are you really faring? Have you been taking care of yourself throughout this stressful process, getting enough exercise, eating well, and having some fun? Depriving yourself of daily self care only results in more problems. Perhaps this is the time to take a breather and pamper yourself with a long walk, a good book, or a dinner out with friends.

✔ How are your partner and partnership doing? Are you spending time doing things other than trying to conceive (whether that be doctor's appointments, required reading, or timed sex)? Consider spending some fertility-free time with each other.

✔ Did your partner or your relationship get a year older with neither of you having noticed? Maybe it's time to shift the focus a little bit.

✔ How does your partner feel about continuing treatments? How do you feel about continuing treatments? Take time to consider your feelings on this topic. Make sure that you're on the same page or at least reading the same book. You're more powerful as a cohesive team. Make sure that all the positions on that team are intact.

✔ How does your banker feel? Now is a good time to also take stock of your finances.

Exploring Some Controversial Fertility Treatments

If standard fertility methods have failed you, you may be interested in moving on to some of the more controversial methods:

✔ Leukocyte immune therapy (LIT)

✔ intravenous immunoglobulin (IVIG)

✔ Enbrel, Remicade, or thalidomide

These methods are considered controversial because only a few doctors support them or because they're considered to be risky in some way. Immune issues are generally believed to be responsible for less than 5 percent of infertility, but some doctors feel that this condition is underdiagnosed because the testing for immune factors is expensive and done only in a few labs.

Leukocyte immune therapy

The idea that some women's bodies reject an embryo isn't a new one, but the methods for overcoming rejection are fairly new. One method, leukocyte immune therapy (LIT), was halted by the U.S. Food and Drug Administration and shows no signs of being reapproved at this writing. LIT was fairly simple: White blood cells from the woman's partner or a donor were washed and injected under the woman's skin. The theory behind LIT is that some women don't have the right amount of blocking antibodies, which keep them from rejecting a growing fetus as a foreign piece of tissue. By giving proteins from your partner or another person, some of the proper blocking antibodies are introduced into your body, and the embryo will hopefully not be rejected.

The FDA currently bans the use of LIT in the United States, but some women have gone abroad to have an LIT done. If you choose this option, you and your partner need up-to-date infectious blood testing.

Some doctors do LIT for anyone with recurrent miscarriages or repeated failure to get pregnant; others give the treatment only if your number of natural killer cells is higher than normal.

Intravenous immunoglobulin

Because LIT has been banned, some doctors recommend intravenous immunoglobulin (IVIG) therapy as a substitute. Unfortunately, IVIG must be administered as an intravenous infusion, which takes two to four hours, and must be done by a doctor or nurse. By way of comparison, LIT is a subcutaneous (under the skin) injection that takes just a few minutes to give.

IVIG has two major drawbacks:

✔ A single infusion may run between $3,000 and $4,000, and if you get pregnant, your doctor will most likely recommend at least two or three infusions.

✔ Unlike the proteins injected from your partner in LIT, IVIG is a commercially produced blood product from strangers, so there is a small chance of transmission of HIV or hepatitis through the infusion.

Use of IVIG therapy in infertility is extremely controversial. Many doctors don't see any benefit at all to IVIG; other doctors believe that good prospective (set up in advance) studies on IVIG treatment in infertility are few and inconclusive.

Side effects of IVIG can be severe; anaphylactic shock is a small risk. Rash, fever, headache, dizziness, and nausea are fairly common side effects.

Enbrel, Remicade, and thalidomide

The newest drugs proclaimed by some doctors to help pregnancies implant are Enbrel, Remicade, and a drug familiar to some from the 1960s, thalidomide. All three are drugs that decrease levels of TNF, or tumor necrosis factor. Because thalidomide is known to cause severe birth defects, it's used mostly in the treatment of leprosy, not for patients trying to get pregnant. All three drugs are used prior to pregnancy, and must be avoided if there's any chance at all of being pregnant.

The FDA states clearly that any woman thinking about becoming pregnant should not take thalidomide, which caused severe birth defects when taken by pregnant women in the 1960s. Be absolutely certain you need this drug before taking it, and *never* take if there's *any* chance at all of being pregnant.

In larger than normal amounts, TNF can cause pain and inflammation seen in autoimmune diseases such as Crohn's disease and rheumatoid arthritis; Enbrel and Remicade help relieve the inflammation and pain by decreasing concentrations of TNF.

Some doctors use TNF fighters to decrease immune responses that may keep pregnancies from implanting and growing. A number of deaths and lawsuits have resulted from patients taking Enbrel and Remicade. To date, Enbrel and Remicade have been implicated in the following:

- Development of lymphoma, a type of cancer
- Neurological damage
- An increase in the development of systemic lupus erythematosus, an autoimmune disease
- Serious infections
- Blood disorders, including severe anemia

Discovering Other Health Problems Along the Way

Most women start infertility treatment in reasonably good health. During an IVF cycle, you'll probably be under more medical scrutiny — at least certain parts of you will — than at any other time during your life. Diseases such as diabetes or lupus sometimes are diagnosed while women are undergoing ultrasounds and blood testing. Women have also discovered ovarian cancer, breast cancer, or cervical or uterine cancer after those areas were under scrutiny for infertility.

If you find out you have another disease in addition to infertility, will it put your conception plans on hold? That depends on the disease and treatment required to cure or control it. Here are some examples:

- If a cancer is found, you may need to put your fertility plans on hold while you receive radiation or chemotherapy. On the other hand, your doctor may allow you to do a cycle of stimulating medications before treatment so that you can have some embryos frozen, especially if your treatment may make you permanently infertile.

- If you're found to have diabetes, your blood sugars need to be controlled before you start treatment. After your diabetes is under control, you should be able to proceed. Your pregnancy will be high risk if you're a diabetic.

- If you're diagnosed with thyroid disease, you'll need treatment to regulate your thyroid. Without treatment, you probably won't be able to get pregnant. Regulating your thyroid can take several months and may require readjustment of your medication if you do get pregnant.

- If you find out that you have an autoimmune disease, such as lupus, you'll need to be evaluated for problems with your kidneys, lungs, or other organs before trying to get pregnant. Your pregnancy will most likely also be treated as high risk.

Gearing Up for More Cycles

A player in the NBA has been known to celebrate missed free throws. After one such incident where a missed shot resulted in high fives and other gestures of excitement, a reporter asked him the reason for this strange tradition. The player responded with the observation that each missed shot brought him one step closer to the successful one. This analogy was particularly helpful to me (coauthor Jackie) in dealing with my many unsuccessful attempts to conceive. Recognizing that I was playing a statistical game, I started to focus instead on the odds that my lucky number, or lucky egg as the case may be, would come up, given enough tries. Obviously, this theory doesn't work for everyone, but it certainly helped me to get back up multiple times and try again.

Another thought process to consider is how you frame your less-than-positive results. Not getting pregnant is not a failure, like flunking a test or messing up an important project at work. It's not your fault, nor is it in your control to will your body to conceive. Reframing your vocabulary may indeed help your spirit. Phrases such as "less than perfect" or "not successful yet" are much better for your psyche than "failed." Remember that your thoughts help dictate your feelings. What are you thinking today?

How many times do most people try before stopping treatment? In the clinic where I (coauthor Sharon) work, patients frequently ask this question. Of course, there is no one right answer. Some patients have tried ten cycles and have finally gotten pregnant, and other patients have changed their game plan and decided to look into adoption or other options after just one failed cycle. Some patients adopted and then got pregnant, and some patients were just getting ready to do an IVF cycle when they had a positive pregnancy test.

When is it right to keep going? Consider these possibilities:

- ✔ When you can afford it
- ✔ When there's still a chance of success
- ✔ When you can't bear *not* to try again
- ✔ When you and your partner are in agreement that continuing is the right thing to do

On the other hand, when might it be time to take a break, temporarily or permanently?

- ✔ When you're out of money
- ✔ When you've been told by a realistic doctor that you have next-to-no chance of getting pregnant
- ✔ When one of you wants to stop
- ✔ When trying has become unbearable

One patient's unstoppable dream

A few years ago, I (coauthor Sharon) had a patient I'll call Jan (not her real name). Jan and her husband, Dean (not his real name), had been trying to have a baby for several years, and had seven or eight embryo transfers. Jan was young, about 30, and there didn't seem to be any reason why she wasn't getting pregnant, but it wasn't happening. In a last-ditch attempt, Jan and Dean transferred eight embryos, something that my clinic had never done for a couple so young. One of the embryos was a blastocyst, an embryo with more than 64 cells; the rest were four to eight cells, normal for an embryo transfer. The miracle finally happened — Jan was pregnant! We were in a panic, worried about how many embryos had implanted. Only one had, probably the blastocyst, but no one knows for sure. Everyone was relieved and very happy when Jan delivered a baby boy — just one! — nine months later.

Giving Up on Fertility Treatments? Considering When to Let Go

"When to say when" may come sooner for some infertility patients because of basic reasons: a lack of money, time, or opportunity. But even for those who've figured out ways to juggle limited resources a little bit longer, knowing when to say when still isn't easy. A good friend of mine counseled me (coauthor Jackie) one day when I felt I couldn't take the fertility treatments anymore.

"When do I give up?" I cried to her over the phone. "When you just can't walk another step," she replied firmly.

I (coauthor Jackie) had moments and even days when I felt that I couldn't take one more blood test or one more ultrasound or answer one more phone call. During those times, the wonderful support of my online network, friends, and family helped me through. It often took what felt like a herculean effort to do the next right thing when it came to fertility. Along the way, however, I also "gave up" in little pieces. By my last cycle (the one that worked after three and a half years), I had put away my extensive filing system in which I cataloged every test result. Instead of comparing my daily results to past results, I stuffed the files into the bottom of a cabinet and just looked at the day in front of me. Was I giving up or letting go? Perhaps a little bit of both. And although the cycle was successful, I realize that it was not *because* I let go. Letting go at the time was my only option in order to continue taking the necessary steps.

For many people, giving up and letting go are one and the same. For me, both actions allow me to take the responsibility and the results off myself, where they don't belong anyway. This attitude allows me to continue without a death grip on every last detail, many of which are truly insignificant in the long run.

Let go if you can, sooner rather than later. Doing so helps you maintain your spirit throughout the process, whether it is short or long. And, if this stops working, and you just can't walk another step, consider your other options.

Part V
The Road Less Traveled . . . So Far!

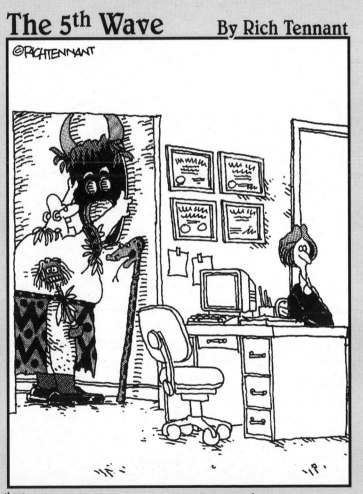

The 5th Wave   By Rich Tennant

"Fortunately for you, Ms. Dobbins, at this fertility clinic we firmly believe in alternative medicine."

In this part . . .

Families today are formed in many ways and consist of many variations on the traditional mom, dad, and bio baby. In this part, we address fertility issues for singles, gays, and lesbians and also look at the use of donor eggs, sperm, and embryos as family-building methods for the traditional family. We also look at adoption and child-free living as alternatives for infertility patients. Finally, we discuss some controversial fertility topics and discuss the future of fertility.

Chapter 16

Third-Party Reproduction: You and You and Me and Baby Make . . . Four!

*T*he traditional happy family picture of mom, dad, and 2.7 children has changed somewhat over the past few decades. Happy families today may contain biological children, adopted children, children born with the help of third parties from donor eggs, sperm, or embryos, as well as children carried through pregnancy by their grandmother, their aunt, or a total stranger.

Although most of the families created through third-party reproduction are perfectly happy ones, the legal and emotional issues involved with using eggs, sperm, or both from someone else can be tricky. In this chapter, we tell you how to decide whether third-party — or even fourth- or fifth-party! — reproduction is right for you, and how to proceed after you make your decision.

Preparing Yourselves for Using a Donor

Deciding to use donor eggs, embryos, or sperm is rarely an elective decision and always a difficult decision. It opens up not only a host of emotional issues but also a host of legal issues. Usually, you make this decision because you have to — because one or both of you has a fertility issue that can't be fixed. Or you make the decision because you're a same-sex couple or a single parent; obviously, you need some type of donor in these cases.

If you're moving to donor eggs or sperm because you have an unfixable problem, you need to come to terms with your loss before moving on. As an infertility nurse, I (coauthor Sharon) have seen couples move too quickly to donor eggs and sperm and then struggle with their feelings about being pregnant with a child not biologically their own. Donor eggs or sperm will always be available; don't jump in before you're sure that you're emotionally ready.

If you decide to use donor eggs or sperm, the child created will be related to *one* of you. Is this fact going to be a problem if you and your partner separate down the road? Is it something that one of you might fling in the other's face if the child has a serious health problem, or ends up in trouble with the law? Will the fact that one of you can see family features in your child's face while the other can't become a source of friction? You need to consider these questions, as well as any others that cross your mind, before you make the leap.

Protecting Yourselves — the Least You Should Do

Before entering into any type of donor situation that we describe in this chapter, whether it involves eggs, embryos, or sperm, you need to do several things:

- **Do some soul searching.** Only you know how you really feel about using another person's eggs, embryos, or sperm. Think it *all* the way through — past the cute baby stage into the teenage years and beyond.

- **Decide who to tell.** You may change your mind later about telling (or not telling) your child and others that you used donor eggs or sperm. If you didn't tell anyone, you don't have to explain anything. If you must tell someone about your decision, make sure that the person or people you tell are supportive and can keep a secret until you're ready for the news to go public.

- **Put things in writing.** If you're using donor eggs, embryos, or sperm, make sure that your clinic's legal documents are thorough. If they're not, get a lawyer to write up a document. Think ahead and consider things such as divorce. You may think that you and your partner will never separate, and maybe you won't, but it's always a possibility. You owe it to yourselves and your potential child to be prepared.

If you're using a gestational carrier or surrogate (see "Borrowing a Uterus for the Next Nine Months," later in this chapter), make sure that everything is in writing. *Everything.* Legally controlling another person's actions is very difficult, so bring up just about any possibility you can think of. Having something in writing may save you from some heartbreak down the road.

Borrowing from the Bank — the Sperm Bank, That Is

Donor sperm has been used for artificial insemination for more than 100 years. About 50,000 children are born each year as a result of donor sperm insemination, also known as TDI (total donor insemination) or AID (artificial insemination donor). The best sperm banks are licensed by the state they're located in, and they have stringent requirements for donors. Sperm banks should be certified by the American Association of Tissue Banks.

Why fewer couples are using donor sperm

Use of donor sperm has decreased since 1992, when it became possible to inseminate an egg with a single carefully selected "ideal" sperm (as ideal as existed in the male's sample, anyway) in a process known as *intracytoplasmic sperm injection,* or ICSI. Men whose sperm counts were very low, or those with poor sperm motility, or movement, could now become biological parents — as long as they could afford to do in vitro insemination.

Many couples, however, can't afford the cost of the treatment, which is about $10,000, so they still use donor sperm. Also, those men who have no sperm at all, such as those with Sertoli cell only syndrome, still depend on donor sperm to become parents.

Picking "dad" from a catalog

In case you were thinking that sperm donation might be a way of making a little extra money, here's a list of requirements for donors from some of the most popular and stringent donor sperm centers:

- ✔ **Height:** Most people request a donor between 5 feet 10 inches and 6 feet 2 inches.

- ✔ **Weight:** The donor's weight should be proportionate to his height.

- ✔ **Age:** The donor should be between the ages of 19 and 39.

- ✔ **Education:** The donor should be a graduate of a four-year college, or at least have completed two years of college.

- ✔ **Sperm specs:** The donor must have 70 percent motile, or moving, sperm, 60 percent with normal appearance (morphology), and a sperm count of 70 million/milliliter. A donor must have better than average sperm because some will be lost in the freeze-and-thaw process.

The donor is tested for all infectious diseases as well as certain genetic diseases, depending on his genetic background. He's also required to fill out a very detailed questionnaire about his background, his family background, his interests, and his likes and dislikes. He may be asked to submit a baby picture.

One center, concerned about donors bringing in a "ringer" to produce a specimen for them, has the donor's hands recorded on a three-dimensional biometric device. The donor then has to "sign in" and match the hand key before he's allowed to produce.

Because the risk of disease transmission is too high, sperm banks no longer use fresh sperm. Instead, sperm are now frozen and the donor retested for infectious disease before the sperm are released for use — usually a waiting period of six months.

Donor sperm can be frozen nearly indefinitely. They're kept in liquid nitrogen containers and shipped out when requested. The cost for a vial of donor sperm runs about $150 to $300, or more if you have specific requests, such as a Nobel Peace Prize winner. Most clinics suggest that you order at least three vials at a time.

The American Society for Reproductive Medicine (ASRM) guidelines suggest that a donor be allowed to father no more than ten children, to hopefully avoid unknowing incest between half siblings 20 years down the road. Sperm banks routinely follow up with questionnaires to centers using donor sperm to ask whether the donation resulted in a live birth.

When ordering sperm, you can choose between sperm that's ready for intracervical insemination (ICI ready) or sperm that's ready for intrauterine insemination (IUI ready). The technique for IUI, which injects the sperm directly into the uterus, is more complicated, but most centers report a higher pregnancy rate with IUI than ICI. Pregnancy rates for women under 35 are about 10 to 20 percent per insemination; rates decrease for women over 40 to 5 to 10 percent per insemination.

Estimates show that only one child in ten is ever informed that he or she is the result of donor insemination, but times may be changing. Some donor clinics now advertise that they have donors open to having some contact with any children born — some say after the child reaches age 18, and others are open to an ongoing relationship. Several recent court cases have questioned the sperm donor's right to remain anonymous, and at least one country, Sweden, has made it illegal to keep the donor anonymous.

Asking someone you know to donate

Some parents-to-be choose a donor they know, perhaps a brother or close friend of the intended dad. In these cases, fresh sperm can be used. However, if the insemination is done by a doctor's office, the doctor probably will insist on having all infectious disease testing up to date.

Fresh sperm have a higher pregnancy rate than frozen, and this fact may be a consideration if you have a relative or friend who's willing to donate. Keep in mind that the donor will need to be tested for infectious diseases, and that there may be a waiting period of six months before the sperm can be used. This gives the clinic time to retest for infectious diseases — many infectious diseases take six months to show up in the blood. Because of the time lag, many centers won't use fresh sperm at all.

With known-donor insemination, of course, the chance that the child will find out the truth about his conception is much higher, because more people are involved in the process. For some couples, the psychological issues may be too complicated for them to handle. However, couples who want a genetic match that's as close as possible, and who can handle the psychological problems, may find this method to be a good solution.

Although such a topic may be difficult to bring up, you really shouldn't go with a known donor until some type of legal document is drawn up. This document should address such issues as how much say the donor will have in the child's upbringing, how much contact he'll have with the child, and whether he'll have legal rights to the child if anything happens to you.

Of course, you may never experience any emotional or legal problems as a result of this donation. The donor may see your child as just another niece or nephew and never give it a second thought. You know your own family best, but covering the possibility of interference down the road is always a good idea.

What if your partner's *father* is interested in being your donor? This happens more often than you might think. He *is* a genetic link, but remember that grandparents in general can be too outspoken about your child's upbringing. (Why do you let that kid have so many cookies? Why do you let him scream like that?) Ask yourself whether his being the silent "parent" as well as the grandparent may cause problems in your relationship.

Using Donor Eggs

Unlike sperm donation, which has been around for decades, the use of donor eggs is a fairly new phenomenon. It required the invention and perfection of in vitro fertilization (IVF) in order to become practical. (See Part IV for complete information about IVF.) Egg donation is a growing national trend, with approximately 30,000 babies born in the United States as a result.

The reasons for using donor eggs are similar to those for using donor sperm. The recipient either doesn't make eggs or doesn't make good eggs. This lack of good eggs may be due to premature ovarian failure or age, or the woman may carry a lethal gene or chromosome disorder that she doesn't want to risk passing on.

Using donor eggs is more complicated than using donor sperm; IVF centers usually try to coordinate the menstrual cycles of the egg donor and recipient so that the recipient can transfer into her uterus fresh embryos that were created a few days before in the IVF lab. This transfer requires monitoring at an IVF center to make sure that the uterus is ready to receive the embryos.

Perhaps you're wondering how you can obtain donor eggs. You have several options:

- ✔ **You can be matched with a paid IVF donor at your clinic.** These women donate all their eggs to one or possibly two recipients for a fee.

- ✔ **You can be matched with a fellow infertility patient at your clinic.** This woman will agree to share half her eggs with you in exchange for your paying her IVF costs. Few women under 35 are infertile because they have "bad eggs." More often, there are sperm problems or blocked tubes, fibroids, or other uterine abnormalities.

- ✔ **Search the Internet.** Type "donor eggs" onto any search engine.

- ✔ **Use a broker.** Brokers can also be found on the Internet by using a search engine, under "donor eggs." One large site is www.eggdonor.com. I (coauthor Sharon) personally like www.awomansgift.com.

- ✔ **Find a willing friend or relative.** If you're fortunate enough to have a friend or relative who agrees to donate eggs to you, you'll both be screened through your clinic for infectious diseases, and then your cycles will be coordinated so that you can have a fresh embryo transfer.

Keep in mind that asking someone to be an egg donor is much more complicated than asking someone to be a sperm donor. Egg donation involves several weeks of injections, blood draws, ultrasounds, and, at some clinics, psychological testing. Plus, you'll need to explore the emotional and legal consequences, just as you would if you were using donor sperm. You'll also need a lawyer to draw up a detailed legal contract; you should do this even if you're using someone you know.

One disadvantage of donor eggs is that, unlike donor sperm, you don't know what you're getting in advance. Because the egg donor is doing a stimulated IVF cycle while you're taking medication to be ready for embryo transfer, you won't know how many eggs you'll get or their quality until a few days before your transfer.

Although you may assume that a 22-year-old donor will make a good number of eggs in an IVF cycle, that doesn't always happen. Clinics usually have rules about what happens if your donor doesn't stimulate well, but chances are that you'll still have to pay.

Finding donor eggs

Most clinics are still doing traditional donor egg programs; seniority on the recipient list gets you first pick at the donor of your choice, all donors being paid the same. However, a search of the Internet reveals a plethora of near genius beauty queens ready to barter their eggs to the highest bidder.

If you really are looking for something very specific — say, a redhead because everyone in your family has red hair or a biracial donor if you're both biracial — the classifieds may be the way to go. Some centers have very few black donors; others have very few Asian donors. A good place to advertise is the campus newspaper or bulletin board in the student union at a large, diverse college campus.

If you're not looking for an exact match, get on the nearest clinic's waiting list. Eventually, you'll have seniority on the list and will be able to find what you're looking for.

The strangest cases I (coauthor Sharon) have seen when it came to picking donors were the couples who picked a donor of another race. I remember standing in a room with one couple, incredulously asking, "You *do* know that this donor is another race, don't you?" Oh yes, they assured me, they knew and they didn't care; a child was a child to them. I made sure that I documented that in their chart. I probably should have made them sign it, too!

Funding donor eggs

The cost of using donor eggs can vary tremendously, depending on what you're looking for. Are you looking for a Harvard grad with blonde hair and blue eyes who stands 5 feet 7 inches tall and weighs 125 pounds and volunteers at the nursing home once a week and bakes cookies for shut-ins in addition to running her law practice and taking care of her adorable twins, picture available upon request? You may be able to find her, but it will cost you. Some Grade-A egg donors are offering to donate eggs for a mere $5,000 *per egg*.

If you're looking for a normal person, like yourself, you'll probably pay about $5,000 to your donor to do an IVF cycle — hopefully with 10 to 15 eggs retrieved.

The cost of the IVF cycle itself is between $5,000 and $10,000 in most clinics, and the medications are an additional $3,000 to $4,000.

A donor egg cycle at your average IVF clinic costs from $13,000 to $18,000, including medications if you don't have insurance. If you're going the designer route, the cost may be much more.

Checking out your donor

Most centers send out donor lists every month or every six weeks. The donor's physical characteristics and family history are listed, as well as education level and current job. Also listed is her childbearing history. Most centers accept anonymous donors only if they're under 35 years old and have no major health issues or inherited family disease. Most centers also have the donor and her partner checked for all infectious diseases, such as HIV, hepatitis B and C, syphilis, and gonorrhea. Some even do psychological screenings to make sure that the donor fully understands the implications of egg donation and is mentally stable enough to handle donating.

If you're bringing a donor that you've found yourself to the clinic, she'll most likely be required to do all the same testing. If your donor is a relative, however, your clinic may allow you to waive some of the testing.

Signing the documents

You and your donor must sign legal consents. The donor signs that she's voluntarily donating her eggs and won't try to claim any parenting rights in the future. This consent is required even if the donor is someone you know.

You sign that you're voluntarily using donor eggs to create a child. You also sign that you and your partner (if you aren't a single parent) agree to be the sole legal parents of the child and assume all costs for bearing and raising the child.

At present, a child born from donor sperm, eggs, or embryos is automatically the child of the recipients and doesn't need to be legally adopted by either parent at birth.

Getting support

You can find numerous support groups on the Internet, not only for egg recipients but also for donors. Go to your favorite search engine, type in "donor eggs," and see what you get! If you have any questions or doubts about donating eggs or receiving donor eggs, you should be able to find plenty of people on the bulletin boards who can help you with your decision. One bulletin board with an active following is found at www.network54.com/Hide/Forum/57451.

If you want a more one-on-one approach, a family counselor who specializes in adoptions or other family situations may be very helpful; the phone book is a good place to look for family counselors, under "Counselors, Human Relations." You can also ask your fertility clinic for recommendations or contact Resolve for suggestions. (We discuss Resolve in more detail in Chapter 8.)

Adopting at the Cellular Level — Embryo Adoption

Some clinics maintain lists of couples who want to donate their embryos to another couple, usually because the donating couple has one or more children through IVF and doesn't want any more. Brokers also match unwanted embryos with prospective parents via the Internet or through organizations dedicated to egg and embryo donation. Screening ranges from no more than infectious blood testing to a full-blown home study done by an adoption agency; you also receive information about the donating parents and usually some type of family genetic history.

When you use donor embryos, you're essentially adopting a child; the difference between this and traditional adoption is that you get to experience the pregnancy and delivery just as if this were your genetic child. Your name is on the birth certificate, and unless you give out the information, no one will know that you used donor embryos. Some couples find it easier emotionally to have a child who's not related to either one of them, rather than using donor eggs or sperm.

Of course, this method again brings up the possibility of legal questions, moral issues, and possible complications a few years down the road. At the time of this writing, no cases have been filed of biological parents going to court to get their children back after their birth. But that doesn't mean that it couldn't happen in the future, despite the paperwork that parents sign when they donate their embryos.

Using donor embryos is fairly simple. The procedure requires doing a frozen embryo transfer at an IVF clinic. This cycle requires minimal medication, usually just estrogen pills before the transfer and progesterone after the transfer to maintain the pregnancy.

One adoption agency, called Nightlight, takes donated embryos and matches them with couples. It coordinates getting the embryos to your clinic, so that they can be transferred to you. This agency requires all the home studies and testing that are required for any traditional adoption.

Borrowing a Uterus for the Next Nine Months

Asking someone for the use of her eggs is one thing; she only has to commit to a few weeks of time and discomfort. Asking someone to commit to your cause for nine whole months by being a *gestational carrier* is quite another.

The use of gestational carriers has exploded with the advent of in vitro fertilization. Women with health issues, women who lack a uterus, and women with a history of recurrent miscarriage are among those who are using friends, family, or total strangers to carry and deliver their biological children.

Finding a willing woman

Some people love to be pregnant, and other people love to be pregnant as long as they're getting paid for it. Either type may be suitable as a gestational carrier. Many women ask immediate family members first, but remember that a "no" doesn't mean that person doesn't love you or want to help. Some women see pregnancy as a nine-month misery and wouldn't go through it if you begged them; others truly enjoy being pregnant and welcome the chance to help you out as well.

If your sister and best friend turn you down, you need to look a little farther. What if your mom wants to do this for you? Would you feel funny about her giving birth to her grandchildren? How would you handle the local press? (You can assume that there might be some, because this type of human interest story is very popular with the press.)

If all possible friends or relatives are out, you may want to look on the Internet, where gestational carriers place ads and, of course, all sound like the salt of the earth. Again, some women love being pregnant and also don't mind the extra money. Others are just looking for the extra money.

Don't sign up with the first wonderful sounding candidate without doing *a lot* of research. Many women have even hired a private agent to check into the carrier's background. That's not a bad idea; it's easy on paper to say that you're something you're really not!

If you want to go with a woman you don't know, visit her home if possible. And make sure that it _is_ her home, not some place that she's borrowed for a few hours to make a good impression. If all this checking sounds sneaky and untrusting, you're right; it is. But the world is full of unscrupulous people who have no problem taking advantage of a desperate couple wanting to have a child.

Another slippery slope that you need to address _before_ a pregnancy occurs is the view that you and your carrier have about genetic testing during the pregnancy and pregnancy termination. Even though the baby is genetically yours, the decision to undergo testing and/or end a pregnancy is that of the carrier, _regardless of legal contract._ Make sure that you and your carrier are on the same page on this difficult and touchy issue. If you're not, consider it a deal breaker.

Going through the process

You'll have to do in vitro fertilization to use a gestational carrier, because you'll be transferring embryos to her uterus. The carrier will usually take Estrace, an estrogen pill, to thicken her uterine lining, for several weeks. The embryos are then transferred to her uterus. You and your carrier can do synchronized cycles, so that the embryos can be transferred to her a few days after your egg retrieval without first being frozen. Or you can do an egg retrieval first, and freeze the embryos to transfer to the carrier a month or even a year down the road.

Legal nightmares: They can and do happen

You may remember the Mary Beth Whitehead surrogacy case. In 1985, Whitehead was a traditional surrogate, meaning that she was the biological mother as well as the gestational carrier. After her daughter was born, she decided not to give her to the biological father. The ensuing court case dragged on for years, dragging all the parties involved through the mud and ultimately giving a type of joint custody to both parents.

Cases debated in the courts in the last few years have involved donor embryos, donor eggs, and gestational carriers, which shows how complicated these cases can be. In one case, a couple used donor embryos and a gestational carrier. The prospective father asked for a divorce several months before the baby was born, and he didn't want to pay child support because he wasn't the biological or adopted father. The courts ruled that he "showed intent" to be a parent when he signed consent forms for the embryo transfer to the gestational carrier.

In another case, the gestational carrier for a couple using the husband's sperm and donor eggs refused to do selective reduction when carrying twins. The couple apparently only wanted one child. The carrier didn't want to keep the children herself but felt she should be allowed to find homes for them. The intended parents found another couple willing to adopt the twins when they were born.

Once the carrier gets pregnant, her pregnancy and delivery will proceed just like any other; there are no additional pregnancy risks to her physically. Most couples are in fairly close contact with the carrier during the pregnancy, so that any problems that arise can be dealt with jointly. If you've hired a carrier rather than using a friend or relative, you should have a payment plan agreed on before doing the embryo transfer.

In most cases, the carrier agrees to let you be present for the delivery, so you can see the baby right away. You'll need to know your state's rules for petitioning to have your names on the birth certificate as the biological parents of the baby. Your lawyer will be instrumental in getting the affidavits you'll need from the IVF center, verifying that the baby is your biological child.

After a short hospital stay, you'll take the baby home with you.

Traditional Surrogacy — the Road Less Traveled

Unlike gestational carriers, surrogates are both the egg donors and the pregnancy carriers. The good thing about traditional surrogacy is that it often doesn't require doing in vitro fertilization. The bad news is that you're asking for more than nine months out of a woman's life — you're also asking for her biological child. Because the child born is the natural child of the surrogate, you could find yourself without a leg to stand on legally if the surrogate decides to keep the baby. Legal agreements, no matter how complete, may not hold up in court if this happens.

If the surrogate is a relative, you may have a greater trust in her to keep her promise to give the baby to you after she delivers. But keep in mind that if she does change her mind, you're looking at a family nightmare that you may never recover from.

States have different laws about the legality of surrogacy, and some states specify that no money may change hands except to cover reasonable expenses. You'll most likely need to go through an adoption process after delivery, which may involve a home study by an adoption agency.

Because of the risks of surrogacy, many couples use donor eggs from one person and hire another to be the gestational carrier, in order to avoid the risks of using a traditional surrogate. This route is more expensive, but it may buy you some peace of mind about the likelihood of your carrier changing her mind and keeping the baby.

No Hallmark cards for this occasion

The most complicated case I (coauthor Sharon) ever remember hearing about involved two sisters, Ann and Sue (made-up names). Ann and Sue were married to two brothers, Joe and Dan (also made-up names). Ann and Joe had children; Sue and Dan didn't. Both sisters had egg retrievals, and then Ann's eggs were inseminated with Dan's sperm, and Sue's eggs were inseminated with sperm from both brothers. Ann's eggs weren't inseminated with her husband's sperm because they wanted all the children to be biologically related to Sue and Dan in some way. The embryos were placed in *both* sisters. Lo and behold, they both got pregnant, and the strangest thing was, they both delivered on the same day! Ann had multiples, and Sue had one baby. Sue and Dan are raising all the children. The birth announcements from the couples were about the most confusing thing you can imagine, because Dan was listed as "dad" on both birth announcements!

Telling the Family or Keeping It to Yourself

Will you tell your family? That depends on you, your family, and a host of other factors that only you know. Some people don't even tell their families that they're doing IVF, much less tell them that they're using donor eggs.

Donor sperm have been utilized for more than 30 years, and evidence shows that most parents *do not* tell the child that his father isn't his biological parent. It seems likely that some families won't talk about using donor eggs, either, although in a recent study, just over half the parents surveyed indicated that they planned to tell the child eventually.

It's possible that somewhere down the line, your child will find out that he's the product of donor eggs or sperm, even if you don't want him to. It may happen in high school biology, where students often test their blood types. Or it may happen when your child develops a rare inherited disease, and you need to go back to his biological family for information.

Keeping a secret like this is difficult, but dealing with negative family reactions, if there are any, is difficult too. If you tell your child, you'll cry inside every time he says, "You're not my *real* mother!" and if you don't tell, you'll cringe every times he says, "I wish I had a different mother!" All children say things like this, whether they're adopted, biological, or whatever; take it with a grain of salt!

Chapter 17

You're Not in Kansas Anymore: Fertility and Adoption for Nontraditional Families

. . . .

In This Chapter

▶ Having a baby as a gay or lesbian couple

▶ Adopting a baby as a gay or lesbian

▶ Having a child or adopting as a single parent

. . . .

*1*n this chapter, we discuss how to achieve parenthood when you aren't a member of a traditional family unit — mom, dad, and junior. Gay, lesbian, bisexual, and transsexual couples are often as eager to build families as their heterosexual counterparts. Others looking to be parents aren't part of a couple at all; they're singles who forgo or just put aside the search for Mr. or Ms. Right in lieu of the quest for a child.

Both gays and singles need a little help to achieve their dream of a family. Welcome to the brave new world where options exist whatever your lifestyle. You're not in Kansas anymore, baby!

For Same-Sex Couples: Examining the Issues That You May Face

As a gay or lesbian couple looking to have children of your own, you need to find an outside source of either eggs or sperm. After you overcome that obstacle, and a child is on the way, you most likely want the child legally to belong to *both* of you.

The biggest problem for same-sex couples who both want to be listed as parents of the child is that not all states acknowledge *both* partners as parents. One partner is considered the legal parent, and the other may or may not be allowed to adopt, depending on the state.

British law doesn't recognize gay couples as legal parents at all, which recently caused an uproar when twins conceived and delivered in the United States through use of a gestational surrogate and egg donor weren't recognized as the offspring of the gay men who fathered them and thus were allowed into the country only on a temporary visa.

Things seem to be changing somewhat in the United States, where a lesbian mother successfully sued her former partner for child support. The courts ruled that both were legally responsible for the child because they had both consented to in vitro fertilization (IVF) to conceive the child.

The supreme courts of California, Pennsylvania, Massachusetts, New York, Connecticut, and Vermont have all voted to approve second-parent adoptions. In addition, second-parent adoptions have been approved by the state legisla-tures in Illinois, New Jersey, and the District of Columbia and have been granted by trial courts in more than 15 additional states. Altogether, second-parent adoptions are generally available in more than half the country.

Unlike their heterosexual counterparts, gay couples will never get pregnant by chance. In other words, having a baby as a homosexual individual or couple can be achieved only through planning and the introduction of a third party, whether known or anonymous. One of the benefits of this necessity to plan ahead is that a gay or lesbian couple has the opportunity to fully weigh and consider all the ups and downs of parenting — something that many "Oops! I'm pregnant" situations that heterosexuals face don't allow for.

Because the issues for gay men and lesbian women are different, in the next two sections, we look at the problems facing each group and some of the solutions couples have come up with.

Support from the establishment

The American Academy of Pediatrics has issued a landmark policy statement supporting legislative and legal efforts to allow for adoptions by a second parent or coparents in lesbian and gay families. Second-parent adoptions have also been endorsed by the American Psychological Association, the National Association of Social Workers, and the Child Welfare League of America.

Gay men

Gay men can be considered "egg-and-uterus-challenged." That is, they lack two of the major necessities of childbearing and, one way or another, will have to "hire out" the pregnancy.

Because of the possibility that a traditional surrogate, a woman who both conceives and carries the child, will decide to keep a child that's biologically hers, many gay men have opted to use both an egg donor and a gestational carrier. The egg donor may be a friend, relative, or someone who has been located by a fertility clinic or private agency. In this new age of technology and the Internet, you may even find egg donors online. (We discuss locating and selecting an egg donor in Chapter 16.) The carrier may also be a friend or someone located through an agency specializing in egg donors and gestational carriers.

After the donor has been tested for infectious diseases or other detriments to pregnancy, she goes through a typical IVF cycle; she's treated with gonadotropins to produce eggs and monitored through the maturation process of the egg follicles until the time of the egg retrieval. However, instead of the eggs being fertilized by the woman's partner or husband or by donor sperm, they're fertilized by sperm obtained from the gay couple. The embryos are then implanted in a gestational carrier who has no biological connection to the child she's carrying, or into the egg donor herself if that's what the couple decides.

The person who'll be carrying the baby will also need to be tested to determine whether her uterus can carry a pregnancy. Most centers want the carrier to do a hysterosalpingogram (HSG) to rule out the presence of any fibroids or polyps that may prevent pregnancy.

Gay couples need to choose how to inseminate the eggs. Will they use sperm from one partner or both? Some gay couples mix sperm from both partners together, choosing not to know who the biological parent is. Others have inseminated half the eggs with one person's sperm and half with the other partner's.

Keep in mind that even if you mix the sperm, the baby will be related to only one of you, unless the result is multiples (twins or more). In this case, one child may be related to one and another to the other partner. Couples wanting to maintain a genetic connection to both partners have chosen an egg donor related to one partner — a sister, for example — and used the other partner as the sperm donor. Laws governing both single men and gay couples vary considerably from state to state, with California currently having the most liberal laws regarding birth certificates and the need to adopt a child born from a surrogate or gestational carrier. Because of this, many gay or single men choose to have their carrier or surrogate deliver in California.

California law allows a gay couple to be named on the birth certificate as parents, or for a single man to be listed alone on a birth certificate. To accomplish this requires a court judgment, which must be filed before the baby's born. Your lawyer will most likely need affidavits from you, your surrogate or carrier, and the clinic involved. Your affidavit states that you are the intended parents, the carrier's affidavit states that the baby she's carrying is yours, and the clinic's affidavit states that, in its best judgment, the child to be born was deliberately conceived to be your child.

Other states' laws are much less liberal than California's. New York, for example, considers surrogacy to be a crime. Arkansas, on the other hand, has fairly liberal policies for listing "intended parents" rather than birth parents on the birth certificate. A large number of states have no regulations for surrogacy. Your best bet is to do your homework before choosing a carrier or surrogate, or at least before choosing where she'll give birth to the baby.

Lesbian couples

Lesbian couples have eggs and uteri to spare — they're merely "sperm-challenged"! They need another part to complete the baby equation, although obtaining sperm isn't nearly as complicated as obtaining an egg and borrowing a uterus.

A quick Internet search reveals various sources through which lesbian women can obtain sperm. You can also get instructions on how to inseminate at home (something that must be done with great care, as discussed later in this chapter).

Some couples have decided to take turns being pregnant, inseminating one partner the first time and the other partner the next time. Legally, this results in children who are considered the child of the partner who gave birth only, unless the couple lives in a state that allows same-sex parents to adopt the other partner's children.

Some couples have used IVF to get pregnant, so that the eggs of one partner can be carried during pregnancy by the other. This way, both partners are involved in the conception and birth of the baby. If one of you is the egg donor and the other is the gestational carrier, you'll need to have your menstrual cycles coordinated by your clinic; this process usually involves taking birth control pills to synchronize your cycles.

Rock-and-roll babies

Singer Melissa Etheridge and her partner, Julie Cypher, opted for a known sperm donor in the conception of both of their children. Cypher's eggs and uterus were used in the conception of both children. The couple later chose to reveal the identity of the donor as singer David Crosby, who remained a close friend to both women but was uninvolved in raising the children that resulted from his donation. The children have been reared with Etheridge and Cypher as their parents, despite the fact that the couple separated not long after the birth of their second child.

Regardless of the method of conception, a third party's sperm is vital to the equation. You can purchase this necessary component through a sperm bank. Some clinics also provide access to donor sperm. One sperm donation agency actively recruits gay and bisexual men who are open to the idea of remaining in their child's life. The agency will also put couples in touch with other lesbian couples whose children are their child's half brothers or sisters, so they can have a relationship as well. The agency, Rainbow Flag Health Services, can be found on the Web at www.gayspermbank.com. Other lesbian couples have chosen to work with known sperm donors, who may or may not retain a role in the life of the baby. If you're using sperm from a friend, it's prudent to have him test for infectious diseases such as HIV and hepatitis before using his sperm. Most prudent of all is to test, freeze a semen specimen for six months, and then test again. If he's still negative for infectious diseases (some take a while to show up in the blood), then you can safely use the frozen specimen.

If you're a lesbian or gay couple with children, you *both* must have wills that are up to date. If something happens to one or both of you, unless you're both listed as legal parents of your child, you could easily end up in a court battle if someone else in your partner's family sues for custody. Same-sex couples have gone to court in the United States and lost custody purely on the basis of their sexual orientation.

Finding the right clinic

You may have to search a little to find the right clinic, one that will treat you with care and respect. You may try the National Center for Chronic Disease and Health Promotion's "Reproductive Health Information Source" (www.cdc.gov/nccdphp/drh/ART99/index99.htm). Don't worry that you're looking at outdated information when you see that the statistics are two years old. It takes that long to assemble information such as live births (which occur almost a year after any assisted reproductive technology cycle). Under the section of "Clinic Services and Profiles," you find information as to whether the clinics work with donor egg patients, gestational carriers, and single women. This information can give you the first insight into how diverse a clinic's clientele is.

Other sources include some of the books that we mention later in this chapter as well as other Web sites, such as www.infertility.about.com. Sites like this one guide you toward a participatory clinic that's hopefully in your area or relatively nearby. If you live in a rural or particularly conservative area, you may have to travel to get the job done.

After you have your list of possibilities, mention your specific circumstances during your first phone call. You want to make sure that your doctor is supportive of your situation before you make an appointment.

Adoption in the Gay and Lesbian Community

So perhaps you and your partner have decided that a biological connection to either one of you isn't particularly important. Or perhaps through your passage of fertility rites, you've discovered that a biological connection requires more medical attention, time, and/or money than you're willing or able to spend. Adoption is often a great alternative, and one that provides a home for a child in need of one.

Adoption, whether domestic or international, comes fraught with its own processes, procedures, and waiting periods. But for a gay or lesbian couple, the red tape may be a little stickier.

It's generally easier for a gay individual to adopt a child than it is for a gay couple to adopt a child together. For many gay couples, one partner adopts the child, and then the other partner asks a court if he or she can also adopt the child through a second legal procedure. Although *second-parent* adoption (also known as *coparent adoption*) does, eventually, accomplish the goal of official parenthood by both partners, it involves more steps and more money than joint adoption. *Joint adoption* allows both parents to have a legally recognized relationship to their child in just one step.

California, Massachusetts, New Jersey, Vermont, and Washington, D.C., explicitly permit joint adoption by lesbian and gay couples. Mississippi is the only state in the country that specifically bars all lesbian and gay couples from adopting, although Utah's ban on unmarried couples effectively bans all gay couples.

Many states have laws or policies that discourage adoption by unmarried couples, and these laws can serve as deterrents to gay couples as well. And of course, states that are generally hostile to gay parents are likely to be difficult places for gay people to adopt jointly. However, in Oregon, joint adoption by lesbian or gay couples is routine in certain parts of the state, although the state as a whole has no written law or policy that supports it. Thus, knowing the "climate" of your area can be as important as knowing its laws.

If you're a single gay or lesbian individual, you'll probably run across the same hurdles that a single heterosexual would face, and then some. Although the state of Florida is the only state with a law that specifically forbids adoptions by any single gay, lesbian, or bisexual person, don't assume that other states welcome these adoptions with open arms. You need to do some research and find out which states are supportive of your desire to adopt and which are unsupportive or even hostile toward the idea.

Another thing to consider is that even though a state may allow you to try to adopt a child as a homosexual single or couple, that state may still give *preference* to married couples, or even to single heterosexuals.

Whatever the state and its stance, you'll most likely find judges and social workers at either extreme when it comes to gay and lesbian adoption, although those in favor may be considerably harder to find.

If you're interested in adopting from a foreign country, you may need to omit your sexual orientation from your adoption application. Many foreign countries with children available for adoption, including China, are adamantly opposed to lesbian and gay adoptions, although they will allow single-parent adoptions. The key here is how much "truthful omission" you're comfortable with. Often, the agency you work with in the United States is aware of your partner but won't state anything about it on your application. After your child is admitted into the United States, the adoption proceeds according to your state's laws, not those of the foreign country.

Going It Alone: Fertility Issues for the Single Parent

If you're a single parent, you're far from alone; 23 percent of American children are raised by their mothers alone, and 3 percent are living with fathers only. If you want to be a single parent, the road may be a little more complicated, but it's far from insurmountable.

It's easier today than it ever has been to adopt as a single parent. And if you want to have your own child, that's easier than ever too, with sperm banks available to single women and the use of gestational carriers and egg donors available to single men.

If you're a woman alone

If you're a single woman, you're going to find it easier to have a baby than a single man — you've got the right equipment! All you need is the sperm, and sperm is something that's readily available, whether you want to use an anonymous donor or a close friend.

If you're considering using a friend as your donor, here are some of the benefits:

- You're most likely aware of the person's personality traits.
- You know what he looks like.
- You probably like the person, or you wouldn't be asking him to do this for you.

Alas, where you find pros, you also find cons. Here are some of the potential complications that come from using a donor you know over one who remains anonymous:

- How involved will he be in your child's life? No involvement, holiday visits, or heavy involvement?
- If your parenting techniques differ, how much input will he have on how you raise your child?
- If something happens to you, will he be the legal guardian?

If you're thinking of using an anonymous donor, consider the following pros:

- You won't have to worry about the father wanting to be involved with the child.
- You can be very picky about physical characteristics and other attributes.

On the con side, consider these issues:

- You'll have to rely on what the catalog says about the donor, with no way of knowing how accurate the information really is.

✔ You won't be able to tell your child much about his paternal heritage.

✔ It may be difficult for your child to be able to contact his birth father, if he wants to.

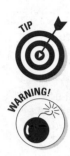

Even if you don't foresee any complications down the road, writing up a legal document to cover your bases is always a wise idea.

If you're using fresh sperm from a known donor, you need to be aware of the risk of contracting an infectious disease such as HIV or hepatitis. It's much wiser to use a frozen specimen after having your donor tested at the time the specimen is frozen, and then tested again six months later. If he's still negative, you can use the frozen specimen.

If you plan to do an insemination at home, you can find home insemination kits that are sold over the Internet that will probably help you get the job done. The kits may contain little more than a small cup, something like a cervical cap, which is placed near the cervix with fresh ejaculate in it. This ejaculate can be caught in a condom, although condoms have been known to break and you may lose some of the sample. If you can get a medical syringe *without* a needle, you can suck up the sperm and place it in the cup. You absolutely positively must *not* try to insert the sperm into the cervix itself or, even worse, into the uterus. Sperm need to be washed before being going into the uterus, and this isn't a do-it-yourself project! You can do yourself some real harm if you try to insert fresh sperm into the uterus.

Never try and do an intracervical or intrauterine insemination at home! You can place the sperm near the cervix but not inside it!

If you're a man alone

Things are certainly more complicated if you're a man trying to have a baby by yourself. You just can't do it alone! If you want to be a father, the first thing you need to find is a mother. You may want to ask a friend, or you may want to hire a surrogate who'll carry the baby for you and then relinquish all parental rights to you. A *traditional surrogate* is both the biological mother of the baby and the person who carries the baby throughout the pregnancy; a *gestational carrier* is not the biological mother of the child, but is only the carrier for the nine months of pregnancy. (You can read more about these options in Chapter 16.)

If you want to use a gestational carrier, you'll have to utilize IVF; the eggs of one woman can be fertilized, and the resulting embryo can be transferred to the gestational carrier. This method, of course, is much more expensive than traditional surrogacy, because you have to pay both the gestational carrier and the egg donor, not to mention the IVF center. You're looking at spending $40,000 or more.

If your surrogate is married, the child, when born, may be presumed to be legally her husband's in some states. You may have to adopt your own child.

Legal issues should be written up by a lawyer who's well versed in surrogacy in the state where the baby will be born, because that state's laws will govern your experience. Many of the laws that govern gay parent surrogacy also cover a single male's use of a surrogate or carrier, with California being the most liberal state.

Your lawyer will need to submit affidavits to the court from your clinic, your carrier or surrogate, and yourself to help establish paternity for the birth certificate. Some states require DNA testing to establish paternity; others don't.

Adopting a child as a single parent

Over the last 20 years, the fastest growing trend in adoption has been the increase in the number of single-parent adoptions. About 5 percent of all adoptions are by single parents, and an even higher percentage — about 25 percent — of all "special needs" children are adopted by singles.

This increase may be due in part to the fact that 20 years ago, many states had laws prohibiting single-person adoptions. Today, it's *technically* legal in every state in the union. However, as is seen by gay and lesbians trying to adopt, just because the law doesn't prevent it doesn't mean that bias doesn't preclude it. Singles trying to adopt may find themselves viewed as second-class citizens to their married counterparts.

Find an agency that specializes in single-parent adoption or consider international adoption as another option. Foster parenting may also be an easier route that's also less discriminating, but in many cases, the state will try to find a two-parent family first before letting you adopt your foster child.

To make yourself as appealing as possible to an adoption agency, prepare some information about yourself and your lifestyle before you start your home study. An agency will typically want to see the following information:

✔ **Financial security.** You don't have to be wealthy, but you do have to have the means to provide for a child.

✔ **A well-thought-out child-care plan.** If you work and will continue to work, this plan is essential.

✔ **Backup plan in the event of your death.** Whom would you leave your child to? Is this designated person agreeable to this?

✔ **A plan for having a "male figure" (or female figure, if you're male) in your child's life.**

However, a formal home visit by a social worker is *not* the best place to trot out your latest beau or, worse yet, beaus. Stability, whether in or out of a relationship, is key, and you don't want to appear as though your home had a revolving door of Mr. or Ms. Rights. If you are introducing a romantic partner into the picture, make sure that he or she is someone who's been a constant in your life for some time. If this person will be a significant other in your child's life, he or she will be subject to the same judgment criteria as you will. The investigation could include finger-printing, background checks, and more — not exactly fodder for a brand-new relationship!

✔ **Evidence of emotional support for both you and your future child.** Letters from potential aunts, uncles, grandparents, or close friends indicate that you have a strong support system.

If you're interested in foreign adoption, be aware that many countries require you to spend two to three weeks in their country. Can you take an extended amount of time off work?

Celebrity adoptions

You've probably seen (and may have been annoyed by) single celebrities adopting babies seemingly without difficulty despite their marital status or sexual orientation. It seems so easy for them to adopt child after child, while you struggle through mountains of paperwork and sometimes spend years only to be turned down again and again as you look for your child with open, yet empty, arms.

But before you consider brushing up on your dancing and singing in order to put yourself in this privileged class of adoptive parents, consider this: Many stars have the benefit of checkbooks with unlimited balances — that is, unending financial resources that can buy them the best legal or professional assistance available. They can afford to register with multiple agencies and/or use their deep pockets to simultaneously pursue all options, be they by way of fertility treatments, domestic or international adoptions, or foster care. Limitless financial resources, rather than fame, do quicken the process. Some celebrities have also opened their homes to slightly older or special needs children, which speeds up the adoption process. Instead of being annoyed with the ease of celebrity adoptions, consider following their methods to some degree: Register with as many agencies as possible, put your information on as many Internet sites for parents looking to adopt as you can find, and spend plenty of time writing your copy to make it as appealing as possible. You may not be able to boast an afternoon talk show on your bio, but undoubtedly you have other appealing qualities to make your application shine above the rest.

If you're considering adopting a special needs child because it's an easier route, really think it through. It takes special people to raise special children, and only you know whether you're really adopting a special needs child for the right reason. If you're interested in a child with a particular handicap, visit other families with a similar child, preferably an older child. Parenthood doesn't end at the baby stage, and handling an infant with a handicap is much different than handling an older child with a handicap. Some people are born to take care of special needs children; make sure you're one of them before jumping in.

If you're interested in a private adoption of a healthy Caucasian newborn, keep in mind that you have an incredible amount of competition. You'll need to be thorough and creative in writing ads to entice women giving their babies up for adoption to choose you. Stress the support system you have and your financial stability, and don't hesitate to make yourself sound like the best potential parent on the planet. You'll have to stand out to be picked!

Line up support in your quest for a child as a single parent. Whether your road is fertility or fostering, support systems are available to help you every step of the way. The International Council on Infertility Information Dissemination (www.inciid.org) has information and chat rooms for a range of fertility and pregnancy-related issues. If your problem is more specific, you may use Google or another search engine to find sites related to your particular condition.

For those choosing the adoption route, the Adoption Family Center (www.adoptionfamilycenter.org) addresses nontraditional adoptions. The National Council for Single Adoptive Parents (www.adopting.org/ncsap.html) may also be an excellent resource. The council also publishes and distributes (through its Web site) "The Handbook for Single Adoptive Parents."

Another good resource is the National Organization of Single Mothers (www.singlemothers.org).

Leaning on the network

If you have an existing network of friends with children, coupled or not, lean on them for advice relating to pregnancy and child care and get their input on the struggles and joys of parenthood. If most of your friends are still footloose and fancy free, now might be a good time to acquaint or reacquaint yourself with people with children, whether you do so through work, social groups, or religious organizations. Your life as a parent will be drastically different than it was as a single person. Make sure that you're familiar with the unique struggles that you'll face when you truly are the sole provider.

Chapter 18

Weighing Other Choices When the Biological Road Is Blocked

- -

In This Chapter

▶ Choosing adoption

▶ Deciding to be happily child free

▶ Finding ways to spend time with children

- -

For some people, the road to biological childbearing closes early. A severe male factor (such as a total absence of sperm), lack of a uterus or ovaries, or other structural problems may make biological parenthood impossible. Other couples invest months or years, along with huge sums of money, seeking biological parenthood, only to end up at the same roadblock.

How you get to this point isn't important. What matters is making decisions about what road to take next. You may choose to adopt, and after you make that decision, you need to make many more. Do you want to adopt internationally, interracially, through a public agency, or a private source? Do you want a newborn or an older child?

You may choose instead to work with children as a teacher or social worker, or as a foster parent. Or you may decide that you can live a fulfilling life without children. In this chapter, we help you evaluate your choices and help you find the path that's right for you — when you're ready.

 Working through the grief process of never having a biological child takes time. You pass through denial, anger, guilt, bargaining, and, finally, acceptance — just as you do with any of life's crises (we discuss the grief process in Chapter 14). After you work through your sorrow, you can be ready to move on.

Opting to Adopt

A life without biological children doesn't mean a life without any children. Many children, both in the United States and abroad, need parents to love and care for them. Adoption is a tree with many branches, and you need to first decide what kind of child you're looking for. Are you open to adopting an older child or one with physical handicaps? Are you interested in a child of another race? Or are you willing to keep all your options open, and try several different routes at one time?

More than 120,000 children are adopted each year in the United States. Nearly half, about 40 percent, are adopted by step-parents or other relatives. Ninety percent of adoptions are domestic, and the other 10 percent come from foreign adoptions. Some adoptions are *open* adoptions, meaning that the adoptive and birth parents meet and continue to have some involvement in one another's lives. Other adoptions are arranged through established public agencies and usually don't include any contact between birth and adoptive families. Adoption can cost anywhere from a few dollars to thousands of dollars. We look briefly at different types of adoption.

Web sites such as www.adoption.com also contain adoption forums, waiting children information, and ads for prospective adoptive parents. The National Adoption Information Clearinghouse (NAIC) can be found at www.calib.com/naic and also contains information on every aspect of adoption.

Traditional domestic adoption

When most people think about adoption, they think about traditional domestic adoption. An old movie, *Penny Serenade,* details the typical scenario: A couple is unable to have children, so they go through the process of adopting a Caucasian infant. The film contains the traditional themes — parents-to-be are evaluated by a strict social worker, and the baby is almost taken away because her father lost his job and income before the adoption was finalized. This type of adoption is becoming rarer today because more birth mothers are choosing to place their children through private adoption, which gives them more control over who will adopt their child. Some agencies still doing traditional adoptions are Catholic charities and county and state adoption agencies. Two well-known established private adoption agencies, Gladney (www.adoptionsbygladney.com) and Spence-Chapin (www.spence-chapin.org), have large Internet Web sites.

In a traditional adoption, the adoptive parents usually have no contact with the birth parents. A social worker conducts a home study to make sure that you're financially and emotionally able to support a child. The children adopted are usually infants, although more older and special-needs children are starting to be adopted, especially through state and public agencies.

If you're older, have any type of criminal record, or aren't reasonably financially secure, the agency may turn you down. The number of people looking to adopt an infant far outweighs the number of infants available, so agencies can afford to be picky.

Private adoption

You've probably seen the ads, and maybe you've even written one: "Loving, financially secure couple wants to give your child a home." Newspapers and many Internet Web sites contain these ads, written to appeal to young women looking to give their children up for adoption. If you really want a newborn, this method is probably your best route to adoption.

These adoptions are handled by a lawyer who may be your source for a baby in addition to being your legal advisor. You may also find an infant through an organization specializing in finding newborns. Your source for a baby may also be your pastor or your doctor.

Private adoption is expensive — you can pay between $8,000 and $30,000 to adopt privately. Legitimate payable expenses in private adoption include lawyers' fees, birth mom's living costs, pregnancy, delivery, and newborn care costs.

Writing a winning ad

Although you may hate to think of private adoption as a contest, it is a contest of sorts. The ratio of hopeful parents to available babies is never in your favor, so you have to stand out and appeal to a birth mother. Here are some ideas that have worked:

- Dress nicely. Avoid anything that's too sexy; you want to look like a mom and a dad.

- Remember that most babies given up are given up by teenagers. Try to look like a mom and dad a teen would be proud of. Ask all the teens you know what a parent should look like!

- Include pets if you have them, but make sure that they sound very warm and fuzzy and non-threatening. Some birth moms may be afraid of dogs and may not want their child in a house with a potentially dangerous animal.

- Stress lots of good times with close family and friends. Birth mothers usually want to picture their baby as part of a warm, loving group.

- Be careful when listing hobbies or interests. If your hobby is collecting ancient druid artifacts, some birth moms may picture you as a strange cookie. Try to list interests that are family oriented.

- Watch how you word religious issues. Again, you don't want to come across as a fanatic of any kind. Stress family-oriented religious events.

- Make your house look kid-friendly and warm in pictures. Stress the hanging swing in your big old tree, the big yard, the inviting kitchen, the adorable nursery.

- If you have other children, include pictures where they look like happy, normal kids, not formal studio shots. You want your children to look like real, lively characters, not cardboard cutouts.

To be successful at a private adoption, tell everyone you know that you're looking. Write the most emotionally appealing ad you can, and send it to as many newspapers as you can afford. (Make sure the state you're advertising in allows this type of ad — not all do.) Many prospective adoptive parents spend up to $5,000 in advertising costs alone. Also, post a Web site on the Internet and make sure that you, your house, and your lifestyle are pictured in as appealing a manner as possible.

Get a good lawyer, even before you start looking. If you find a baby, you want to have all the legal issues taken care of as soon as possible.

After you find a possible candidate, keep your guard up all the time. Go slow, and don't commit to anything right away. And, most importantly, don't give anyone money without having a lawyer review everything.

A private adoption can be as open as you want it to be. Some couples have the birth mother live with them before she delivers; others just have a few meetings at a neutral location. Some never meet the birth parents at all. You may be able to be at the delivery and take the baby home from the hospital, if the birth mother agrees. Many experts today argue that open adoption is better for the adopted child and his family, because his origins are never hidden and are often well known. However, you must do what you feel is best for all involved.

If you're normally a trusting person, you'd better learn to be wary and cautious during this process. We've heard of many cases of women pretending to be pregnant, taking money from more than one couple, or just reneging on the deal after the baby is born. You can't be too careful.

For information about the legalities of adoption, check the Web site www.adoption.about.com.

Harry Holt became an adoption pioneer when he and his wife headed off for Korea to help find families for the mixed-race children of the Korean War. (The sidebar "Molly's adoption," later in this chapter, tells you one of his success stories.) Now, Holt is one of many agencies placing children from Korea, China, Russia, South America, and India, among others. (His Web site can be found at www.holtintl.org.)

Ten percent of adoptions (or more than 10,000) each year are international adoptions. Not all are done through agencies; some are private. The cost of adopting internationally is seldom less than a domestic adoption and, sometimes, is much more. Besides the costs for a home study, lawyers' fees, and agency services, there's the cost of travel and doing business in a foreign country.

Some parents feel more secure with a foreign adoption, because the chances of the birth parents showing up and asking to take their child back are perceived as lower than with a stateside adoption.

Some of the children up for adoption are younger than 6 months, but the red tape of international adoptions means that your baby may be closer to a year by the time you get him or her home. Some countries want you to stay in the country for several weeks; others let you pick your child up at the airport.

PERSONAL STORY

Molly's adoption

My husband and I (coauthor Sharon) adopted our Korean daughter Molly through Holt International when she was almost 3 years old. We already had four sons, ages 4 to 12, when Molly arrived.

We lived in military base housing when Molly arrived, so of course we worried about the home study. Our typical four-bedroom military row house was anything but spacious. And it wasn't that easy to keep clean, either, with four young boys running around!

We'd originally requested a girl whose age was between the ages of our two youngest sons, but the agency felt that she should be the youngest child. We didn't need a baby — we'd had enough of those! It took about six months for our home study to be completed and all our documents to be in order. I called the social worker at least once a week, and more often if I thought I could get away with it. Finally, a referral came for us. Being too impatient to wait for the social worker to bring it to us, I jumped in the car and raced to Trenton to pick it up myself. Inside the package were two tiny pictures of the most adorable Korean child on the face of the earth. And she was waiting for us.

Then the situation turned into a waiting game. We memorized every word in her scanty history and every detail of her face in the pictures. I remember typing some horrendous document for the Immigration and Naturalization Service

(INS), which could have *no* typing mistakes, because having the INS type it would've cost more than $100. I made at least three separate trips to the Newark, New Jersey, INS office with the stacks of paperwork.

Finally, everyone in our home study group had an arrival date — except us! We think that Molly must have gotten the chicken pox and had to wait for the next group, although no one ever told us this. It was horrible watching everyone else in our group with their new children, but our turn finally came on April 7, 1982. And wouldn't you know it — a freak blizzard hit! We drove up to the airport on the deserted turnpike and waited and waited. The plane finally arrived — the only plane to land that night — around 4 a.m. And there was Molly, sweaty and exhausted with vomit in her hair. She'd obviously had a rough flight. She spoke no English, but on the way to the car, she tried without success to tell us that she'd lost one of her shoes (little yellow moccasins with flowers painted on them) in the parking lot. Imagine how we felt when we got a letter from Alaska a few weeks later from a wonderful woman who'd taken care of Molly at the airport there. In her letter, she wrote, "Molly loved her new shoes. She kept looking at them and stopped every few feet to dust them off." Imagine what *she* thought of her new parents, losing one of her most prized possessions right off the bat!

Children adopted from foreign countries may arrive sicker than those adopted from the United States. Medical care ranges from excellent to nearly nonexistent, depending on where your child came from. More countries are trying to place children in foster care rather than keep them in orphanages, to help their social and emotional development. Some children come with serious attachment disorders, and others may have undiagnosed medical conditions.

Adopting a special-needs child

Plenty of children up for adoption, in this country and abroad, are classified as *special-needs children*. Usually, they have a physical handicap, but they may also have a mental or emotional handicap. Some children are classified as special-needs kids because they're not infants or toddlers, or because they're members of a racial minority.

Back in the heyday of adoption, before abortion was legal and having a child out of wedlock was a social stigma, children were plentiful, and older children (older being anyone over a year back then), racially mixed children, and handicapped children were rarely adopted. Now, parents are applying to adopt Down syndrome babies, children with serious emotional and physical disabilities, and children of a different race.

Sharon's advice: Do's and don'ts for adoptive parents from someone who's been there

Even though my daughter, Molly, arrived more than 20 years ago, I still remember some of the feelings I had and some of the difficulties we went through. Hopefully, this list will prevent you from making some of the same mistakes that we did.

Do:

✔ Set up some parts of your new child's room; doing so helps make everything seem more real, and passes the time!

✔ Get involved with a group of waiting parents. This support helps beforehand, when you're waiting together, and afterwards, when you're frustrated together!

✔ Start a journal of everything you're experiencing. In one of our many moves, I lost the journal I kept before Molly arrived, and I really regret not having my written impressions of our waiting time and her first days here.

✔ Read up on whatever age group your new child fits into, especially if you don't have any children yet. You'll get a better idea of what to expect.

✔ Buy some outfits ahead of time, if you know whether you're getting a boy or girl. Hang them in the closet, where you can take them out and imagine your new child wearing them.

✔ Learn a few words of your child's language, if she's coming from a foreign country. Your pronunciation may be terrible; I know ours was. Molly never understood a single word we said, due, I'm sure, to our atrocious accents! But we were able to make out some of what she said, which was helpful.

✔ Make tapes of your child speaking in her native language. Again, in a move, we lost tapes of Molly singing in Korean — the one and only time we ever heard her sing in Korean. Make sure that you make backups!

Don't:

✔ Expect instant love on either side. These days, many children from foreign countries are in foster homes before they arrive here, and they may be mourning the loss of their foster mother. An older child may not be quite sure who you are. For example, Molly called me "big sister" (in Korean) for several weeks after she arrived.

✔ Buy too many clothes ahead of time. Your child may be *much* smaller than you're expecting.

✔ Buy too many toys ahead of time. Wait until you know your child a little better and have a better idea of what he or she will like.

✔ Be surprised by temper tantrums, backsliding in toilet training, and other acting out behaviors. Lots of older children need to act out a little to make sure that you're going to keep them. Babies' schedules may be in complete turmoil, and they may take several weeks to adjust.

✔ Neglect to take your child to a doctor soon after he or she arrives, especially if you've adopted from overseas. Pinworms, head lice, ear infections, rickets, and other not-so-pleasant illnesses or parasites may arrive with your new son or daughter. Molly had had a constant ear infection in Korea. Her preflight report said that her "ear keeps draining, so keeps taking the medicine." Whatever she was taking, it obviously didn't help at all. When she was 6 years old, she needed a large part of her eardrum replaced.

✔ Get discouraged. *All* parents, no matter how they became parents, have moments when they just plain don't like their kids and wonder for a few moments why they ever did this to themselves! This too shall pass!

✔ Deny having a real problem. Not all adoptions end successfully; if things aren't going well, talk to your caseworker as soon as possible. She's probably seen it all.

Sometimes, people are tempted to adopt special-needs children because they're more easily available. Other couples are drawn by a picture of a child on a TV program or in a magazine. I (coauthor Sharon) remember thinking seriously about adopting a child with handicaps while we were waiting for our referral; *OURS Magazine* had pictures every month of hard-to-place children who were waiting for homes, and every one of the pictures appealed to me. However, I realized that our family wasn't really emotionally prepared to handle a child with serious problems.

WARNING!

Although it's easy to be caught up emotionally in the idea of raising a special-needs child, look realistically at your lifestyle and personalities before making a decision.

Social workers in the United States are still somewhat hesitant to place an African American or Native American child in a family of a different race. Many Native American groups are vehemently opposed to their children being placed in white families, and many African Americans feel the same way, saying the children won't develop a proper racial identity if they aren't raised by parents of the same race.

Foster parenting first?

Some couples look at foster parenting as a way to get a foot in the door, so to speak. Although you may possibly be allowed to adopt a foster child, the majority of children in foster care aren't available for adoption.

However, some foster children are released for adoption. If they do become available for adoption, 64 percent will be adopted by their former foster family, so in some cases you may be able to adopt your foster child.

Foster parents usually need to take classes to qualify. They're also subject to home inspections and supervision from social workers. Foster parents receive a monthly stipend of anywhere from $300 to $700 a month, depending on where they live.

Foster parenting can be very rewarding, but it can also be heartbreaking to see children you've come to care about go back to environments that were harmful to them in the first place. However, there's a real need for good foster parents, and if you want to be truly instrumental in the life of a child — or more than one — foster parenting can be a good place to start.

Finding support systems for adopted families

Parents wanting to adopt or foster a child can find many support groups to help them. Most large towns have several groups that meet once a month or more; if you can't find anything listed in the phone book or your paper, call a local adoption agency and ask if it knows of any groups meeting near you.

If you go to any of the "get to know us" meetings that some agencies hold, talk to other couples there. Exchange phone numbers and start your own group if one doesn't already exist.

If you live in the wilds of East Jipip, get on your computer and type in "adoption," and you'll come up with a lot of discussion groups. Sometimes, these groups are even better than face-to-face meetings because you can be very open and candid with people you can't see and will probably never meet.

You may be very involved with a group before and right after your child arrives, and then find yourself not wanting to spend so much time online or in meetings. The good thing is, the Internet is always open, and when you're having a really frustrating experience with your child, you may find yourself back with the group, in person or online. And now *you'll* be the expert everyone else is listening to!

At some point, you may find yourself needing psychological help for your child, especially if your child is a bit older and/or from a foreign country. Adoption is hard work, just like biological parenting is, but adopted children may have additional issues with abuse or abandonment. Many children have psychological baggage that new parents and three square meals a day can't erase. Be realistic about asking for help when things are beyond control.

Interesting reading for adoptive parents

You can find many how-to books on adoption, but I (coauthor Sharon) always found personal adoption stories the most interesting. They usually present both the good and bad aspects of adoption. Here are a few that you may find interesting as well. Many of these books are out of print but can be found in secondhand bookstores and on the Internet. Great sources for old books include eBay (www.ebay.com) and www.alibris.com.

A few years ago, I read an excellent book written by a woman who had three biological kids when she and her husband adopted two sisters, ages 2 and 4. The book, called *The Limits of Hope,* by Ann Kimble Loux (University Press of Virginia), chronicles in a brutally honest way the impact the two children had on the family, and the impact they continue to have as adults. Anyone interested in adopting an older child would do well to read the book, if only to hear the other side of adoption, the story of a family who had a very hard time with their adopted daughters.

For a more traditional view, you may want to read *At Sixes and Sevens,* by Maia Pederson.

This book is long out of print, but I found it on the Internet. Her family adopted 6-year-old twins, and the book follows their first two years in their new family.

They Came to Stay by Marjorie Margolies describes her adoption first of a 6-year-old "perfect child" from Korea and then a 6-year-old "terror" a few years later from Vietnam.

Patchwork Clan by Ann Lund chronicles the adoption of a large, diverse family, including foreign and severely handicapped children.

The Family Nobody Wanted by Helen Doss (Northeastern University Press), the story of a minister's family who adopted 12 children, is a timeless one.

Another classic is *The Children,* by Jan de Hartog, which describes his and his wife's adoption of two Korean sisters.

Ten Thousand Sorrows was written by a Korean adoptee, Elizabeth Kim, and it describes her life in Korea and in the United States after her adoption. This book is an interesting story from the viewpoint of the adoptee.

Deciding to Live Child Free

So here you are. You've tried and tried to conceive your child, and you've run out of money, time, hope, or all the above. Third-party reproduction (donor eggs or sperm) isn't an option for you. Adoption is neither financially nor emotionally feasible at this time. What do you do?

Allow us to start by telling you a few things *not* to do:

- ✔ **Don't blame yourself or your partner.** Your bodies have done the best they could to cooperate with your childbearing plans. You have no more control over your reproductive capabilities than you do over your ability to digest food. This is not anyone's fault. You're dealing with biology, not punishment.

- ✔ **Don't harass your doctor or his staff.** Even if they have appeared to be rushed, doubtful, or just plain insensitive, they, too, wanted to see you succeed at this. Chances are, by now, you've probably sought out a second opinion as well (and if you haven't, go to Chapter 10 and consider doing so!). The medical teams are on your side! They feel your disappointment, albeit with a bit more detachment. They have seen cases better and worse for years, and sometimes, this experience may cause them to arrive at conclusions long before you do. Let this mix of care and practicality guide you in your decisions.

- ✔ **Don't commit yourself to a life of misery.** Whether you have a child or not, happiness is still your power *and* your responsibility. It's up to you to make it one way or the other.

Okay, so now that you're in the right frame of mind, what do you do next? Take stock in your life as a child-free individual or couple. Think that living a life without children sounds depressing? Well, consider a few benefits of being child free:

- ✔ **Extra money.** Can you figure out a fun way to spend $250,000? We thought so! We discuss the costs of child rearing at the beginning of this book, but, in short, child-free couples have a "spare" quarter million to play with. Maybe you've always wanted a second home, for winter or summer, or maybe you'll decide to take a trip around the world. And maybe you just like the idea of being able to go out to dinner whenever you want and not worry about whether you can afford the extra appetizer or bottle of wine.

- ✔ **Extra time.** Most parents today find themselves in a time crunch that forces them to skip many former activities, such as hobbies and working out.

Former pleasures, such as putting your feet up after a long day at work or enjoying a relaxing dinner with your partner, quickly become a thing of the past for most parents, new and old. And sleeping in on Saturdays? Forget about it!

One of my (coauthor Jackie's) favorite pastimes is to sit in a warm bath on a cold winter day. Add to this a spirited phone conversation with a friend, and I'm in heaven. I expressed this pleasure to my friend Vivian one day last year as she tried desperately to carry on a conversation while her two young sons ran to and fro with a vacuum cleaner and a dog. "A bath?" she squeaked. "The last time I had a bath was after giving birth to my youngest son. It was doctor's orders." Vivian also doesn't spend much time curled up with a good book or parked in front of a classic movie on a Sunday afternoon. Consider some of these joyful pleasures of solitude as another perk to child-free living.

✔ **Spontaneity.** Are you the type who enjoys a last-minute vacation or even a last-minute movie? Spontaneity of this sort doesn't fit in well with raising children, particularly when they're young. Child-free living, however, leaves plenty of room for spur-of-the-moment plans and quick turn-arounds. Whether you're talking about a romantic interlude in the living room or a decision to chuck dinner and eat out instead, as a child-free adult, you can freely indulge in these whims.

Even after considering the extra money and time, along with the ability to be spontaneous, your mind may still be filled with 101 romantic notions of life with baby. Do you dream of watching your young charge score the winning touchdown for your collegiate alma mater? Consider that the chances of your child becoming a star athlete are probably about equal to him or her spending time in prison. Do you dream about you and your partner sharing blissful moments with your baby? Keep in mind that many couples spend far more time fighting over child rearing than they do reveling in it.

We're not trying to say that having a child is not a miraculous experience. Rather, it's best seen as a long, arduous process that's interspersed with moments of joy, along with moments of terror. If your life is to be child free, remember that although you may have your work cut out for you in realigning your thoughts and dreams, you also aren't enduring some of the painful moments that make up parenthood. Nothing is all good or all bad, and child-free living does have its high points. Make it a point to figure out all the positives of the situation and go on from there.

And also keep in mind that not having children of your own doesn't mean that you have no children in your life whatsoever. You probably have nieces or nephews or friends' children to spoil and care for. And the best part is, at the end of the day when they get tired and grouchy, you can give them back!

Working with Children

Of course, you can work with children as a teacher or a social worker, but there are other, less known ways of becoming important to the life of a child. Here are some other options that you may want to consider:

✔ **You can volunteer at a hospital.** Inner city hospitals may need committed adults to hold neglected or abandoned babies, or read to frightened children.

✔ **You can become a *guardian ad litem*.** These volunteers represent the child's best interest in the legal system. A training period of 25 to 30 hours is required. Volunteers are expected to spend at least four hours per month in this position.

✔ **You can be a coach, a music teacher, part of a children's theater group, or a school volunteer.**

✔ **You can work with Special Olympics or any number of other organizations that work with special-needs children.**

✔ **You can volunteer at your church or synagogue, work in the nursery, or teach a Sunday school class.**

✔ **You can be a Big Brother or Sister to a child in need.** You can be as involved as you want to be with your child and his family. You may see your child as many as several times a week or as little as once or twice a month.

✔ **You can become the best aunt or uncle in your family.** If your siblings have children, become involved with them. Oftentimes, a special aunt or uncle can be a child's mentor or confidant for life.

Chapter 19

Hello, Dolly! New Advances, New Concerns in Fertility

*Y*ou probably remember hearing about Dolly, the famous cloned sheep who had to be put to death in 2003 at the age of 6 as the result of a progressive lung disease. (For more on Dolly, see the sidebar "The creation of Dolly," later in this chapter.) Now, if you believe the tabloids, cloned human babies are already a reality. Every week you see a story about one wealthy person or another harboring a little "Mini Me" created by scientists working secretly in some exotic place.

Whether or not you believe the tabloids and all the hype, one thing is certain: Technology is a double-edged sword. With every advance comes questions about what technology *can* do versus what it *should* do. Some of the newest advances — sex selection, preimplantation genetic diagnosis, and stem cell research — have come under heavy fire by ethicists and others concerned about the consequences of tinkering with potential human beings.

In this chapter, we look at some of the hottest fertility debates and how they affect you now; we also put on our visionary glasses to see what new advances may be available ten years from now.

Looking Down the Road: Long-Term Health Effects of Fertility Medication

Fertility medications, or *gonadotropins,* are powerful stuff. Anyone who takes them through even one cycle can attest to the physical and emotional effects of having one's hormones surging at a much higher level than nature ever intended. Do people suffer long-term effects 2 or 20 years down the road? No one knows for sure, but here are the most recent conclusions on the safety of taking gonadotropins.

Effects on the mother

At this time, experts have no solid proof that taking gonadotropins has any long-term effect on women. Some studies have shown a possible link to fertility medications and ovarian cancer, but other studies have not supported these findings.

One thing most studies have agreed upon is that the risk of ovarian cancer is higher in all women who've never become pregnant, regardless of whether or not they've taken fertility medications. So if you've taken fertility drugs for any amount of time and never had a child, make sure to do your yearly gynecological checkup — no skipping a year or being a few months late. This is especially important if other women in your family have had ovarian cancer because doctors have established a genetic link for this type of cancer, among others.

Effects on the baby

No one is sure whether fertility medications will have a long-term effect on the children conceived through their use — the children born through high-tech methods such as in vitro fertilization (IVF) aren't old enough yet. The oldest IVF baby, Louise Brown, is only in her twenties. Techniques such as ICSI (intracytoplasmic sperm injection) and assisted hatching are even newer; they've only been used extensively since the 1990s.

Because research is ongoing even as children are being born, high-tech treatment has an element of risk, simply because the jury's still out on long-term effects. Some studies have indicated that high-tech babies have lower birth weight and developmental delays.

However, more twins and triplets are born to moms using fertility meds, and multiples more commonly have low birth weight and developmental delays. Also, more babies are born to older mothers through high-tech treatment, and older women tend to have more complicated pregnancies than women under age 35.

Because some men who need ICSI to conceive have part of a chromosome missing, which results in their infertility, some of their sons may have the same chromosomal abnormality and may also need to do ICSI (or whatever high-tech methods are available in 30 years) to have children.

Sex Selection: When You Absolutely, Positively, Want a Boy (Or a Girl)

There are lots of old wives' tales about having a boy versus a girl — where to sleep, what to eat, what to wear, and so on. But if you already have five boys and would dearly love a girl, or if you carry a genetic link to a sex-determined disease, such as hemophilia, you're probably looking for something a little more scientific. Until recently, 50-50 odds were the best you could do, but newer advances have made it possible to increase the odds of taking home the boy or girl you're hoping for.

The Percoll method and the swim-up method are two of the most used methods of sperm separation in the lab; MicroSort is the newest sex selection method on the market.

The Percoll method and the swim-up method both utilize the fact that female sperm (the Xs) are heavier (they contain 2.8 percent more DNA) and slower swimming than male sperm (the Ys). Both can be used either with IVF or with intrauterine insemination (IUI).

If you want a girl, you use the *Percoll method*. The sperm are placed on a layer of media in a sterile container. Because the females are heavier, they sink faster, so more females are on the bottom layer, which is used for insemination. This method gives you about a 75 percent chance that you'll have a girl.

The *swim-up method* uses the top layer of sperm to select male sperm. The sperm are placed on the bottom of a sterile container, and media is layered over top. Because male sperm swim faster and are lighter, you find more male sperm on top, so the top layer is used for insemination. This method delivers a baby boy about 65 percent of the time.

The trouble with statistics like these is that they're a bit misleading. You have to remember that nature gives you odds of about 53 percent to 47 percent in favor of males, so a 65 percent chance of a boy is only 12 percent more than nature gives you already.

The newest kid on the block is MicroSort, first done at Genetics and IVF in Fairfax, Virginia. Creating one vial of MicroSorted sperm costs about $3,000, and one vial is enough for only one IVF cycle. And don't forget to add travel costs to the deal. This is one package the post office can't deliver. The sperm sample must be produced on site, although after it's washed and processed, you can take it back to your local clinic for insemination purposes. One disadvantage of MicroSort is that some doctors feel that it lowers the number of sperm available, so you may need to do IVF, although IUI can also be used.

After choosing baby's sex, what next?

At the moment, the only absolute way to determine a baby's sex is to do *preimplantation genetic diagnosis* (PGD), in which a cell taken from an already created embryo can be analyzed to see if the baby will be a boy or a girl. Right now, PGD is mainly used to screen for genetic diseases or to check for sex if the parents are carriers of a disease that affects only a child of one sex.

However, the technology is there to determine the sex of the potential infant, although it's still very expensive. One can imagine PGD being used routinely in a few years for couples who want only a boy or a girl.

Currently, PGD can test for a wide variety of genetic diseases, including hemophilia, Huntington's, muscular dystrophy, sickle cell disease, and Tay-Sachs, as well as chromosomal defects, such as Down syndrome and Turner syndrome.

As genetic mapping advances, it's not hard to imagine parents screening embryos not only for sex or genetic diseases but also for hair and eye color, intelligence, and personality traits. Although it's possible that none of these traits

will ever be able to be accurately determined by PGD, they may be. This possibility has ethicists concerned about where PGD is headed.

Ten years from today, will parents be routinely selecting the child of their choice, picking height, IQ, hair and eye color, and left or right handedness? Or will they even go one step farther and have the potential to insert genes that they themselves don't possess into their children, with short parents having tall children, or brunettes having blondes?

The potential for gene tinkering is limitless, after certain traits have been mapped out and identified. The positive aspect of such manipulation could be the elimination of certain diseases or handicaps.

The negative side is that we could end up with populations skewed in one direction only, such as a nation full of tall, blonde, genius baseball players. Or we could find the male to female ratio off balance, as is happening in China with its one-child-only rule.

Although the potential for using gene selection for good purposes is high, the potential for abuse is just as high.

MicroSort uses the fact that female sperm contain more DNA and are larger than males; the sample is stained with a fluorescent dye that binds to the DNA. The males show up green, and the females show up red/pink. The sample is sorted using an instrument called a flow cytometer.

Female MicroSorted sperm will result in a girl 90 percent of the time, and male MicroSorted sperm will give you a boy about 75 percent of the time. Of course, the merchandise is nonrefundable.

You can have a cell taken out of your embryo and sent for genetic testing, which can definitely tell you whether the embryo has X or Y chromosomes, along with a lot of chromosomal information. Of course, this procedure requires doing IVF, which is a little inefficient, because an IVF cycle is expensive (about $10,000) and may give you only a few embryos to test.

Selective Reduction: Making the Hardest Choice

Selective reduction is the elimination of one or more fetuses in a multiple pregnancy. It's a wrenching decision to make, and few couples make it lightly, especially when they've tried so hard to get pregnant in the first place.

One of the best parts of my job as an infertility nurse (coauthor Sharon) is making the phone call to tell people they're pregnant. When receiving this call, almost everyone asks the same question: "Do you think it's more than one?"

Some women ask this question with real fear in their voices. They're the ones who've had a multiple pregnancy — usually triplets or more — and ended up losing all three babies because they were unable to carry so many to term.

Nature never intended women to have more than one baby at a time. Most women can carry two without serious complications, but triplet and higher pregnancies can be a disaster.

Selective reduction isn't done too early in the pregnancy because it's possible that some of the fetuses won't continue to grow past five or six weeks. Usually, doctors wait until ten weeks or so to see what happens. Reduction is usually performed only to reduce triplets or higher, although some women with medical conditions, such as a smaller than normal uterus, may reduce to a single baby.

Courage and mercy

I (coauthor Sharon) will never forget a couple who lost triplets around 20 weeks. I'll never forget them because they were one of my favorite couples and because we at the clinic all felt so bad for them. They'd lost twins the year before around 14 weeks. When it came time to try again, they brought up the subject of selective reduction. "We'll do it," she said. "Last time, we said no, but now we know what will happen if we try to continue the pregnancy." This decision was a very hard one for the religious couple, and even as they said it, I wondered what they would do if the time actually came. Fortunately, it never did. They got pregnant with one baby and were spared making a decision that I was sure would haunt them no matter what they decided.

The process in done under ultrasound guidance; the doctor tries to pick the fetus that appears least likely to grow well, such as the smallest. He or she also tries to pick a fetus that's farthest away from another, to avoid losing both babies.

Potassium chloride is injected into the sac, and the fetus dies and is absorbed in the body. The miscarriage rate after reduction is low, less than 5 percent. Some studies have shown that the remaining babies are born slightly earlier than the norm.

Dividing Up the Leftover Embryos

A few years ago, England found itself with more than 3,000 embryos in storage tanks that weren't being used or paid for by the people who created them. Because English law stipulated that frozen embryos must be used within five years, unless the parents are granted an extension, the embryos were destroyed.

In the United States, an estimated 100,000 embryos are frozen in storage tanks. Some will be used for another pregnancy attempt by their parents, but others will be left frozen, unpaid for and unused. In the United States, clinics who have documented proof that they tried to contact parents can destroy embryos after five years, according to guidelines from the American Society for Reproductive Medicine (ASRM).

Frozen embryos have survived and created healthy children after a ten-year freezing period, so most centers aren't anxious to destroy embryos after five years.

In an ideal world, couples would use up all their embryos, having one baby initially and then one or more a few years later. However, for various reasons, that often doesn't happen. Leftover embryos then become a huge emotional and legal headache for most IVF centers. It takes space to store them and costs money to maintain the storage tanks. Few centers want to make decisions for potential human beings without some input from their parents, even if the parents haven't been seen or heard from in years.

When parents separate or divorce with embryos still in storage, frozen embryos can become a bitter battleground. In more than one case, divorcing couples have fought publicly over what should be done with their unused embryos. One ex-husband wanted to implant the embryos in his new wife!

The United States still has no hard and fast rules for frozen embryos. Each state rules differently when the cases go to court.

Infertility centers try to prevent these types of lawsuits by having couples sign a form at the time of egg retrieval stating what they want done with their embryos if they die or are divorced. Recently, though, a judge ruled that the decisions made at the time of retrieval were meaningless under changed circumstances.

Frozen embryos have been at the center of other types of lawsuits. Even in 1983, when IVF was a brand-new technology, frozen embryos made the news when their wealthy parents were killed in a plane crash, leaving no heirs. Technically, their only offspring were two frozen embryos. Of course, many women offered to carry the embryos and raise them — as long as their inherited fortune came with them! In the end, the embryos were treated as property and were destroyed.

Even if parents don't divorce or die, the decision of what to do with frozen embryos is a tough one, because the choices are limited. Parents can donate the embryos to research, donate them to another couple, or have them destroyed. Not liking any of the choices, many parents just keep the embryos in storage, postponing any decision on what to do with them.

Catching "Snowflakes"

A Christian agency called Nightlight has recently begun adopting out frozen embryos donated to them in a program called "Snowflakes." The prospective couples go through an adoption process, including a home study. Many clinics also run an embryo adoption program, but the parents donating the embryos have no input into who gets their embryos, which is a deterrent for some couples.

Freezing Eggs: The Next Big Technology?

Sperm have been frozen for decades. Embryos have been frozen for 20 years. Eggs haven't caught up yet, although a lot of clinics are working on it. And the demand is there: One California clinic has more than 60 women on a waiting list who want to freeze eggs for nonmedical reasons.

Egg freezing would be a boon for women, whose eggs are all present at the time of birth and age along with their carrier. Many women are marrying later and/or deciding to have children later — in their 30s and beyond — only to find that their eggs have used up their expiration limit. Although it's possible to create embryos at a younger age and freeze them for later, the sperm used in your 20s may not be the sperm you want in your 40s.

The perfect answer would be to freeze unfertilized eggs. Women who want to delay childbearing or who haven't found the perfect partner yet, as well as women with diseases harmful to eggs, would benefit from egg freezing.

The trouble is, eggs don't freeze well. They contain a lot of water, which crystallizes when it freezes. Ice crystals can damage the chromosomes or ruin the outer shell, the *zona pellucida*. Antifreeze solutions could be used to prevent the water inside from freezing, but antifreeze agents tend to be *cytotoxic*, which means damaging to cells, and will damage the egg. Also, frozen eggs can only be fertilized by using ICSI, which adds to the cost of doing an embryo transfer.

Programs in Italy and Korea are claiming high success rates for freezing eggs by using a new technique called *vitrification*. Using this technique, the eggs freeze so quickly that crystals don't have time to form.

Right now, the best you can hope for with frozen eggs is a pregnancy rate of less than 10 percent. You'll also have to go through a full IVF cycle, using stimulating medications and having an egg retrieval.

Other experimental techniques that may hold promise for freezing eggs for future use involve freezing a portion of the ovary. The hope is that the tissue can be replanted later and that the eggs it contains will mature normally.

Putting Old Genes into New Skins: Cytoplasmic Transfer

Because egg freezing isn't all that successful yet, enterprising scientists a few years ago tried a different tack. They took the egg of an older woman and injected a small amount of cytoplasm from a younger donor into the egg.

Cytoplasm is found inside the shell of the egg but outside the part (the nucleus) that contains the genetic material. So a woman who gets pregnant after cytoplasmic transfer will have her own biological child.

Cytoplasm contains *mitochondria,* which is the energy cell of the body, and the spindles along which genes separate and divide. Some doctors believe that older eggs need extra "energy" to divide and grow, and that their older spindles allow DNA to separate abnormally. So by injecting cytoplasm, they hope to energize and normalize call division in the egg.

Cytoplasmic transfer has a few downfalls. First, the egg injected with cytoplasm has to be genetically normal, and the reason that many women over 40 don't get pregnant is that their eggs contain abnormal genetic material. The cytoplasm injected won't fix a genetically abnormal egg.

Second, the mitochondria transferred carries a little DNA from the donating mom with it, so the resulting baby has DNA from three people instead of two. Proponents of cytoplasmic transfer say that the extra DNA isn't harmful and occurs frequently in nature as spontaneous mutations. Opponents are concerned that the children created, even though they look normal at birth, may develop problems down the road from the extra DNA.

About 30 children have been born after cytoplasmic transfer. The main genetic problem found in the pregnancies was the rate of Turner syndrome, a genetic abnormality where the female has only one X chromosome. It was about six times higher than the normal rate.

Currently, the U.S. Food and Drug Administration has banned cytoplasmic transfers until more studies can be done to assure that the children born won't suffer any negative effects from the technique.

Posthumous Conception: Legal and Ethical Issues

It's not difficult or expensive to do. It creates a child. It usually helps heal wounds that come from the death of a loved one. So why is there so much controversy over posthumous conception?

Posthumous collection of sperm — removing sperm from the testes after a man has died — has been done on just about every continent. The legal issues have been discussed almost as much as the ethical issues. And there's still little legal or moral consensus about using a deceased man's sperm to create a child.

The person using the sperm is usually the spouse or partner of the dead man. Sometimes, but not always, she has advance written permission to collect and use the sperm at the time of his death. Legal issues have revolved around inheritance of the dead man's property and the payment of Social Security to the children who are born after a man's death — more than 300 days after his death.

The waters become murkier when the man has given no written permission for the sperm extraction. Can a spouse or partner legally request this be done? How does she know that it's what the man would want done? Does it matter?

One widow used a videotape in which her husband, who had been killed in a car accident, expressed a desire to have children someday as support for her request to have sperm removed at the time of his death.

Most recently, a case in which a man left frozen sperm to his fiancée came under scrutiny because she didn't want to use the sperm, but the man's parents did. They wanted to use donor eggs and a gestational carrier to create a child of their child, which they presumably would then raise.

In England, a widower is trying to find a surrogate to carry embryos created right before his wife's death; she had an egg retrieval done while she was waiting for a heart-lung transplant.

In another case of motherhood after death, the parents of a dead woman were searching for a gestational carrier to give birth to their dead daughter's children, created from their daughter's eggs and donor sperm.

Cases like these and even more complex ones will be popping up in courts all over the world in the next few years.

Cloning and Human Concerns

People talk about cloning as if all cloning is the same thing. In reality, there are three different types of cloning; some have been successful, some have been partially successful, and some haven't been done at all yet as far as we know. We discuss all three in this section.

The cloning causing the most controversy is the type that produced Dolly the sheep. It involves taking a healthy embryo, removing its DNA, and putting the DNA from another person into the embryo. Any cell contains DNA, so obtaining

DNA isn't difficult. If the embryo continues growing normally, it can be placed into a host uterus to grow for nine months.

There are numerous concerns about cloning. Many of the offspring cloned so far have had serious abnormalities. There is also concern that cloned individuals might age much faster than normal because their DNA was obtained from a mature adult.

People wanting an exact copy of themselves may be disappointed because cloned animals aren't totally identical. Environmental influences can change certain characteristics and alter appearance.

Another type of cloning that could be used to create human beings has been done pretty successfully in animals. It involves taking a cell from an embryo and allowing it to grow into a second, identical embryo. This is how identical twins occur in nature.

It would be possible to give birth to identical twins several years apart by using this technique, which is done frequently in farming. It would also be possible to do genetic testing on the "cloned" embryo while freezing the original. If the clone passed the genetic tests, the "original" could then be thawed and implanted.

Animal cloning from an adult hasn't been very successful, but separating cells at an early embryonic stage has worked fairly well. The trouble with this technique is that it doesn't have much practicality in humans. Although identical twins, triplets, or more could be created, few families are looking to have an army of identical children.

The creation of Dolly

The cloning technique that created Dolly, the well-known cloned sheep, involved taking a cell from another sheep and putting it into a sheep embryo. The genetic material was removed from the embryo, so that the only DNA was from the donor sheep, which was about 6 years old at the time. Dolly was the only successful clone born out of about 300 original attempts. Dolly started to develop arthritis when she was almost 6 years old, causing concern that she was aging faster than normal. In early 2003, Dolly had to be euthanized at the age of 6 after being diagnosed with a progressive lung disease. Sheep usually live to be 12 to 14 years old. Calf cloning has been mildly successful; 73 percent of pregnancies end in miscarriage, and 20 percent die soon after birth. Some are born oversized, with enlarged tongues, with immune deficiencies, or with diseases such as diabetes.

Saving Stem Cells for Research: Raising Ethical Concerns

Stem cells are cells that can be grown into any type of tissue or organ. In other words, they're not specific.

Human embryos are a good source of stem cells, and it could be possible to substitute DNA from a living person into a human egg after the egg's DNA was removed. The egg could then be "shocked" to get it to grow, and after two weeks or so, the stem cells would be removed, and the embryo would die.

The stem cells would then be grown into whatever the adult needed — organs, skin, or other tissue. Because the genetic match would be exact, the person's body wouldn't reject the new organ or tissue. People needing organ transplants or new skin after a burn may find this type of science valuable.

Some doctors feel that the surplus of embryos destroyed every year should be used for stem cell development. Others feel that the potential life of the embryo shouldn't be sacrificed to save an already living person. Many people with frozen embryos would like to see something positive done with embryos that they donate for research, and would rather have them used for stem cell development than just be destroyed.

Parents with sick children have already been in the news for trying to create embryos for the specific purpose of donating stem cells to their living child. Others have had a baby specifically born for the purpose of donating blood or tissue to a sick child. Whether it's morally and ethically acceptable to give birth to a child so that that child can save another's life is a question that's still under debate.

Forcing Clinics to Decide Who's Fit to Parent

If you're fertile, you can become a parent anytime you want. No one is in your bedroom rating your ability to raise children. And after children are born, they're taken only from parents who've crossed far over the line of normal parenting behavior.

People who do IVF are no better or worse as parents than anyone else; the potential for child abuse or neglect exists just as it does in any other population. Some clinics require psychological screening for their patients, trying to weed out those who are psychologically unprepared to raise children; others do not.

Cutting the cord — but saving it

Stem cells can be obtained from other places besides human embryos. Many parents are now banking blood from their child's umbilical cord in case the child needs stem cells at a later date.

Not long ago, a father was arrested for beating his infant son to death. The father had used IVF with donor eggs and a gestational carrier to create his son. This case raised questions about how aggressive clinics should be in evaluating patients for parenthood. Should potential parents be turned away because they don't fit a typical social mold? In Australia, for example, gay women aren't allowed to do IVF. Should IVF parents be required to have a certain income level or be of a certain intelligence level?

At this time, most clinics set their own rules for evaluating patients. One prime example is the use of donor eggs or embryos for older women — older as in over 55. Many centers use 55 as an arbitrary cutoff age. Why 55 and not 65? Some centers do strict testing on patients over 40 to make sure that they're healthy enough to carry a pregnancy. Yet some 45-year-olds are much healthier than some 25-year-olds.

IVF isn't well regulated in the United States. Although most centers follow guidelines set by ASRM and the Society of Assisted Reproductive Technology (SART), guidelines are only that. A patient denied treatment at one center may be accepted at another. Should IVF centers be in the business of choosing who will be good parents? Are they guilty if an IVF parent harms his child?

Making Mistakes in the Lab: When Saying You're Sorry Isn't Enough

Black children born to white couples. Embryos misplaced while in storage. A clinic in California charged with more than 100 cases of taking one woman's eggs and giving them to another and of selling embryos left in storage. These are just a few of the mistakes (whether accidental or intentional) that fertility clinics have made.

Most clinics are careful not to work on eggs or embryos belonging to two different people at the same time. They label everything that they're working on to prevent mix-ups, yet mix-ups do sometimes occur.

When a clinic makes these kinds of mistakes, saying sorry isn't nearly good enough. Most of the highly publicized cases of parents ending up with the wrong children have come to light only because the parents and children were of different races. It's hard to say whether similar errors have been made and not discovered because parents and children were all of the same race.

In one instance involving black children and white parents, the error was made in the andrology lab; sperm from a black man was used instead of the sperm from the Caucasian spouse. In this case, the birth mother was also the biological mother, making the children genetically hers.

In another case, embryos from a black couple were implanted along with a white couple's own embryos. The woman gave birth to one biological child and one unrelated child, who was then returned to his biological parents by the courts.

It's hard to safeguard yourself against errors like these. The errors aren't made purposely; they're the result of fallible human beings making mistakes. You can help keep mistakes to a minimum by reading everything you're given to sign, and making sure that your name is properly spelled on everything. When you leave a semen specimen, make sure that it's labeled properly. When the embryologist hands your embryos over for transfer, make sure that she says your proper name.

If you have questions at any point about your eggs or embryos, ask them at that time. If there's any question of error, getting to the bottom of it right then is much easier than getting to the bottom of it nine months later. Monetary compensation is never going to be adequate enough to fix the heartbreak caused by an error in an embryology lab.

That's not me!

One of the scariest things I (coauthor Sharon) remember happening during and after an embryo transfer involved a foreign couple whose name was not pronounced properly by an embryologist. Amazingly enough, they said nothing at the time, but when their pregnancy test was positive, they made a point of telling us that they would do genetic testing on the baby because they were sure that they'd been given someone else's embryos because the name pronounced by the embryologist "wasn't their name."

Where Is All This Leading?
New Fertility Frontiers

There's always new ground to be gained in infertility treatment. Twenty some years ago, when the first IVF baby was born, egg retrievals and embryo transfers were major surgical procedures. Now, patients who have egg retrievals and transfers go home the same day and are back to work the next.

Ten years ago, the perfection of ICSI (see Chapter 13) brought new hope for fatherhood to thousands of men. A few years later, assisted hatching (also see Chapter 13) seemed like it would greatly increase the chances for embryos to implant. Now, hatching and ICSI are routine, and the focus is on determining which embryos are most likely to implant, decreasing multiple pregnancies, and improving the chances of women over 40.

Preimplantation genetic diagnosis (PGD), discussed earlier in this chapter, may be routine in the next ten years. When only the best embryos are implanted, the pregnancy rates will increase, and fewer embryos can be transferred back. This advance will bring new concerns about destroying "not so perfect" embryos.

If egg freezing becomes routine, women who wish to delay having children a decade or two will have no problem waiting. For those women who are already over 40, some new variation on cytoplasmic transfer may be developed in the next ten years. (We discuss egg freezing and cytoplasmic transfer earlier in this chapter.)

Blastocyst transfer (see Chapter 13) will certainly be perfected in ten years, if not replaced by something else altogether. In ten years, men may even be carrying pregnancies to term!

The fertility centers of ten years from now will almost certainly be more regulated than centers are now. Although most clinics in the United States follow guidelines written by ASRM, the fact is that guidelines are only that. No one is enforcing them — no one is allowed to. Questions also exist about whether clinics have a legal responsibility to screen their clients better to make sure that they're psychologically prepared for parenthood.

Insurance for fertility coverage may correct the huge variation in what centers can charge for their services; it may also force some profit-driven clinics out of business.

We're living in a brave new world, indeed! We can only imagine what the future will bring.

Part VI
The Part of Tens

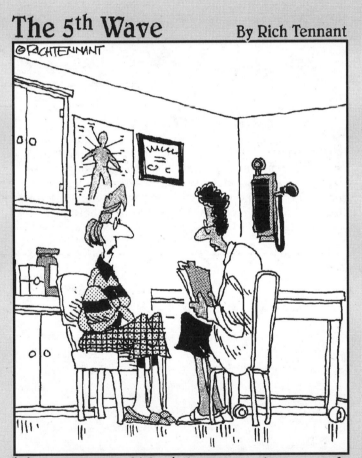

The 5th Wave   By Rich Tennant

"Actually, I didn't become dizzy and nauseous until I started inhaling the scent strips in the waiting room magazines."

In this part . . .

In this part, we prepare you for some annoying things that well-meaning people will say to you while you're trying to get pregnant. On the more serious side, we describe the medications typically used in infertility treatment and also give you a list of mail-order pharmacies specializing in infertility treatment.

Chapter 20

The Ten-Plus Most Annoying Things to Hear When You're Trying to Get Pregnant

As if trying to get pregnant wasn't stressful enough, anything to do with reproduction seems to be fair game for comment by friends, relatives, and complete strangers. In this chapter, we list some of the most common and most annoying things you'll hear on the road to pregnancy. Feel free to tear this chapter out and throw darts at it!

Helpful Hints

"Just *relax,* and you'll get pregnant." (Who hasn't said this to you by now?)

"My friend Bootsy adopted a child and got pregnant the next day. Have you considered this?"

"Have you tried . . . ?" "Have you read . . . ?" "Have you heard . . . ?" (These questions all usually refer to harebrained schemes for getting pregnant.)

"Dr. Perfect has the best stats around. He can get anyone pregnant, well almost anyone." (Of course, you usually hear this after your first, second, third, or later unsuccessful attempt.)

"I Know How You Feel"

"I know how you feel. It took us *four* months to conceive our third child." (There should be a law against comments like this.)

"I can't believe you're having such a tough time! I get pregnant every time my partner walks in the door!" (See response to preceding comment.)

"Things could be worse." (No, really?)

"I bet this experience has brought you and your partner a lot closer." (Of course, brain surgery would, too, but I'm sure there's an easier way.)

Comments You Can't Believe You Heard

"Are you pregnant yet?"

"You're *still* not pregnant?" (Yes folks, people really *do* say the dumbest things!)

"Do you have a good doctor?" (Actually, I'm using a vet, but thanks for asking.)

"Trying to conceive is *really* hard work." (You may hear this from your spouse, whose contribution involves monthly ejaculations while watching and/or reading pornography in your doctor's office.)

"Plenty of people live happy lives without children." (Thanks for sharing!)

Straight from Your Doctor's Mouth

"Your chances of conceiving are 2.6786 percent, about the same as getting hit by lightning." (This statement is obviously taken from the table of famous statistics that doctors pull out of thin air.)

"You're not having much of a response, are you?" (Doctors generally say this when you're lying in a prone position with an ultrasound wand in position.)

"You need to be very aggressive, considering your age."

"Maybe you shouldn't have waited so long to start trying." (Hmmm, let's spend some time flogging ourselves over that!)

"Guess you and your partner will just have to keep 'practicing' (wink, wink, nudge, nudge)." (From the doctor who continues to "practice" his skills, or lack thereof, on you!)

Leaving You Speechless

"God has a reason/plan/purpose for putting you through this."

Chapter 21

Ten (Okay, Seven) Groups of Fertility Medications and Where to Find Them

Although fertility medications come with a bewildering array of names, these medications fit into only a few categories. The different names are brand-name-only differences, in most cases. In this chapter, we describe the different categories and list the most common brand names of each.

Sorting the Medications

Fertility medications are generally sold in boxes of five or ten vials or ampules. The ones that come with rubber stoppers on the top are called *vials,* and the ones that have a glass "nipple" that you need to break off are called *ampules.*

There's no logical reason for fertility medications to be sold in multiple units; the main reason, of course, is profit. Pharmacies that specialize in fertility medications will break up a box and sell you one or two, but usually your local Cost-Cut Pharmacy won't.

Gonadotropins

These drugs are the mainstay of fertility treatment. Gonadotropins (gonad = reproductive organ; tropin = hormone) stimulate follicle growth. Gonadotropins can be *recombinant,* which means manufactured in the lab, or made from human proteins. In addition, they can be nearly pure follicle-stimulating hormones (FSH) or a 50/50 mixture of luteinizing hormone (LH) and FSH. Side effects of gonadotropins include bloating, headache, and mood swings.

Recombinant gonadotropins

Recombinant drugs are 100 percent lab created; they contain no human proteins, so they're considered to be nearly 100 percent free from impurities. These drugs are follicle-stimulating drugs; they contain nearly pure FSH, so they encourage the growth of many follicles rather than just one in an in vitro fertilization (IVF) or stimulated cycle. Because they're pure and unlikely to cause a skin reaction, they can be given subcutaneously, with a very small needle; women with a body mass index over 30 should give the drug intramuscularly for best absorption. Two brands are currently available: Follistim and Gonal-F.

Follistim

Follistim is made by Organon, a large manufacturer of several fertility medications. It comes in 75 IU vials, with a freeze-dried cake (powder vial) and a 5 cc vial of sterile water. Each box of Follistim contains five powder vials and five water vials. The main disadvantage to Follistim is that the water vial contains more water than should be used; the recommended amount of diluent is 1 cc, or ml (ml and cc equal the same amount).

Gonal-F

Gonal-F is produced by Serono Labs, another large manufacturer of fertility medications. Gonal-F is sold in two types of packaging:

- **In boxes with five ampules, each containing 75 IU of freeze-dried powder with five 1 cc ampules of sterile water:** The main disadvantage of the single-dose ampules is the glass ampule itself. Some people have a hard time breaking off the top without cutting themselves, and others are concerned that small pieces of glass will fall into the powder. However, even if you break the glass, you probably won't draw any glass up into the thin needles used for injection.

- **In a multidose vial containing about fourteen 75 IU injections:** The advantage is that you mix it with a small amount of water and have only a tiny amount to inject at a time; plus you have to mix a new batch only every couple of days. The disadvantage is that you can't save the unused portion for another cycle. As a result, you may waste a lot of medication or have to buy a combination of multidose and single-dose vials.

Urinary FSH

Two nearly pure FSH products made from urine are available. One is fairly new, and the other isn't being made any longer, but if you bought your medications a while ago, you may still be using it.

Bravelle

Bravelle is made by Ferring, another large manufacturer of fertility medications. Although Bravelle is made from purified urine, it's nearly as pure as recombinant FSH and is somewhat cheaper. It comes in 75 IU vials and is given subcutaneously with a small needle.

Fertinex

Fertinex is no longer being produced, but you may still have some left from a previous cycle; it was made by Serono. It also is nearly pure urinary FSH and comes in 75 IU vials; it too is injected subcutaneously.

Urinary LH/FSH

These were the earliest gonadotropins on the market. They're made from purified urine from menopausal women and contain nearly equal amounts of LH and FSH. Some doctors now believe that some LH is helpful in a stimulated cycle and may prescribe these along with a pure FSH product.

Humegon

Made by Organon, Humegon comes in 75 IU vials and must be injected intramuscularly due to irritation from the proteins it contains. It's mixed with 2 cc of diluent, also included in the packaging.

Pergonal

Made by Serono, Pergonal comes in 75 IU glass ampules and must be given intramuscularly. Pergonal is mixed with 2 cc of diluent packaged with the powder.

Repronex

Manufactured by Ferring, Repronex is the easiest of the three in this category to find in the United States. Some centers give Repronex subcutaneously, but others have found skin rashes to be very common unless given intramuscularly. It comes in 75 IU vials and is mixed with 1 cc diluent if given subcutaneously, 2 cc if given intramuscularly.

GnRH agonists

Leuprolide acetate, more commonly known as Lupron, is a gonadotropin-releasing hormone agonist, meaning that it suppresses hormones such as LH and FSH. It's manufactured by TAP Pharmaceutical Products and sold in a 14-day kit, which contains a 2.8 ml multidose vial of premixed Lupron and 14 syringes. Lupron first causes a stimulation of the ovaries and then after a few days starts to suppress them. This shuts off your normal menstrual cycle, which matures only one egg at a time, and allows many follicles to be stimulated with gonadotropins. If taken for more than a few weeks, Lupron can cause hot flashes, headaches, and bone pain.

GnRH antagonists

A newer category of medication called GnRH antagonists was designed to keep women from releasing eggs early during an IVF cycle without the suppressing effects of Lupron. It's manufactured by Organon as Antagon and by Serono as Cetrotide. Cetrotide is manufactured as a 3 mg one-time injection and also as a 25 mg daily injection; Antagon is sold as a daily 250 mcg injection. The daily injection usually starts around day six of an IVF cycle. Antagon is sold in a prefilled syringe that requires no mixing. Cetrotide comes with a syringe prefilled with diluent, which needs to be injected into a powder; the mixture is then drawn back into the syringe and injected.

hCG (human chorionic gonadotropin) intramuscular

Several different brands of hCG are sold; all contain 10,000 IU of hCG. They're packaged with more water than is needed for a single injection, usually 10 cc; the hCG is generally mixed with 2 cc of water and then injected intramuscularly. Common brand names are

- ✔ Novarel (Ferring)
- ✔ Pregnyl (Organon)
- ✔ Profasi (Serono)

HCG subcutaneous recombinant

Ovidrel is a lab-manufactured subcutaneous dose of hCG packaged as 250 mcg equivalent to 10,000 IU; it comes with a 1 cc vial of water for mixing. Serono makes Ovidrel.

Progesterone

Progesterone can be given in intramuscular injections (the best absorbed), vaginal suppositories, vaginal gel, or pills (the least absorbed).

- ✔ **Injections:** The intramuscular injection form of progesterone comes in multidose vials of 50 mgm/ml. Progesterone in oil needs to be mixed under a special hood, so it's made only by pharmacies that compound medications; these are usually pharmacies that specialize in fertility medications, such as those found at the end of this chapter.

✔ **Vaginal suppositories:** These suppositories are made in several strengths and must be made by the pharmacy, so they can be hard to find; they're not commercially manufactured. They're little bullets that must be inserted manually and come in 100 mgm, 200 mgm, and 400 mgm strength.

✔ **Gel:** Crinone is a gel manufactured by Serono; it comes in prefilled applicators of 90 milligrams. Some patients have fewer problems with yeast infections and irritation with Crinone than with vaginal suppositories.

✔ **Capsules:** These are manufactured as Prometrium by Solvay and are available in 100 and 200 mg. Compounding pharmacies also make their own micronized progesterone capsules.

Clomiphene citrate

Clomiphene citrate is more commonly called Clomid even though it's sold as Clomid by several manufacturers and Serophene by Serono Labs. Clomid is a 50 mg pill that stimulates the ovaries and increases the release of follicle-stimulating hormones. Side effects include hot flashes, bloating, headache, and blurred vision.

Mail-Order Pharmacies

Although medications such as Clomid and hCG are fairly easy to find at your local pharmacy, gonadotropins and progesterone can be harder to find. A whole industry of mail-order pharmacies that specialize in fertility drugs has evolved. They take insurance, have lower costs than most pharmacies, mail the medications directly to your home, and offer overnight delivery. In addition, some pharmacies produce injection instruction tapes and have hotlines you can call with medication questions. They're usually available 24 hours a day. This list of mail-order pharmacies is by no means complete; the area you live in may have similar pharmacies that your clinic deals with on a regular basis.

What do they call this drug in Europe?

Various medications available in the United States are sold under different brand names in other parts of the world. Here are some examples:

✔ Follistim and Gonal-F type medications are sold as Puregon outside the United States.

✔ Fertinex-type medications are sold as Metrodin or Fertinorm outside the United States.

✔ Humegon, Pergonal, and Repronex type medications are sold as Menogen, Pertisol, and Meronal outside the United States.

✔ **Alexander's Twin Pharmacy:** Trenton, New Jersey; 1-877-750-7222

✔ **Apthorp Pharmacy:** New York, New York; 1-800-775-3582

✔ **BioPlus:** Altamonte, Florida; 1-888-292-0744

✔ **FertilityMeds:** Alpine, California; 1-800-346-9660

✔ **Franklin Drug:** Philadelphia, Pennsylvania; 1-800-537-3788

✔ **Freedom Drug:** Lynnfield, Massachusetts; 1-800-660-4283

✔ **IVPcare:** Carrollton, Texas; 1-800-483-8001

✔ **King's Pharmacy:** New York, New York; several locations in the city; 1-800-RXKINGS

✔ **Metro Drug:** New York, New York; several locations in the city; 1-212-627-2300

✔ **Poet's Pharmacy:** Freehold, New Jersey; 1-800-427-POET

✔ **Reses Pharmacy:** Pomona, New Jersey; 1-609-646-3600

✔ **Schraft's:** Livingston, New Jersey; 1-800-876-4545

✔ **Stadtlander's:** Pittsburgh, Pennsylvania; 1-800-218-6315

Appendix

Fertility Stories from Both Sides of the Glass

••

*E*verybody has a story. In this appendix, the authors tell their real-life story — as patient and as fertility nurse, from both sides of the glass.

Is This Over Yet? Jackie's Final Hurrah

My neighbor called it a goat rodeo — you know, something you just can't get your arms around. That would have been an adequate description of in vitro cycle #3. My husband (affectionately known as DH, also known as Darling Husband, Darn Husband, or whatever works on the chat room boards that I frequented) and I had been through this process before, and it was no surprise that my 39-year-old ovaries had a response that was neither fast nor furious. My protocol was anything but common. I had two failed attempts at in vitro fertilization (IVF), the first a high stimulation approach using six amps of Gonal-F per day for a total of 13 days, 52 temper tantrums, and as many crying fits; followed by a low stimulation approach of two amps per day, which yielded far fewer emotional repercussions, but also a lot fewer eggs. Now we were going to try the middle road: three amps per day along with the drug Estinyl to keep my sometimes fluctuating follicle-stimulating hormone (FSH) in line. By the time my period made its regular appearance, I had arranged the drugs neatly on the kitchen table. I generally looked forward to beginning a cycle, but this time I was a bit battle worn. The past three years had taken their toll, but I still hoped, beyond hope, that I would miraculously produce the golden egg (or 20 of them of them, no less, for good measure).

As an out-of-town patient at a large East Coast clinic, I am in the unenviable position of monitoring my cycle locally and then boarding a plane for the ultimate retrieval and transfer. As you can imagine, the local doctor, whose job it is to do the grunt work of ultrasounds and blood work, with none of the glory (or money) of the actual IVF procedure, views me as a less than desirable patient. Although I am certainly accommodated, it is generally after the regular patients, and often with a bit more disdain.

Through this, I had come to know and dread the "tsk, tsk" of the sonographer when she measured the few proud small follicles that I produced. She was skeptical both of my out-of-town doctor and my own ability to produce.

Thursday, Cycle Day 2: Time for blood work. There's always a hurdle to leap over. It is time to measure the dreaded FSH again. Dreaming of low numbers, all the while a measurable estrogen level, I am in the phlebotomist's chair at 8 a.m. sharp, hoping to get the jump on my aging hormones.

The envelope, please: FSH of 4.6 and estrogen less than 20. While managing to limbo the FSH bar, my estrogen remained low, but I hope that a few days of gonadotropins will fix that. I start shooting up that night.

Monday, Cycle Day 6: First ultrasound and blood work to check on the progress of what I have termed the third-time-is-a-charm cycle. I hold my breath and stare expectantly at the screen.

The sonographer quickly moves past the right ovary. "Empty" she declares. I can't believe it. Could 20 follicles be hiding on the other side? That question is quickly answered. The left ovary yields two small follicles, both less than 10. I am off to a very unimpressive start. The sonographer looks at me and comments, "It's what to expect without meds." I decline to tell her that I am on meds. I drive crosstown to the monitoring lab for my blood work and then back home to wait for the results. Every phone call seems an interruption until the nurse calls with my results: "Estrogen still less than 20." I'm crushed. My body is not responding.

We are coming upon a holiday week, and the chance to track my cycle will be limited. I receive instructions to stop the injectible drugs, continue on the Estinyl alone, and come back in five days for repeat ultrasound and blood work. The doctors are hoping my body will begin to produce on its own. I am thinking that if the best of science has failed me, my own efforts will be futile.

Tuesday, Cycle Day 7: I wake up with a bout of the flu that has actually made me thankful that I don't have to contend with hormones as well. I drag myself to the doctor's and then home to bed. It's turning out to be quite the holiday.

Saturday, Cycle Day 11 (AM): Despite nausea that won't quit, my husband and I manage to travel to Chicago for a few days to salvage what's left of our days off. Still feeling a little sickly, I'm up bright and early on a Saturday morning to revisit my innards, wondering if my brief illness has roused my ovaries to action. The waiting room is full. A woman next to me tries to engage me in conversation with the opening line of "Didn't I see you here last May?" It is not an invitation that I want to accept. I fight off waves of nausea and manage to remain vertical until I'm called in to the dark little room with the machine that reads my reproductive fate. "Still nothing on the right side," the sonographer calls out as I feel my insides tighten up. "Let's see, there are two little ones on the left, not growing much though." I fight back tears. Luckily, I'm in time for the blood draw on site, so my next stop is home. My husband greets me with the usual trepidation reserved for post-monitoring mornings. "How did it go?" he asks nervously. That's all I need to burst into tears. When will they call me with the blood work?

Cycle Day 11 (PM): Luckily, my favorite nurse is on duty and on the phone with my blood work results. "Estrogen at 34. Well, it's going up," she says with the optimism reserved for the terminally ill . . . and fertility patients. "Do I start meds again?" I ask excitedly, wanting to feel like this cycle is actually going somewhere. "Are you nuts?" she asks, all pleasantries aside. "What? And risk sending your estrogen back down again? Go back on Monday and repeat ultrasound and blood work." I hang up, trying to imagine what my ovaries will do on this rare day off. With two follicles, I want my estrogen to be at least 400 prior to the hCG trigger. I'm hoping it uses the brief respite to begin the long journey upward.

Sunday, Cycle Day 12 (AM and PM): I scour the bulletin boards looking for cycle buddies and their progress. Most of the women who started the cycle with me are getting ready for the hCG shot and retrieval. I am wondering if I will end up with two sets of cycle buddies, one for each half of my never-ending cycles.

Monday, Cycle Day 13 (AM): I call around to another fertility clinic to see whether I can monitor elsewhere, thereby eliminating any unnecessary "tsking" from the staff. As luck would have it, the first place I ever went, when I began my fertility wars long ago, will monitor out-of-town patients and file with insurance on my behalf. Most reproductive endocrinologists' offices require cash upfront, which puts patients in a wish and a prayer scenario for getting reimbursement. This new arrangement, albeit about 15 minutes farther, seems like a dream.

Cycle Day 13 (PM): Dream over. My two follicles have morphed into one, which is just barely greater than 10. But the nurse performing the ultrasound is encouraging. "It's still early," she says. "Anything can happen." That's what I'm afraid of. By the time I get home, my blood results are on my answering machine: estradiol of 72 to match my slow-growing follicle. Instructions are left to return the next day for repeat ultrasound and blood work. I am not starting my meds yet. It's shaping up to be a long week.

Cycle Day 13 (bedtime): My husband asks if we're going to Philadelphia for in vitro. "I have to plan my schedule." This is a rare moment when I feel like killing my darling husband. I try to explain again that there is no way of knowing when or if this cycle will mature enough to warrant in vitro. "Well, when will you know?" he asks again. This has been a long day.

Tuesday, Cycle Day 14: My husband and I are both self-employed. Many wax enviously of our flexibility. That we do have. However, wrapped in that package of "make your own hours" is the greater reality of financial insecurity, clients that demand much and guarantee little, and none of the amenities that the working public take for granted, including employer-paid and -provided health insurance, paid vacation, and retirement plans. So with all this in mind, I get to my desk by 6 a.m. the next morning to try and get a half day in before my ultrasound at noon. Don't let anyone fool you: Infertility is a full-time job with no benefits. I use the Internet to quickly scan the available flights to Philadelphia. I am hoping that my follicle will spawn others in its likeness and that they will grow, steadily and evenly . . . by Sunday. If my body cooperates, we will be able to benefit from the weekend getaway airfares . . . you know, "See the world through long distance in vitro." I haven't yet figured out how I am going to take the next week off so that I can remain in Philadelphia for the time it takes for the embryos to divide and then be transferred back into my uterus. I will need a minimum of six days away. I figure all this out before my morning cup of coffee.

Cycle Day 14 (noon): There are two follicles today — the "big guy" at 12, and a late bloomer, making an appearance at 7, still small but a contender no doubt. "Some meds would help," says the nurse tentatively. I am thinking the same thing, but obviously my doctor in Philadelphia is not. When Favorite Nurse calls back and reports an estradiol of 105, I cradle the phone on one shoulder and begin to unpack my stash of fertility drugs for what I assume will be the evening dosage. "No meds yet," Favorite Nurse announces. "What?! Are you sure?" Apparently the doctor is and has left me with nothing more than a pat on the back and orders to repeat the same tests again . . . tomorrow.

Wednesday, Cycle Day 15: As I wait for my ultrasound, I try and strike up a conversation with the pregnant women who are there to see one of the group's obstetricians. I poll them on their ages, seeing if anyone falls in range of my 39 years. There is a 37-year-old who is pregnant with her second, a 35-year-old, and a blushing young thing whose silence seems to affirm an age of under 30. Later, in the darkness of the ultrasound room, the machine reveals modest growth of the "top gun," the lead follicle, now at 13. The also-ran, however, is not running too well and has remained at 7. Back at the ranch, the blood work comes in. The estradiol has crawled up to 126. This is not looking like a winner. "Good news," chirps Favorite Nurse. The doctor says to start boosting. "Use two amps tonight." The pendulum has swung. The cycle is looking like a bust. I'm wondering about the sense of throwing good hormones after bad. My husband comes home, and we decide to alter the good doctor's advice. We do one amp. If the follicle progresses, we will carry on.

Thursday, Cycle Day 16: The nurse at the monitoring office looks at me like I'm crazy. I have been their most consistent patient. This consistency is wearing on my nerves. I am tired of monitoring, tired of getting stuck for blood, tired of my slow growth, tired of putting my life on hold, tired of planning around infertility, tired, tired, tired. I become even more exhausted when the follicle appears on the screen at a mere 14. The second follicle is now shrinking and measures in at 6. This looks like a one-partner dance.

Favorite Nurse calls a few hours later with my blood results. "Wellllll," she draws the word out, giving me a good indication that things aren't so good.

My estradiol is 146, another small hop from the day before. The results put me over the edge. "Please," I beg her, "just give me hCG so that I can release this follicle and put both of us out of our misery." Patiently (easy for her to be patient), she turns down my request. "You can always stop monitoring if you want," she offers. I have gone too far for that. I either want the follicle to release, preferably now, or else continue on. To just try and ignore the rest of the cycle seems impossible to me. Actually, today, *everything* seems impossible. Favorite Nurse instructs me to do another two-amp boost and — who would have guessed it? — return for blood work and ultrasound in the morning.

In my office, I pore over my charts, the records I have meticulously kept since we began our quest three years ago. Usually, I compare and contrast results every day. Not today. I feel beat. Instead, I collect all of my records and deposit them in the bottom of my filing cabinet — out of sight and hopefully out of mind. I can't take this anymore.

That night, my husband and I decide to go along with the doctor. We do the two-amp boost as instructed. I long for the ability to take a vacation and leave my ovaries at home.

Friday, Egg Hostage Crisis Day 17: The nurse asks me if I will need monitoring this weekend. I tell her that I am unsure as to anything I will need, or not need, forever more. I'm not much help. Thar she blows! My solo follicle is up to 16, which is a decent day's growth. My lining, however, is the wrong pattern, HH instead of triple lined. This cycle seems determined to come out all wrong. The kind monitoring nurse regales me with a story of how she coaxed a patient along for three long weeks with one follicle. Said patient is now pregnant. All I hear, however, is the three weeks part. I am horrified.

A bit of good news at home! Estradiol has gone up to 258! Favorite Nurse says it's time to decide: IVF or not. If we decide to go for it, we need to do hCG tonight and be in New Jersey by Sunday morning. This isn't exactly the fore-warning that my husband was planning on. I call him excitedly to tell him the news. "I can't go tomorrow," he moans. "I've got a deadline on Monday." Kill, kill, kill! I check with the clinic in New Jersey. They do have my husband's sperm on ice, so I can go alone — for one egg. It's too much to do for one egg. I realize if I ovulate prior to getting there or if one egg doesn't fertilize, I'm still out the plane fare and the $2,000+ for the procedure. I talk to Favorite Nurse. She recognizes the risk but is unwilling to make the decision for me. I put in a call to the doctor. He is cautiously optimistic. "This could be a good egg," he says. I call my husband. He is as unsure as I am. I call back Favorite Nurse. "You have four hours to decide," she says. The plan is that if I do IVF, I am to take the hCG shot at 3:30 a.m. for a Sunday morning retrieval. If I'm not going to do IVF, then I take hCG at 10 p.m. and schedule an insemination locally for Sunday at noon. After a week of waiting, this sudden flurry of activity is overwhelming. I look over my calendar, trying to figure out how to take the next week off work. Maybe I'll freeze the egg. I call the monitoring nurse "Go for it!" she says. I hold an airline reservation. To IVF or not to IVF?

At 6:00, I decide. I'm too (pick one) nervous, cheap, unsure to travel 1,000 miles to do IVF on one egg. I try desperately to reach the local clinic to set up the intrauterine insemination (IUI) for Sunday. Here on the edge of the Bible Belt, Sundays don't lend themselves to readily available medical care. I am told to try back in the morning. I feel (somewhat) at peace with my decision, particularly after we do the hCG shot at 10 p.m. We can't turn back now.

Saturday, Cycle Day 18: After many attempts to reach the local clinic by phone, I finally get a call back from the doctor herself. She is not amused. "What do you mean you want an IUI at 2 p.m. tomorrow?" she says. I try and explain that my doctor wants to wait 40 hours after hCG, even though the usual time is 36. She isn't budging. "I'll do it at 9 a.m., not a minute later," she says. "Besides, I wouldn't have triggered you until tonight anyway. Your follicle was only 16 yesterday." I had wondered the same thing, and now I have a physician wondering along with me. Why is nothing in fertility ever easy or straightforward?

Sunday, Cycle Day 19: Our big day. I imagine what it would have been like had I decided to pursue IVF with this cycle. I am almost sick of thinking about it. We arrive on time, and I ask the doctor to do an ultrasound to confirm that I have indeed released the follicle. "We'll do it after the IUI," she says "We're not waiting around if you haven't." Her message is clear. She comes back with my husband's sample and comments about odd shapes (morphology). She suggests a male infertility specialist. My husband is very obliging. I am not. I am spent, not only with this crazy cycle, but with the whole process. After the IUI, I tell my husband that after this one fails, I need a few months off. We decide to wait until at least October. I can't imagine more waiting, but I also can't imagine another month like this one.

Monday, Cycle Day 20: I go in for another ultrasound. The follicle has released, probably sometime after yesterday's IUI. We decide against a repeat IUI. "You've done your best," says the monitoring nurse.

Tuesday, Cycle Day 21: What should be my first day for progesterone and estrogen support begins with a horrible bout of nausea and vomiting. I often have a bad reaction to the hCG shot. Today is worse. We go to the emergency room, where the doctors ply me full of fluids and antinausea medicine. It barely relieves my discomfort. Back at home, I decide not to start progesterone and Estrace . . . yet. I can't imagine putting anything into my body at this point. I don't.

Thursday, Cycle Day 23: Another bad morning. By late that night, we are back in the emergency room. The staff looks at me like I'm crazy. All I feel is sick. The nurse on our case comments that fertility drugs can make anybody sick or crazy or both. I am thankful that I did not travel to New Jersey. Being sick at home beats being sick on the road any day.

Sunday, Cycle Day 26: Still haven't started the progesterone or the estrogen. I think I've resigned myself to giving up this ridiculous cycle. I've also resigned myself to feeling sick most of the time. After a weekend of more nausea, my internist gives us orders to have an endoscopy done to check for ulcers. I don't wonder for too long what the cause of that might be.

Tuesday, Cycle Day 28: I check into the outpatient area to have an endoscopy done. I have lost 10 pounds in the last week, unable to keep food down or to do much else for that matter. The nausea wakes me from deep sleep yet keeps me in bed all day. Although I am not one to readily volunteer to have a tube stuck down my throat, I welcome a diagnosis and a treatment for whatever ails me.

My husband has accompanied me to the hospital, and a friend joins us to keep him company. The doctor saunters over to introduce himself. "Could you be pregnant?" he asks as part of his report. I snicker. "Doubtfully," I respond, unwilling to launch into the litany of how or why. "Well, we have to run a pregnancy test just to make sure, so it'll be about 45 minutes once we draw the blood." I quickly calculate how long it has been since I took the hCG shot, which is the same hormone measured in a pregnancy test. I tell the doctor it is possible that the shot may not have cleared my body, thus giving me a low positive. He nods. "We'll see." They take me back and prep me, insert an IV, and take my blood. I doze a bit as I wait. I have not had a decent night's sleep in a week. I wake up to the nurse pulling the IV out of my arm. "What are you doing?" I ask. The doctor appears. "Well, you were right. The pregnancy test shows a low, very low positive, but nonetheless, we can't do the procedure." For the umpteenth time this month, I lose it. I try and explain to the doctor how that number will drop by tomorrow. He will not budge. He recommends retesting the next day and rescheduling for later in the week. Then he dismisses me. I lie there and cry for a while. I am now sick and tired.

Wednesday, Cycle Day 29: I wake up feeling just as sick as I have the past week. The month of July is now safely on record as one of my worst months ever. My husband is exhausted as well. I am waking up two to three times per night feeling horribly ill and then am up for the duration by 5 a.m. This morning, we take a long walk at 6 a.m. My nerves are frayed, and I cry most of the way. I don't tell my husband, but I have given up on the fertility course completely. I just want to regain the health I had one short month ago.

I call the doctor to see when I can reschedule the endoscopy. The nurse fits me in on Friday but reminds me to get my blood drawn today. How could I forget? I run a few errands and by late afternoon drag myself over to the lab for the blood work. I make it home and lie down to see if I can fall asleep. The nausea has subsided a little, but sleep doesn't come. One of my bulletin board friends calls and asks me to report back with my blood work. I tell her it's a waste of time and money. I already know the test is negative. It's just a formality.

My husband calls and tells me he is going to the gym. "Did you get the results yet?" he asks. I repeat myself. "It's only a formality."

The phone rings again. I hear the background noise of my doctor's office. Despite what I've said, my throat closes up. In a moment, I hear Favorite Nurse on the phone. "It's positive," she screams. "The number tripled . . . you're pregnant." After all that time, I'm only one day late.

Sharon's Response to Jackie's Goat Rodeo

After I read Jackie's story, I just had to write mine. My patients never listen to me. Well, they do listen, but they don't do what I tell them. Or they don't do it *when* I tell them. Jackie is certainly a prototype patient in both respects. Here's my view of Jackie's saga.

Jackie wanted to do a stimulated IVF cycle, to make as many eggs as possible. I told her this wasn't a very good idea, because the last time (six months before) she used a lot of medication, for which she was paying dearly out of pocket, and made only a few eggs. Most likely, she would do just about as well taking only a small amount of medication on a "natural" cycle. "Uh-huh", she said, just as if she believed me and was actually going to do as I (and the doctor) recommended, but of course, she wasn't.

First, she got on the computer and asked all her fertility friends what she should do. I know most of her fertility friends firsthand (and they don't listen to me either), so I knew that this exchange would be a combination lovefest, cheerleading conference, and conflicting information session.

Jackie called back and said she just had to try one more time with stimulating medications. "Okay," I said, as if this were a good thing to do, even though I was pretty sure it wasn't.

So she started her meds, and nothing happened. No estrogen rise, no follicle growth, nothing. I hate to say, "I told you so," so I didn't say it. But I thought it, of course.

Jackie started back on Estinyl, which brought her FSH back down, and with excruciating slowness, her estrogen started to rise. "Should I start some meds?" she asked eagerly, and I was pretty sure I could hear her already breaking open the vials. "Are you nuts?" I asked nicely. (I know Jackie well, so I can talk to her this way. Some of my patients would be very upset if I asked them if they were nuts.) "The doctor said no meds yet."

We went on this way for several days, with Jackie growing the slowest egg known to man and calling daily (or more than daily) wanting to inject something, anything. When the doctor finally gave her the go-ahead to inject one vial, she of course injected two, after checking with her all her fertility friends to see if that was okay.

After what seemed like a year, her lone follicle was ready for retrieval. I called, very excited, to give her the good news. "Does he *really* think I'm ready?" she asked, more than once. "Don't you think I need another day?" "Isn't my follicle too small?" "Should I do a retrieval for just one?"

I answered yes, no, no, and yes, but I could tell that these were not the answers she was looking for. Nevertheless, we scheduled her retrieval and told her what time to take the hCG.

The next day, she was on the phone bright and early, to tell me that she hadn't taken the hCG when I said (surprise, surprise) and had decided to do an IUI in her hometown instead of flying all the way to New Jersey for just one egg. I was disappointed (I was looking forward to seeing her in person to work on this book), but I could understand the economics. I still felt her best chance of pregnancy was with a retrieval.

So she had her IUI. Then she wanted to know when to start her progesterone and estrogen, so I asked the doctor and told her what he said. Of course, she didn't do it, because now she was feeling sick. She told me she was sick, but she never told me she wasn't taking progesterone.

After listening to all the details of the emergency room visits from Jackie and her long-suffering husband, I wasn't at all hopeful about the outcome of the IUI, especially when she finally confessed that she wasn't taking any progesterone.

Then came the day of her endoscopy. It was her DH (Darling Husband), not Jackie, who wanted to know whether they should tell the doctor she might be pregnant. I knew she wouldn't be but didn't tell him that. "Yes, tell him" I said, and the pregnancy test came back a very low positive.

Probably from the hCG shot, I thought, and Jackie was ready to kill me for interfering with her endoscopy. The doctor refused to do the test, Jackie went home to bed, and I wondered how we'd ever finish this book if she never got out of bed again.

Three days later, she tested her beta again, and it had gone up. After the worst cycle in the history of IVF, she was pregnant, and all I could think was, "It's a good thing my patients don't always listen to me."

Index

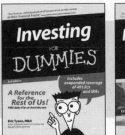
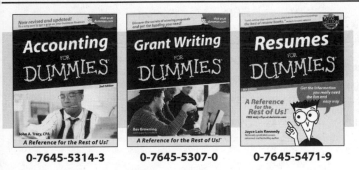
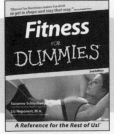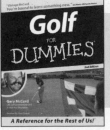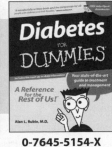
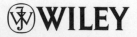

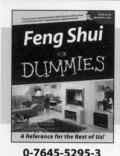
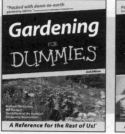
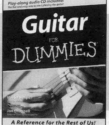
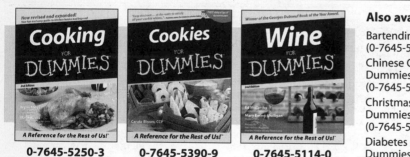
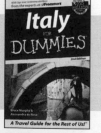
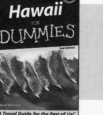
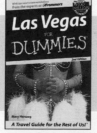

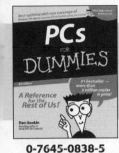
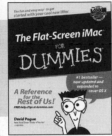
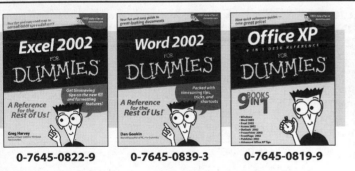
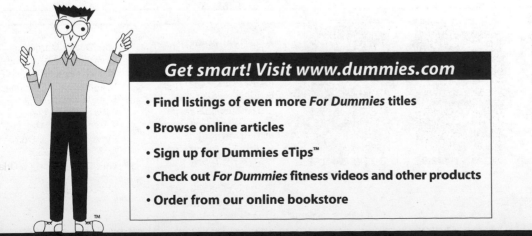

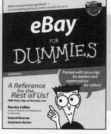
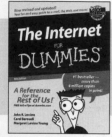
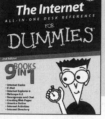
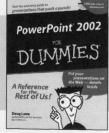
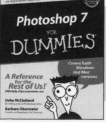
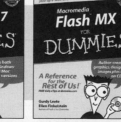
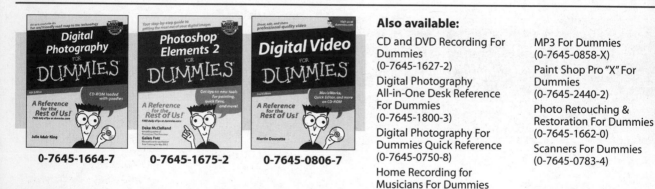

FOR DUMMIES®

The advice and explanations you need to succeed

SELF-HELP, SPIRITUALITY & RELIGION

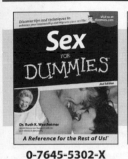 **Sex** FOR DUMMIES
0-7645-5302-X

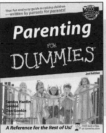 **Parenting** FOR DUMMIES
0-7645-5418-2

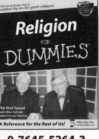 **Religion** FOR DUMMIES
0-7645-5264-3

Also available:

The Bible For Dummies
(0-7645-5296-1)

Buddhism For Dummies
(0-7645-5359-3)

Christian Prayer For Dummies
(0-7645-5500-6)

Dating For Dummies
(0-7645-5072-1)

Judaism For Dummies
(0-7645-5299-6)

Potty Training For Dummies
(0-7645-5417-4)

Pregnancy For Dummies
(0-7645-5074-8)

Rekindling Romance For Dummies
(0-7645-5303-8)

Spirituality For Dummies
(0-7645-5298-8)

Weddings For Dummies
(0-7645-5055-1)

PETS

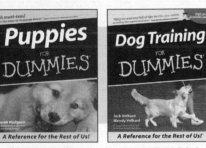 **Puppies** FOR DUMMIES
0-7645-5255-4

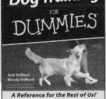 **Dog Training** FOR DUMMIES
0-7645-5286-4

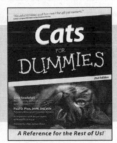 **Cats** FOR DUMMIES
0-7645-5275-9

Also available:

Labrador Retrievers For Dummies
(0-7645-5281-3)

Aquariums For Dummies
(0-7645-5156-6)

Birds For Dummies
(0-7645-5139-6)

Dogs For Dummies
(0-7645-5274-0)

Ferrets For Dummies
(0-7645-5259-7)

German Shepherds For Dummies
(0-7645-5280-5)

Golden Retrievers For Dummies
(0-7645-5267-8)

Horses For Dummies
(0-7645-5138-8)

Jack Russell Terriers For Dummies
(0-7645-5268-6)

Puppies Raising & Training Diary For Dummies
(0-7645-0876-8)

EDUCATION & TEST PREPARATION

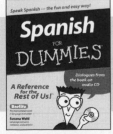 **Spanish** FOR DUMMIES
0-7645-5194-9

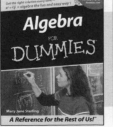 **Algebra** FOR DUMMIES
0-7645-5325-9

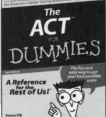 **The ACT** FOR DUMMIES
0-7645-5210-4

Also available:

Chemistry For Dummies
(0-7645-5430-1)

English Grammar For Dummies
(0-7645-5322-4)

French For Dummies
(0-7645-5193-0)

The GMAT For Dummies
(0-7645-5251-1)

Inglés Para Dummies
(0-7645-5427-1)

Italian For Dummies
(0-7645-5196-5)

Research Papers For Dummies
(0-7645-5426-3)

The SAT I For Dummies
(0-7645-5472-7)

U.S. History For Dummies
(0-7645-5249-X)

World History For Dummies
(0-7645-5242-2)

Available wherever books are sold. Go to www.dummies.com or call 1-877-762-2974 to order direct.

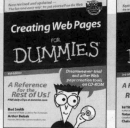
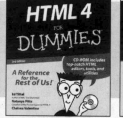
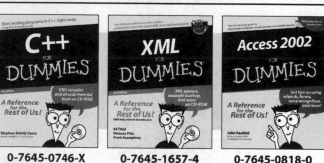
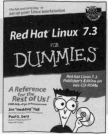
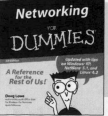
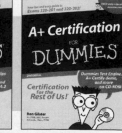
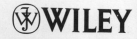